T0218468

Fundamentals of Operating Department Practice

Fundamentals of Operating Department Practice

Second Edition

Edited by

Daniel Rodger
Senior Lecturer in Perioperative Practice, London South Bank University

Kevin Henshaw
Senior Lecturer in Perioperative Practice, Edge Hill University, Ormskirk

Paul Rawling
Senior Lecturer in Perioperative Practice, Edge Hill University, Ormskirk

Scott Miller
Consultant Anaesthetist, St Helens and Knowsley Hospitals NHS Trust

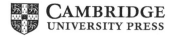
CAMBRIDGE
UNIVERSITY PRESS

CAMBRIDGE
UNIVERSITY PRESS

University Printing House, Cambridge CB2 8BS, United Kingdom

One Liberty Plaza, 20th Floor, New York, NY 10006, USA

477 Williamstown Road, Port Melbourne, VIC 3207, Australia

314–321, 3rd Floor, Plot 3, Splendor Forum, Jasola District Centre, New Delhi – 110025, India

103 Penang Road, #05–06/07, Visioncrest Commercial, Singapore 238467

Cambridge University Press is part of the University of Cambridge.

It furthers the University's mission by disseminating knowledge in the pursuit of education, learning, and research at the highest international levels of excellence.

www.cambridge.org
Information on this title: www.cambridge.org/9781108819800
DOI: 10.1017/9781108876902

© Cambridge University Press 2022

First published 2000

This Second Edition 2022

A catalogue record for this publication is available from the British Library.

ISBN 978-1-108-81980-0 Paperback

Cambridge University Press has no responsibility for the persistence or accuracy of URLs for external or third-party internet websites referred to in this publication and does not guarantee that any content on such websites is, or will remain, accurate or appropriate.

....

Every effort has been made in preparing this book to provide accurate and up-to-date information that is in accord with accepted standards and practice at the time of publication. Although case histories are drawn from actual cases, every effort has been made to disguise the identities of the individuals involved. Nevertheless, the authors, editors, and publishers can make no warranties that the information contained herein is totally free from error, not least because clinical standards are constantly changing through research and regulation. The authors, editors, and publishers therefore disclaim all liability for direct or consequential damages resulting from the use of material contained in this book. Readers are strongly advised to pay careful attention to information provided by the manufacturer of any drugs or equipment that they plan to use.

Contents

Contributors

Hannah Abbott
Head of School, Health Sciences
Birmingham City University
Birmingham, UK

Will Angus
Consultant in Intensive Care Medicine and
Anaesthesia
Aintree Hospital
Liverpool University Hospitals NHS Trust
Liverpool, UK

Suzanne Arulogun
Senior Clinical Research Fellow
Department of Haematology, Cancer
Division
University College London Hospitals NHS
Foundation Trust
London, UK

Robert Ayee
Clinical Fellow in Intensive Care Medicine
Royal Liverpool University Hospital
Liverpool, UK

Tahzeeb Bhagat
Consultant Anaesthetist
Guy's and St Thomas' NHS Foundation
Trust
London, UK

Paul Bond
Patient Safety and Quality Support Officer
The Association for Perioperative Practice
Keswick, UK

Sarah Brady
Lecturer in Perioperative Programmes,
Allied Health Professions (ODP Team)
Edge Hill University
Ormskirk, UK

Victoria Cadman
Senior Lecturer in Operating Department
Practice
Sheffield Hallam University
Sheffield, UK

Brian Corrin
Anaesthesia Associate
Sheffield Teaching Hospitals NHS
Foundation Trust
Sheffield, UK

Michael Donnellon
Former Senior Lecturer in Operating
Department Practice
University of Central Lancashire
Preston, UK

Joanne Fielding
Lecturer in Operating Department
Practice
London South Bank University
London, UK

Anne Followell
Senior Lecturer in Perioperative Practice
Buckinghamshire New University
High Wycombe, UK

Nathan Gamble
Senior Resident Physician, Internal
Medicine
University of Alberta
Edmonton, Alberta
Canada

Laura Garbett
Senior Lecturer in Operating Department
Practice
Birmingham City University
Birmingham, UK

Craig Griffiths
Senior Lecturer in Operating Department
Practice
University of South Wales
Pontypridd, UK

Efua Hagan
Workforce Lead
Croydon University Hospital
Croydon, UK

Jo Han Gan
Consultant Anaesthetist
Royal Brompton Hospital
London, UK

Heather Hartley
Manager, Perioperative Services
Trenton Memorial Hospital
Quinte Health Care Corporation
Ontario, Canada

Mark Hellaby
North West Simulation Education Network
Manager
NHS Health Education England (NW)
Manchester, UK

Kevin Henshaw
Senior Lecturer in Perioperative
Practice
Edge Hill University
Ormskirk, UK

Edmund Horowicz
Lecturer in Healthcare Law and
Bioethics
School of Law and Social Justice
University of Liverpool
Liverpool, UK

Senthil Jayaseelan
Consultant in Anaesthesia and Pain
Management
St Helens and Knowsley Teaching
Hospitals NHS Trust
Prescot, UK

Sarah John
Specialty Registrar in Anaesthesia
Liverpool Women's Hospital
Liverpool, UK

Lindsay Keeley
Patient Safety and Quality Lead
The Association for perioperative Practice
Harrogate, UK

Martin Kiernan
Visiting Clinical Fellow
University of West London
Brentford, UK
and
Conjoint Fellow
University of Newcastle
New South Wales
Australia

Roger King
Senior Lecturer (Retired)
University of West London
Brentford, UK

Vicky Lester
Consultant Anaesthetist
St Helens and Knowsley Hospitals NHS
Trust
Prescot, UK

Rebecca Helen Lowes
Learning and Development Manager
Sheffield Teaching Hospitals NHS
Foundation Trust
Sheffield, UK

Faye Lowry
Head of Resuscitation
Alder Hey Children's NHS Foundation
Trust
Liverpool, UK

Jamie MacPherson
Senior Lecturer in Perioperative Studies
Edge Hill University
Ormskirk, UK

Scott Miller
Consultant Anaesthetist
St Helens and Knowsley Hospitals NHS
Trust
Prescot, UK

Mark Milligan
Lecturer in Operating Department Practice
London South Bank University
London, UK

Steve Moutrey
Senior Lecturer (retired)
University of Portsmouth,
Portsmouth, UK

Karim Mukhtar
Consultant in Anaesthetia
St Helens and Knowsley Hospitals NHS
Trust
Prescot, UK

Kathryn Newton
Specialist Registrar
Mersey Deanery
Liverpool, UK

Jane Nicholas-Holley
Matron, Nuclear Medicine
Guy's Hospital
Guy's and St Thomas NHS Foundation
Trust
London, UK

Dominic Nielsen
Locum Consultant Paediatric Anaesthetist
Cambridge University Hospitals NHS
Foundation Trust
Cambridge, UK

Rebecca Parker
Psychiatric Senior Registrar
Northern deanery
UK

Julie Quick
Senior Lecturer in Operating Department
Practice

Birmingham City University
Birmingham, UK

Paul Rawling
Senior Lecturer in Perioperative Practice
Edge Hill University
Ormskirk, UK

Shane Roadnight
Associate Professor in Perioperative
Practice
Buckinghamshire New University
High Wycombe, UK

Daniel Rodger
Senior Lecturer in Perioperative Practice
London South Bank University
London, UK

Kully Sandhu
Consultant Interventional Cardiologist
Liverpool Heart and Chest Hospital NHS
Foundation Trust
Liverpool, UK

Rebecca Sherwood
Senior Lecturer in Perioperative Practice
London South Bank University
London, UK

Patricia Smedley
Education Lead
British Anaesthetic and Recovery Nurses
Association
UK

Sally Stuart
Senior Lecturer and Programme Lead for
MSc in Surgical Care Practice Edge Hill
University
Ormskirk, UK

Peter Turton
Specialist Trainee in Anaesthesia and
Intensive Care Medicine
St Helens and Knowsley Hospitals NHS
Trust
Prescot, UK

Cheryl Wayne-Kevan
Senior Lecturer in Perioperative
Studies Edge Hill University
Ormskirk, UK

Paul Wheeler
Senior Lecturer in Perioperative practice
Buckinghamshire New University
High Wycombe, UK

Amy Williams
Associate Tutor in Healthcare Law and
Ethics
Edge Hill University
Ormskirk, UK

Chris Wood
Anesthetic and Intensive Care Registrar
Northern deanery, UK

Foreword

For educators in operating department practice like myself, the previous edition of this book has always been recommended reading for my students. Those involved in editing and contributing to it played a significant role in the education and development of the profession. Since then, the profession has been through many changes, which have included registration with the Health and Care Professions Council (HCPC), moving from a National Vocational Qualification (NVQ) to a degree award which will become the new threshold for qualification as an operating department practitioner.

Operating department practitioners became eligible to join the HCPC register in 2004 and with these changes came greater legal responsibility and accountability regarding controlled drugs, for instance. Among other changes in practice, we also saw the introduction of terms like 'never event' and the World Health Organization Surgical Safety Checklist, and a greater emphasis on patient safety. It was therefore time for a new team to inform and prepare the current and future generation of operating department practitioners and nurses wishing to embark on a career in perioperative care.

This new edition takes the reader on a helpful journey through the attributes, knowledge, and skills required to excel in the perioperative environment. Perioperative care is sometimes viewed as very technical, where patients for the greater part, are unconscious and require very little 'care'. However, from the offset, we are informed that caring perioperative practitioners are essential to the well-being and safety of the patient. The inclusion of evidence-based practice is a sign of maturity within the perioperative professions – no longer are our actions based on 'ritualistic practices' but on 'a sound evidence base'. The discussion of healthcare ethics, the law, health and safety, operating department design, and infection prevention form the foundations on which the other chapters are built. They are subjects that are factual and can be very dry; however, the contributors cite examples that help to relate each subject to healthcare and the perioperative setting. Although fundamental, these chapters can be revisited as greater experience and understanding is achieved.

Those delivering perioperative education to more experienced students can also use many of the chapters in this edition as the basis for interactive workshops, debates, and discussion. From exploring ethical and legal dilemmas in perioperative care to redesigning an operating department, meeting the increased demands of surgical provision, and exploring how to cope emotionally after the death of a patient in the operating theatre. If the above chapters form a foundation, the chapters on physiology create a base layer. It is important to understand that alongside anaesthetists and surgeons, perioperative practitioners need to be knowledgeable and be experts in their own area. These chapters will also be very useful to those extending their practice to critical care areas, something that is becoming more common and will only increase in the future.

Operating department practice has evolved since the publication of the first edition in 2000. Many of the chapters in this book make up the core components of operating department practice which have existed for decades, and this edition blends this history and unchanging principles with updated practices based on up-to-date evidence. Previously, 'human factors' were rarely a consideration within the perioperative setting; however, they now underpin our actions, behaviour, and professional practice when caring for patients. There are greater challenges encountered relating to patients' health and lifestyle, and so today's perioperative practitioners are required to understand and plan the care of these patients. The multidisciplinary team has always been present within the operating department. However, the ongoing flattening of hierarchy has meant that the non-medical members of the team are or should be more empowered to influence best practice and have an obligation to do good in so far as possible.

It could be argued that, aside from management and education, career progression was limited, certainly for operating department practitioners 20 years ago. However, this is increasingly no longer the case and there are now many new opportunities, both outside and within the space that operating department practitioners have historically resided. For instance, there are several extended and advanced clinical roles that have been created within the operating department itself. Moreover, these roles are being undertaken by registered operating department practitioners and nurses who have completed the required programmes of study.

Operating department practice has continued to evolve and adapt along with the environment and demands. This new edition will be of interest to, and a valuable resource for, operating department practice students, post-registration nurses, student midwives, and anyone else looking to work in the operating department and I highly recommend it.

John Dade
President of the Association for Perioperative Practice

The Caring Perioperative Practitioner

Julie Quick

Introduction

Care, defined as the process of protecting someone and providing what that person needs [1], is a fundamental principle at the centre of operating department practice, which subsequently links to every chapter of this book. Care is not a single event and therefore the definition of the word can be more complex, as care is provided in several different settings including the pre-, intra-, and postoperative phases of the patient's journey. The care provided depends upon several factors including the needs of the patient, the setting where care is provided, and who provides the care.

The principle of care should not be considered in isolation. As one of the '6Cs' (see Table 1.1), care should form one of the foundational values inherent in all healthcare professionals [2]. To provide care without compassion or commitment simply becomes a task, and without competence it may be unsafe. Poor communication skills or the lack of courage to speak up could put patients at risk. Consequently, the provision of high-quality care delivered by compassionate and competent practitioners and aligned to all the 6Cs forms part of the UK's National Health Service (NHS) Constitution that puts the patient first and ensures the care they receive is safe and effective [3].

Perioperative Care

There are several prefixes associated with the word 'care' and this is often confusing, particularly when some terms appear to be associated with different disciplines. Nursing care is a term usually associated with the care nurses provide due to the historical role of nurses as the main caregivers in hospitals or community settings. With the emergence of the operating department practitioner (ODP), perioperative care can be defined as the care provided by any practitioner working within the operating theatre. However, care does not always have to be delivered by registered practitioners. Theatre support workers (TSWs), other theatre team members such as students, apprentices, nursing associates, and other caregivers such as family members may also provide certain aspects of care within the patient's journey. Those who

Table 1.1 The 6Cs [2]

Care	Compassion
Courage	Commitment
Competence	Communication

provide care often have an instinct to care but healthcare practitioners learn additional skills required to care for patients through experience, training, and education [4]. In this chapter, care is explored in relation to that provided by perioperative practitioners whether they are ODPs, nurses, or non-registered members of the team. Supervised students within the disciplines of operating department practice and nursing may also find this chapter useful to identify the fundamental principles of perioperative care.

Theories of Care

A theory is a set of ideas and concepts that attempt to explain or predict something, often formulated by people who are experts in their field. Several theories have been put forward to explain concepts of care in health and the social sciences. The majority of these emerged in the mid-twentieth century, derived by nurses to develop an evidence base to move away from the myths and ritualistic practice often seen in nursing at the time [5]. To examine each theory in depth is beyond the remit of this chapter and so overviews of some of the more well-known frameworks and their models are provided within Table 1.2.

Models of Care

While theories of care examine the wider concepts of care delivery, models of care are deeper, multi-layered concepts, which provide a detailed view of how care is delivered [7]. At their broadest sense, models of care refer to where care is delivered, as seen in the new care models programme for the NHS [8]. This programme aims to improve care and coordinate services. Within this model, surgery and, consequently, perioperative care, are often provided in a purpose-built operating theatre although patients requiring minor procedures such as excision of a skin lesion may be offered the option to have their surgery performed in a primary care setting such as general practice.

At a clinical level, models of care identify who will provide the care. Historically, care was often based upon the disease the patient presented with rather than their individual needs. Even today, treatment still follows this medical model of care, using disease-specific evidence-based clinical guidelines [9]. In the nineteenth century, Florence Nightingale identified that nursing care should be assessed on an individual basis and all care provided should be holistic in nature [10]. Holism can be defined as the recognition that all aspects of an individual – the physical, social, psychological, and spiritual needs – are attended to with equal importance [10]. Therefore, perioperative practitioners need to consider the patients' physical, psychological, and emotional needs (while respecting their social and cultural beliefs), rather than just the surgery or procedure that the patient is undergoing.

As identified earlier, care is not a one-off episode but a process whereby patient needs are identified, planned, and managed [11]. This process is often called the 'nursing process' since the concept of a methodological approach was established by nurse theorists in the 1950s. This has since been developed to reflect the complexity of care requiring critical thinking and decision-making skills and to acknowledge the inclusion of practitioners from other disciplines in caring for the perioperative patient. Within the perioperative environment, care is delivered in three, often separate, phases: the pre-operative, intraoperative, and postoperative phase. Patients' needs will differ in each stage, with each one often determining care required in the next. Aspects of care will also vary depending upon whether the surgery is elective, urgent, or an emergency. Any episode of perioperative care should be assessed, systematically diagnosed, planned,

Table 1.2 Nursing models (adapted from [6])

Model	Main concept	Aspects of care assessed	Framework through which care is assessed
Peplau's interpersonal model	Emphasised the nurse–client relationship as the foundation of practice	Orientation Identification Exploitation Resolution	Observation Description Formulation Interpretation Validation Intervention
Orem's self-care model	Encourages independence	Model looks to identify the needs that patients have or acquire	History taking Planning care Intervention Evaluation
Roy's adaptation model	Person is constantly adapting to surroundings	Physiological Self-concept Role function Interdependence	Assessment Nursing diagnosis Goal setting Intervention Evaluation
Roper, Logan and Tierney's activities of daily living model	Looks to assess how well a person performs each of the 12 activities of daily living	Breathing Eating and drinking Eliminating Mobilisation Sleep/rest Washing/dressing Temperature control Hygiene Maintain safe environment Communication Death and dying Working/playing	Assessment Planning Implementation Evaluation

implemented, rechecked, and evaluated. This is called the ASPIRE process of care and is an adaptation of Yura and Walsh's assessment, planning, implementation, and evaluation (APIE) process [5]. Using this process allows perioperative practitioners to identify and document patient care needs, justify why that episode of care was carried out and provide an evaluation of that care [5]. This process is carried out using the framework of a nursing model such as those detailed in Table 1.2 and forms the basis for a care plan [12].

Due to the critical nature of surgery, care planning in the operating theatre may appear buried in the urgency of the practitioner's work or even appear to be non-existent [13]. The perioperative practitioner has a short timeframe to establish a rapport with the patient and must assess their care needs quickly. Within the operating theatre, practitioners become experienced in prompt care planning to ensure that the care delivered is not only safe and effective but also efficient and responsive.

Assessment

The assessment of the surgical patient can take place in several different settings, such as the preoperative assessment clinic a few weeks before the planned operation, on the day of surgery, or in the anaesthetic room. Assessment involves collating information about the patient by talking to them or a family member, reviewing medical records, performing baseline observations, and liaising with the ward and medical staff. This first stage of the nursing process allows the identification of an individual patient's needs by using a problem-solving approach to allow the assessment of existing or potential problems a patient may have.

Assessment in the perioperative setting is often carried out in the form of risk assessments to ensure patient safety and prevent complications [13]. The use of the National Patient Safety Agency (NPSA) *Five Steps to Safer Surgery* documentation incorporating the World Health Organization (WHO) Surgical Safety Checklist [14] also allows for the assessment and identification of potential problems that can be communicated to the whole team. Using these tools, the perioperative practitioner can ascertain the care that will be required during anaesthesia, surgery, and postoperative recovery. For example, on hand-over from the ward nurse, the anaesthetic practitioner (ODP or nurse) is informed that the patient is worried about the surgery and so she introduces herself to the patient with the aim of forming a therapeutic relationship and takes the time to explain her own role in the procedure in a calm and gentle way. Developing this type of interpersonal relationship where the perioperative practitioner demonstrates empathy and a genuine interest allows the opportunity to help the patient navigate their care [15]. When baseline observations are taken in the anaesthetic room, they confirm patient anxiety – his heart rate and systolic blood pressure are above normal limits. The anaesthetic practitioner identifies that anxiety may also be a potential problem during the surgery due to the planned spinal anaesthetic, as the patient will be awake for the procedure.

Systematic Diagnosis

Once all pertinent information is gathered in the assessment stage, this is documented in the patient's care plan, allowing them to consider this information and diagnose the care that is required for the patient. The anaesthetic practitioner in the above example detects that the patient's anxiety levels may well worsen due to the nature of the surgery and anaesthetic. She records this on the care plan and considers how she and the team can plan care to help reduce the patient's anxiety. Having carefully looked through the patient's notes she identifies that the patient has chronic obstructive pulmonary disease and reasons that the patient is not being sedated due to the increased risk of respiratory complications. She shares this information with the anaesthetist who confirms this is the case.

Planning

When the assessment and diagnosis stages have been completed, the perioperative practitioner plans the exact aspects of care required and communicates this to the patient and appropriate members of the team. The anaesthetic practitioner in the example above suggests to the patient that he may like to listen to some music during the procedure to reduce the amount of noise the patient hears when the surgery is underway. She also suggests to the team that background noise is kept to a minimum in theatre to avoid causing additional patient anxiety.

Implementation

After planning the care required for each patient, the next stage is to implement the planned care. Who delivers that care will depend upon what aspect of care needs to be implemented and the role and responsibility of the specific practitioner. All members of the team should be trained to nationally recognised standards, which means that only practitioners who have undergone a university-accredited training programme can perform the role of the anaesthetic practitioner [16]. Following additional training, some practitioners may go on to provide aspects of enhanced or advanced care within the perioperative setting, practicing as surgical first assistants, surgical care practitioners, or anaesthetic associates (see Chapter 39).

In some instances, a team approach may be required, such as when positioning the patient for surgery. After the patient is positioned on the operating table, the anaesthetic practitioner asks the circulating TSW to access some headphones and an electronic tablet, ready for when the surgery commences. The TSW asks the patient what music he would like to listen to and then helps the patient select his choice for the duration of the procedure. During the surgery, the patient asks if everything is fine and the scrub practitioner and surgeon relate that all is progressing well. The patient is reassured, further alleviating his anxiety.

Recheck and Evaluation

In these final two stages of the care process, the care that is being delivered is initially rechecked. Using the same example, during the procedure the TSW checks that the patient is still listening to the music and is comfortable. The anaesthetic practitioner rechecks the patient's heart rate and blood pressure to ensure that they are stable, indicating that his anxiety has reduced. When the surgery has finished, the surgical team reassures the patient that the surgery went well. The Sign Out stage of the WHO Surgical Safety Checklist is utilised in this stage of the care process to ensure all key information is collated and handed on to other team members now taking over the patient's care. In this example, it is handed over to the recovery practitioner, who is made aware that the patient was anxious preoperatively but his fears have been alleviated with reassurance and the use of music therapy. In the post-anaesthetic care unit, the recovery practitioner introduces himself to the patient and evaluates the patient's anxiety level by checking with the patient. He reports that he feels much better and the practitioner notes that his baseline observations are within the normal physiological range. At this point in the patient's journey, the practitioner also performs an initial postoperative assessment to identify any new or potential problems; and so the perioperative care process commences again until the patient meets the discharge criteria to return to the ward.

Recording Care

Within the perioperative setting, several different documents are used to record individual aspects of care at different times in the patient's perioperative journey by different members of the team. This includes but is not limited to the surgical checklist, consent form, theatre care plan, theatre register, operation notes, and discharge checklist. In some departments, these documents are collated together to form one document, which specifies and records key aspects of care. Often used for patients undergoing surgery, this model is often known as an integrated care pathway (ICP) and allows the assessment of individual patient's needs and identification of the care that has been planned, implemented, and evaluated through each step of their journey [7]. Documentation of care is a legal and professional requirement [17–19]. If any aspect of care is not recorded, then it may be deemed not to have been performed and, subsequently, care plans and ICPs may be used as evidence when investigating a complaint regarding care or if required during a court case. It is therefore essential that documentation is completed to provide an accurate, legible, and contemporaneous record of the assessment, management, and evaluation of the patient's needs [20].

Scope of Practice

The scope of practice describes the limits of a registered practitioner's knowledge, skills, and experience. As identified in the implementation stage, the care provided in the operating theatre will depend upon both patient need and the boundaries of a perioperative practitioner's knowledge, skills, and prior experience. Working within their professional scope of practice ensures that, while responding to the needs of patients, practitioners only carry out aspects of care that they are trained and experienced to undertake [17, 18]. The role and responsibilities of a perioperative practitioner will vary depending upon what is outlined in an individual's job description, contract of employment, and organisational policy. Providing patient care that falls within their role remit, training, and scope of practice ensures the care provided is safe and of a high standard, and protects practitioners against litigation.

Monitoring Care

The monitoring of care is essential to protect those receiving it. For any health and social care organisation the provision of care is regulated by four independent bodies in each of the countries of the United Kingdom. The Care Quality Commission, Care Inspectorate, Healthcare Inspectorate Wales, and the Regulation and Quality Improvement Authority are responsible for ensuring care meets national standards in England, Scotland, Wales, and Northern Ireland, respectively. Each independent regulator inspects, monitors, and rates healthcare services, publishing findings to facilitate patient choice. When care is judged to fall below the expected standard, the regulator takes action to help the organisation improve services to ensure that care provided is patient centred, dignified, and safe [21]. Furthermore, health organisations monitor care through a framework known as clinical governance that includes audit and research [7].

The provision of care is also monitored by professional regulatory bodies such as the Nursing and Midwifery Council (NMC) and Health and Care Professions Council (HCPC), who set the standards for education and practice ensuring that each registered practitioner provides care that is safe and effective, safeguarding high standards of care [17, 18]. Non-registered practitioners such as the TSW are not regulated by a professional body. However, like registered practitioners they are responsible through a duty of care to their employer and the patient for the care they deliver [19]. Perioperative practitioners also have a professional obligation to monitor the care they provide through reflecting on their practice [22, 23]. Reflection is an integral part of professional development that can help practitioners gain a deeper understanding of themselves and the care they provide [24].

Summary

This chapter has defined the principles of perioperative care delivered by registered and non-registered practitioners within the operating department. Perioperative care is a systematic, cyclic, and dynamic process whereby the current and potential needs of each patient are assessed, managed, and evaluated on an individual basis at each stage within their perioperative journey. Ensuring that perioperative care is safe and effective is monitored by healthcare organisations, regulatory bodies, and independent regulators across the UK. Adhering to their scope of practice ensures that the care a practitioner provides within the operating theatre is safe and delivered to a high standard.

References

1. *Cambridge Dictionary* [online]. Available from: https://dictionary.cambridge.org.

2. Department of Health. *Compassion in Practice: Nursing, Midwifery and Care Staff: Our Vision and Strategy*. London: Department of Health, 2012.

3. Department of Health. *The NHS Constitution for England*. London: Department of Health, 2015.

4. J. Baughan and A. Smith. *Compassion, Caring and Communication Skills for Nursing Practice*, 2nd ed. Harlow: Pearson Education, 2013.

5. B. Wilson, A. Woollands, and D. Barrett. *Care Planning: A Guide for Nurses*, 3rd ed. Harlow: Pearson Education, 2019.

6. H. McKenna, M. Pajnkihar, and F. Murphy. *Fundamentals of Nursing Models, Theories and Practice*, 2nd ed. Hoboken, NJ: Wiley-Blackwell, 2014.

7. H. Lloyd, H. Hancock, and S. Campbell. *Principles of Care*. Oxford: Blackwell Publishing, 2007.

8. NHS. *Next Steps on the NHS Five Year Forward View*. London: NHS, 2017.

9. J. Phillips. *Care*. Cambridge: Polity Press, 2007.

10. W. McSherry. *The Meaning of Spirituality and Spiritual Care within Nursing and Health Care Practice*. London: Quay Books, 2007.

11. C. Hurley and J. McAlveay. Preoperative assessment and intraoperative care planning. *Journal of Perioperative Practice* 2006; **16**: 187–190.

12. B. Williams. The Roper–Logan–Tierney model of nursing: a framework to compliment the nursing process. *Nursing* 2015; **45**: 24–26.

13. A. Coulsey and D. Martin. *The Perioperative Model and Framework for Practice*. Keswick, M&K Publishing, 2016.

14. World Alliance for Patient Safety. *The WHO Surgical Safety Checklist*. WHO, 2008.

15. R. Kornhaber, K. Walsh, J. Duff, et al. Enhancing adult therapeutic interpersonal relationships in the acute health care setting: an integrative review. *Journal of Multidisciplinary Healthcare* 2016; **9**: 537–547.

16. Association of Anaesthetists. *Guidelines: The Anaesthesia Team*. London: Association of Anaesthetists, 2018.

17. Nursing and Midwifery Council. *The Code: Professional Standards of Practice and Behaviour for Nurses, Midwives and Nursing Associates*. London: Nursing and Midwifery Council, 2018.

18. Health and Care Professions Council. *Standards of Proficiency: Operating Department Practitioners*. London: Health and Care Professions Council, 2014.

19. R. Griffiths and I. Dowie. *Dimond's Legal Aspects of Nursing*, 8th ed. Harlow: Pearson Education, 2019.

20. B. Smith and L. Field. *Nursing Care: An Essential Guide for Nurses and Healthcare Workers in Primary and Secondary*, 3rd ed. Harlow: Pearson Education, 2019.

21. The Care Quality Commission. How we do our job. Available from: www.cqc.org.uk/what-we-do/how-we-do-our-job/how-we-do-our-job.

22. Health and Care Professions Council. *Continuing Professional Development and Your Registration*. London: HCPC, 2017.

23. Nursing and Midwifery Council. Revalidation. Available from: www.nmc.org.uk/revalidation/.

24. B. Bassett. *The Reflective Journal*, 2nd ed. London: Macmillan International Higher Education, 2016.

Evidence-Based Operating Department Practice

Paul Rawling

Introduction

Safe and effective healthcare underpinned by a sound evidence base is considered the gold standard of quality and compassionate patient care. For example, before any new practice, surgical technique, drug, or technology are used in the operating department it is essential that their implementation is based on high-quality evidence that has been critically appraised [1]. Evidence-based practice (EBP) is commonly assumed to be reducible to empirical research. Despite its value, it should also be integrated along with clinical experience and expertise to enhance clinical performance and ensure effective clinical decision making [2, 3]. The roots of EBP can be found in the desire to move away from unsystematic and ritualistic practices [4, 5] and towards an approach to patient care that is systematic and supported by a sound evidence base. EBP can easily just become a buzzword and so it is vital that perioperative practitioners clearly understand what it is, what it demands, and what can hinder its implementation.

What Is Evidence-Based Practice?

In 1996, David Sackett et al. [6], defined EBP as the 'conscientious, explicit and judicious use of current best evidence in making decisions about the care of individual patients'. This provided a broad definition of what EBP was that included the best available evidence at the specific point in time, and acknowledging that this could change over time, in conjunction with clinical expertise and experience, and the inclusion of patient preferences and values.

EBP can be summarised as having three core elements [7, 8]:

- the integration of the best available evidence from accepted robust and reliable research;
- professional expertise; and
- patient choice and values.

In perioperative care the three core elements of EBP are readily seen, although practitioners are often required to presume that patient preferences have been discussed prior to their arrival in the operating department. It is never ideal practice to start considering changes to care or consent following the patient's arrival.

Why Is Evidence-Based Practice Important?

EBP is important because it is the primary means of ensuring that patient care is effective, safe, and improving. All practitioners from the most junior to the most senior should be willing and able to question current practice because this is the primary means by which the standards of care will continue to develop and improve [9]. One way that EBP can be utilised is to promote standardisation of practice that leads to a reduction in the variance of care [10]. An example would be the National Safety Standards for Invasive Procedures (NatSSIPS), which are standards all practitioners are tasked with meeting to reduce the incidence of never events and other serious incidents. A further example would be the use of the World Health Organization (WHO) Surgical Safety Checklist. These strategies do not just appear from the ether, they are based on evidence and are developed to improve patient outcomes and ensure patients are kept safe. EBP is essential to continue improving the quality of patient care and to ensure it is safe.

Where Can Evidence Be Found?

It is important to understand where evidence can be found, what it looks like, and how valuable it may be. In real terms there is a clear hierarchy of evidence, which places different forms of information and knowledge into a broad list from high- to low-quality evidence. The higher up the hierarchy something is, the more likely it is that the methodology and study design will have reduced the likelihood of bias affecting the findings of the study. Systematic reviews provide a comprehensive and careful summary of all the available empirical evidence in response to a clear research question. They use explicit and transparent methods to reduce bias and provide replicable findings that can then be used to assess the effectiveness of the intervention and inform recommendations and changes to practice. It is rare that a single research study provides enough evidence to justify a change in practice. Therefore, a good systematic review can provide a sound basis for clinical decision making because there is a lower risk of being misled, which can happen when only considering the findings from one study. A basic evidence hierarchy [11] is set out below:

There are numerous sources of evidence that can be readily accessed. Importantly, evidence should always be critically appraised to ensure that it is not accepted at face

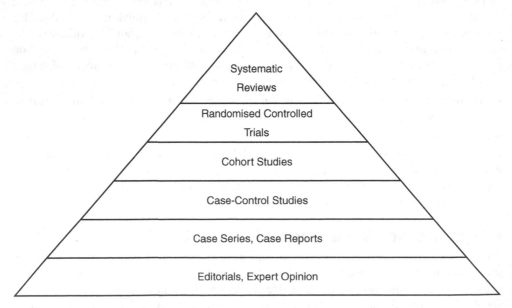

Figure 2.1 Basic hierarchy of evidence

value. Critical appraisal is a key aspect of evidence-based practice that describes the process of carefully and systematically assessing the relevance, trustworthiness, validity, quality, and findings of a research study. Important national and international organisations such as the UK's Department of Health and Social Care, the WHO, and the National Institute for Health and Care Excellence provide guidance and policies within healthcare [12]. Academic journals and textbooks are available for multi-professional groups and this information can be easily disseminated. Electronic journals are now easily accessible within clinical areas and, for example, most staff in the UK National Health Service (NHS) are provided with a national Open Athens account that allows them to access to a range of online journals and databases. Databases provide access to a wide range of valuable research and include the Cochrane Library, who develop and publish systematic reviews of the strongest evidence available on healthcare interventions. Many other healthcare-related databases are available including PubMed, Cumulative Index of Nursing and Allied Health Literature (CINAHL), Medline, and Embase. Other sources of evidence can be from professional bodies and organisations; for example, in the UK, the College of Operating Department Practitioners, the Association for Perioperative Practice, the Royal College of Nursing and the Medical Royal Colleges. Lastly, information and evidence can be gained from reliable news and media sources along with podcasts, blogs, and websites. No published information, irrespective of its source, should ever be received uncritically but is merely the initial step to using the evidence for the benefit of patients.

Why Do We Need Evidence to Support Our Practice?

The development of new knowledge in perioperative practice is crucial to the improvement of clinical decision-making processes. It is important to be aware that the current best evidence may be superseded later in the light of subsequent evidence. This is how safe, individual care adapts and improves across time. Practitioners must be willing to update and employ new practices once the balance of evidence has shifted. However, as already noted, changes to practice should not usually be amended based on evidence from a single study. An example of such evidence would be the research carried out by Andrew Wakefield and colleagues in 1998, which claimed to link the measles, mumps, and rubella (MMR) vaccine with autism. This research appeared credible, was published in a highly respected scientific journal and led to widespread public concern. The research was later discredited, retracted by the journal that published it, and Wakefield was struck off the medical register by the UK's General Medical Council, having been found guilty of ethical and scientific misconduct.

Consider what would happen with clinical decision making, pharmaceutical development, and surgical techniques while trying to promote patient safety if no evidence was ever sought, found, and implemented [13]. How would it be determined which treatment or intervention was effective, for whom, when, and for how long? This is what can be learned from the best evidence and experience of professionals, combined with a critical evaluation of the evidence available. This does not mean that the complete picture will be available but there should be sufficient evidence to make safe and reliable clinical judgements.

Evidence allows practitioners to practice in a more guided and legitimate manner with more confidence and with a rationale to support informed decision making. All practitioners, regardless of their professional group, owe every patient a duty to ensure that their care is safe and effective. The evidence required will be dependent on the situation and the type of decision to be made. The kind of evidence needed to solve the problem should include credible empirical research, professional expertise, personal experience with expert opinion, and the patient's personal preferences, which must be ascertained quickly [14, 15]. Unfortunately, clinical practice is still not always evidence based, and frequently remains based upon ritual and intuition. It has been estimated that 30–40% of patients do not receive evidence-based care and of these patients 20–30% of the care provided is not required or is even potentially harmful [16].

Barriers to Evidence-Based Practice

There are several significant barriers to the implementation of EBP. These include a lack of knowledge, understanding, and awareness of the relevant evidence base and how it can be incorporated into clinical practice [17]. This can be exacerbated by a lack of time and motivation within busy clinical schedules [12, 17]. These barriers are similar across professional boundaries and have been discussed for many years and are not easily resolved [18].

A relatively recent shift to overcome some of these barriers has been the introduction of a research and critical appraisal component imbedded in many undergraduate allied health and nursing courses so that new graduates possess these skills. There are also numerous postgraduate courses and free online training available for practitioners to enhance their existing research skills and understanding of EBP. A functional understanding of research, critical appraisal, and statistics can help practitioners apply evidence to practice [19]. It is no longer acceptable for practitioners to harbour negative attitudes towards EBP [20]. Although it is not necessary for every practitioner to become research active, to effectively implement EBP it is vital that they are research aware and capable of assessing the credibility of published research findings [10, 21].

Professional workload and staffing shortages will always add to the limitations felt by practitioners in relation to becoming effective consumers of evidence. Access to research outputs and resources may be linked directly to a lack of knowhow around finding and evaluating research and then implementing it. The organisation itself can be an additional barrier if, for instance, practitioners find themselves working in an environment where EBP is not prioritised. It is essential that an organisational culture is based on the beliefs and behaviours of the people working within the environment [13, 18]. If this culture leans towards supporting EBP, then practitioners will be more likely to become involved in and embrace the values associated with EBP. Open and honest exchange of ideas is required within a multidisciplinary environment to engage more practitioners in research and the development of EBP. Research findings should be shared at staff meetings and on audit days and small wins should be recognised and rewarded. Some practitioners might be encouraged to engage with research and the role of EBP by starting a monthly journal club where a particular study can be read, discussed, and collaboratively appraised. This can function as a means of introducing practitioners to the value of EBP and to encourage those who need to be supported as they begin to critically explore research and how to apply evidence.

Perceptions of Evidence for Future Practice Development

EBP is not new, and it remains a dynamic concept of which practitioners are broadly aware but do not always understand. EBP will continue to develop and facilitate changes in practice. Professionals are obliged to do this, it fits with the current approach to lifelong learning, and it is necessary to ensure that perioperative practice will continue to develop and improve [13, 19]. Practitioners must be aware of individual situations including local processes, guidelines, and policies from within the organisation, and be aware that any form of change will never be linear in implementation. EBP should be an easy concept to understand, but unfortunately it is surrounded by the complexities of practice and the ongoing changes in medical science [22].

New treatments and technologies drive increasing patient expectations, and a rapidly aging population (which is showing few signs of slowing) creates increased demand. Furthermore, the internet has increased the accessibility of healthcare information, evidence, and knowledge of alternatives, and patient choice is a key component of EBP. In short, patients are now often more knowledgeable, informed, and have higher expectations about their care; they expect to receive care that is safe, effective, and evidence based. This has many benefits but also has the potential to cause conflict as not all or perhaps most patients will know how to discriminate between trustworthy and untrustworthy sources and its evidence base.

Supporting practice with evidence enables practitioners to feel that they are providing their patients with the best possible care and as the values of EBP are embraced there will likely be a continued increase in the standardisation of practice. This will help provide a safer, more efficient, effective, and less questionable approach to clinical practices. This chapter is based on the premise that practitioners should be doing the right things, for the right people and at the right and appropriate time [9], in the most efficient and effective way they can. This means practitioners must develop the habit of challenging what they do, how they do it, why they do it, and change it if there is an evidence-based alternative.

Summary

The ability to make appropriate clinical decisions in perioperative practice requires the practitioner to link their individual experience with the strongest evidence base. Moreover, it is necessary to be able to effectively judge the credibility of the available evidence and to be discerning enough to avoid accepting evidence at face value. Critically appraising literature is a skill that requires practice, and it is important not to let these skills go to waste; effort should be taken to ensure that these skills are honed, developed, and applied. The evidence hierarchy can be a useful guide to assess what weight to ascribe to the evidence and effort should be taken to become proficient at reading and understanding the implications of the evidence to practice.

References

1. L. Spruce. Back to basics: implementing evidence-based practice. *AORN Journal* 2015; **101**: 106–112.

2. A. Mackey and S. Bessandowski. The history of evidence based practice in nursing education and practice. *Journal of Professional Nursing* 2017; **33** : 51–55.

3. J. Rycroft-Malone, K. Seers, A. Titchen, et al. What counts as evidence in evidence-based practice? *Journal of Advanced Nursing* 2004; **47**: 81–90.

4. Evidence-Based Medicine Working Group. Evidence based medicine: a new approach to teaching the practice of medicine. *Journal of the American Medical Association* 1992; **268**: 2420–2425.

5. F. Davidoff, B. Haynes, D. Sackett, et al. Evidence-based medicine: a new journal to help doctors identify the information they need. *British Medical Journal* 1995; **310**: 1085.

6. D. L. Sacklett, W. M. C. Rosenberg, J. A. M. Gray, et al. Evidence based

medicine: what it is and what it isn't. *British Medical Journal* 1996; **312**: 71.

7. P. Moule and G. Hek. *Making Sense of Research: An Introduction for Health and Social Care Practitioners*, 4th ed. Sage: London, 2011.

8. M. Hervey and L. Land. *Research Methods for Nurses and Midwives*. Sage: London, 2017.

9. J. A. Muir-Gray. *Evidence Based Healthcare: How to Make Health Policy and Management Decisions*, 2nd ed. Edinburgh: Churchill Livingstone, 2001.

10. K. Gerrish and J. Lathlean. *The Research Process in Nursing*, 7th ed. Chichester: John Wiley & Sons Ltd., 2015.

11. S. Mantzoukas. A review of evidence-based practice, nursing research and reflection: levelling the hierarchy. *Journal of Clinical Nursing* 2008; **17**:214–223.

12. P. Ellis. *Evidence Based Practice in Nursing*. Exeter: Learning Matters, 2010.

13. J. V. Craig and R. L. Smythe. *The Evidence-Based Practice Manual for Nurses*. London: Churchill Livingstone, 2002.

14. J. Hewitt-Taylor. *Using Research in Practice*. London: Palgrave-Macmillan, 2011.

15. P. Cronin, M. Coughlan, and V. Smith. *Understanding Nursing and Healthcare Research*. Sage: London, 2015.

16. H. E. Breimaier, R. J. G. Halfens, and C. Lohrmann. Nurses' wishes, knowledge, attitudes and perceived barriers on implementing research findings into practice among graduate nurses in Austria. *Journal of Clinical Nursing* 2011; **20**: 1744–1756

17. P. Abbott, R. McSherry, and M. Simmons. *Evidence Informed Nursing: A Guide for Clinical Nurses*. London: Routledge, 2002.

18. C. E. Brown, M. A. Wickline, L. Ecoff, et al. Nursing practice, knowledge, attitudes and perceived barriers to evidence-based practice at an academic medical centre. *Journal of Advanced Nursing* 2008; **65**: 371–381.

19. C. L. Macnee and S. McCabe. *Understanding Nursing Research: Reading and Using Research in Evidence-Based Practice*. London: Lippincott, Williams and Wilkins, 2008.

20. H. Sadeghi-Bazargani, J. S. Tabrizi, and S. Azami-Aghdash. Barriers to evidence-based medicine: a systematic review. *Journal of Evaluation in Clinical Practice* 2014; **20**: 793–802.

21. L. D. Hickmann, M. DiGiacomo, J. Phillips, et al. Improving evidence based practice in postgraduate nursing programmes: a systematic review, bridging the evidence practice gap. *Nurse Education Today* 2018; **63**: 69–75.

22. K. Parahoo. *Nursing Research: Principles, Processes and Issues*, 3rd ed. London: Palgrave Macmillan, 2014.

Chapter 3

Healthcare Ethics and Professional Regulation in Operating Department Practice

Edmund Horowicz and Amy Williams

Introduction

At the core of the provision of safe, effective, and high-quality healthcare is competent and ethical decision making on the part of healthcare professionals. Ethical values traditionally inherent in healthcare practice, such as avoiding harm and promoting the welfare of the patient, remain central features of modern perioperative practice. Yet we should accept that it is impossible to avoid questions as to how these should be weighed or applied in individual cases. In addition, the increasing complexity of perioperative practice, advancements in medical technology, and social developments continually give rise to new ethical and professional issues. It is essential to the provision of diligent care that patients trust that those caring for them will act in their interest and maintain their confidence. This is further reinforced through professional regulation which provides a means of holding healthcare professionals to account for their conduct through formalised ethical codes and standards. This chapter has been designed to support all perioperative practitioners in developing a better understanding of ethics and professional regulation relevant to patient care in the operating theatre. It includes a discussion of some of the key moral theories and frameworks that may be used to guide reflective, ethical decision making, before moving on to consider the role of professional codes and regulation in prescribing and enforcing standards of professional conduct and directing ethical decision making.

Ethics in Healthcare

Although clinical competence is essential to the provision of effective treatment and care, many of the dilemmas that perioperative practitioners face in practice concern moral questions to determine the right course of action. Reference and adherence to professional codes, the law, and policy are important and necessary in both determining standards of care and establishing the boundaries for decision making in practice. However, these cannot always determine precisely what ought to be done in each case and issues can arise when a situation causes a conflict between two competing professional principles or where the law and regulations do not provide an answer to a specific question.

The perioperative practitioner must exercise their professional judgment and engage with decision making in a way that draws on an informed understanding of the relevant legal, regulatory, clinical, and moral issues. This will often involve a careful navigation of the assumptions, values, priorities, and interests of healthcare professionals, patients, their families, and society. It is therefore important for the perioperative practitioner to develop an understanding of ethics in healthcare and how key ethical perspectives can support decision making in practice and the provision of competent, principled care.

Ethical Dilemmas and Moral Theory

Ethics is the concern of moral philosophy and involves examining questions about what is morally right, what is the morally correct thing to do, and how or whether this can be determined. Healthcare ethics, otherwise referred to as medical or clinical ethics, is a form of applied ethics [1]. That is, the application of ethical theories or principles to healthcare and the use of critical moral reasoning to identify and scrutinise ethical dilemmas that arise in day-to-day healthcare practice [2].

Ethics is important because it challenges us to tackle issues and dilemmas that arise in the development of healthcare practices and the subsequent provision of care.

Consider the following:

- When can the withdrawal or withholding of life-sustaining treatment be justified?
- How should healthcare decisions be made for a person who is unconscious and therefore unable to decide for themselves?
- What should a healthcare practitioner do if a patient with HIV refuses to disclose their condition to their intimate partner?
- When can surgical innovation in the treatment of a patient be ethically justified?
- Is it ethically acceptable for healthcare practitioners to give a teenager a life-saving blood transfusion against their wishes and where their parents have refused consent due to their religious beliefs?
- Should perioperative practitioners be required to participate in a surgical abortion if it contravenes their religious or ethical beliefs?

These are distinct issues but what they have in common is that they each involve questions of morality and, in practice, these types of issues will often present the healthcare professional with a moral dilemma. Beauchamp and Childress define a moral dilemma in the following way [3]:

> moral dilemmas are circumstances in which moral obligations demand or appear to demand that a person adopt each of two (or more) alternative but incompatible actions, such that the person cannot perform all the required actions.

There is likely to be more than one way to approach the issue, with competing views on what is acceptable and the underpinning rationale. There may be good arguments for and against taking a particular action, or the individual might feel morally obliged to take two competing courses of action [3]. Moral dilemmas present a particular challenge for the healthcare professional because despite there being no obviously 'correct' answer, they must reach a decision as to the course of action to be taken, either individually or as part of a team. Ethical reasoning can help healthcare professionals to understand and clarify the issue in question and highlight relevant considerations that they may not have otherwise considered. Furthermore, the ability to critically reason supports individual practitioners and clinical teams in exploring issues that arise in practice and enable them to reach reasoned decisions in difficult cases [2, 4–6].

Given that healthcare professionals commonly face moral dilemmas in practice, it might be argued that these dilemmas exist in part because these professions are subject to moral expectations; the implication being that their actions must be ethically justifiable. The application of ethical reasoning within a specific situation requires the perioperative practitioner to move beyond their own intuitive reactions to reach a decision that takes into account all the relevant circumstances and morally relevant matters, in order to reach a carefully reasoned conclusion [5].

Understanding the role of ethics in healthcare and how to recognise moral dilemmas is a helpful starting point from which to begin the important exercise of developing an understanding of how to approach and construct reasoned moral arguments. Once the relevant facts of an issue have been ascertained, reference to moral theories and frameworks can help to identify relevant moral considerations and to explore arguments and counter-arguments relating to the possible courses of action [2, 4] (see also [7]).

There are numerous moral theories and frameworks but here we will provide a brief overview of four of the most common approaches to be found in healthcare practice: consequentialism, deontology, virtue ethics, and principlism. Consequentialism and deontology are the predominant moral theories in healthcare ethics and are often discussed in contrast to each other [8].

Consequentialism

Consequentialism considers that an action is right or wrong depending on the consequences that result. In other words, the end justifies the means and nothing other than the outcome is relevant to the morality of the action [9]. Choosing actions based on consequences is common in healthcare, for example the provision of surgery may be considered the right course of action where it brings about positive outcomes or an overall 'good', such as improved health and well-being for the patient, despite there being some harm caused, as well as the potential for risks and complications.

There are difficulties, however, in applying a consequentialist approach to decision making in practice because consequences are not definite and can only be predicted on the best available evidence or opinion as to what will be the likely outcome [10].

One of the most well-known forms of consequentialism is utilitarianism. Utilitarianism states that the morally right action is the one that maximises the amount of happiness or well-being overall [11, 12]. A utilitarian approach is relevant in a publicly funded healthcare system, such as the National Health Service in the UK, where allocating limited resources usually involves consideration as to how benefits can be maximised for the population. Consider, for example, innovative and costly surgery, where there already exists a less expensive alternative.

There are issues with consequentialist/utilitarian approaches:

- Maximising benefit may mean that the interests or rights of the individual are overridden by the good of the majority, which may not always feel intuitively right.
- Who decides what is a good outcome or what consequences should be considered?
- It may disregard motive or intent which, at times, we may feel is morally relevant.

Deontology

In contrast, deontology considers whether an action is itself right or wrong based on fundamental moral rules, rather than on the consequences [6]. Deontology is concerned with moral obligations or duties. According to deontological theories, individuals have a moral duty to carry out morally right actions and should refrain from undertaking morally wrong actions, even where this may result in harmful consequences [2, 13, 14].

The philosopher Immanuel Kant developed a theory for determining whether an action was right or wrong with reference to what he called categorical moral imperatives. He also argued that certain actions were always wrong, such as lying [15, 16]. Critics of deontological approaches argue that while moral rules are important, they can in some cases be too broad and therefore fail to take into consideration the specifics of a situation.

If we consider the issue of lying, an ethical dilemma may arise where telling the truth risks causing a patient unnecessary and avoidable distress. For example, responding to the requests of a person recovering postoperatively from emergency surgery, asking about the welfare of their loved one, unaware that they have died in the same accident. The deontological position would be that it is always wrong to lie but a consequentialist may argue that telling the truth in that moment and letting the patient know their loved one has died could negatively impact their immediate recovery.

Virtue Ethics

Another way of thinking about the morality of a decision is to consider the moral character of the person making the decision, known as virtue ethics. In virtue ethics, rather than focusing on the action itself, a decision is justified based on the characteristic or attitude motivating the individual. For virtue ethicists, the morally right action is the one a virtuous person would choose [10, 17, 18]. Perhaps the easiest way for healthcare professionals to think about this is through the expected attributes found within professional codes, such as being trustworthy, compassionate, and acting fairly [19].

Principlism

Arguably, the most common or influential approach to ethical decision making in contemporary healthcare practice is principlism. This approach was most famously developed by Beauchamp and Childress [3] as a framework of four principles which can be applied by healthcare professionals to a moral dilemma [20]. The four principles are [3]:

(1) **Autonomy**: respect for a competent individual's 'right' to make decisions in relation to their bodies and how they live their life, free from interference.
(2) **Beneficence**: the positive moral obligation for healthcare professionals to do good in so far as possible.
(3) **Non-maleficence**: the moral obligation that healthcare professionals should avoid causing unnecessary harm.
(4) **Justice**: healthcare professionals should treat people equally and fairly.

The four-principles approach has attracted criticism, with some arguing that the approach is too narrow or simplistic [21, 22]. However, they do provide a set of ethical principles that share widespread agreement across religious and philosophical lines.

Paternalism

Paternalism can be explained as acting or making a decision on behalf of another 'against their will; and defended or motivated by a claim that the person interfered with will be better off or protected from harm' [23]. Healthcare professionals have been subject to much criticism for historically acting in a paternalistic way. Medicine, for example, has had to shift away from the tenet that 'the doctor knows best' [24]. We will see this when we explore the legal changes that have taken place in relation to informed consent in the following chapter. However, it is important to highlight that, in healthcare, paternalism is generally considered to undermine the empowerment of the patient by restricting their autonomy. An example here may be that a surgeon decides to use a product in surgery derived from animal constituents because they offer the best clinical outcome, even though the patient is an ethical vegan who refused the use of animal-derived products in any part of their care [25].

The most common justification for paternalism is that some patients are unable to make decisions for themselves, such as young children or those with serious brain injuries. This is often referred to as 'soft' paternalism because the patient lacks the competence to make autonomous decisions for themselves. While we will see later that the law in many cases allows paternalistic decision making by parents, carers, or healthcare professionals, providing there is agreement that it is in the best interests of the individual unable to make the decision, this does not mean that these decisions are not subject to ethical criticism. A more controversial situation arises in the case of 'hard' paternalism where a person has sufficient competence to decide, but their wishes are overridden to protect their welfare [23]. Generally, these cases are much more difficult to justify as they involve interfering with a person's autonomous decision.

The increased prioritisation of patient autonomy and rights in healthcare practice has driven a change in approach to one of shared decision making between healthcare professionals and their patient. This involves a subtle shift in emphasis, with the principle of beneficence seen to underpin support for patient autonomy and requiring the meaningful involvement of the patient in deciding what is best for them overall, rather than decisions based on what the healthcare professional considers to be purely in their medical interests [26].

Ethics and the Law

Healthcare professionals are also subject to the law and it is widely accepted that law and ethics in healthcare are intertwined, with one never far from the other. That is to say that healthcare law ought to reflect accepted and established moral principles and, at the least, should not require the perioperative practitioner to act in a way that is generally considered immoral. However, there is a distinct difference between law and ethics in that ethics considers what we ought to or should do, while the law sets out the threshold for what must be done and what is prohibited for public protection. As Goold and Herring explain, 'the law tells you how not to be a devil, while ethics often asks what it means to be an angel' [27].

Professionalism

Alongside legal and ethical obligations, the healthcare professional must also work in accordance with professional regulations and professional ethical codes of conduct and behaviour. The remainder of this chapter will consider operating department practice in the context of a professional regulatory framework.

Before considering the significance of professional regulation and professional ethics, it is necessary to consider what it means to be a 'professional' and to obtain professional status. While the concept of a profession has no singular definition, the recognition of an occupation as a profession or the attainment of professional status within society is likely to involve the following characteristics and qualities identified by Creuss et al. [28]:

> An occupation whose core element is work based upon the mastery of a complex body of knowledge and skills. It is a vocation in which knowledge of some department of science or

learning or the practice of an art founded upon it is used in the service of others. Its members are governed by codes of ethics and profess a commitment to competence, integrity and morality, altruism, and the promotion of the public good within their domain.

This personal and professional commitment to competent, ethical, and altruistic practice is understood to form the basis of trust upon which professions are afforded the privilege of self-regulation and the right to practise with considerable autonomy [29]. It is perhaps the central feature of our understanding of professional and ethical healthcare practice. Membership of a profession typically involves accountability for the exercise of one's professional skill and conduct through registration with a professional regulatory body. It is, therefore, important for perioperative practitioners to understand the regulatory framework in which they and other professionals in the operating department undertake their respective roles.

Professional Regulation

A defining feature of the role of the registered nurse, nursing associate, and operating department practitioner is that of professional regulation. In the UK, nurses became a regulated profession with the establishment of the General Nursing Council by the Nurses Registration Act 1919. This council, now called the Nursing and Midwifery Council (NMC) maintains a register of qualified nurses and midwives in the UK, and it welcomed nursing associates to their register as a newly regulated profession in 2019. Operating department practitioners became a regulated profession in 2004, joining a register maintained by the Health and Care Professions Council (HCPC). Professionalisation of the surgical team continues apace with the announcement, in 2019, that physician associates and anaesthesia associates will soon become regulated professions under the auspices of the General Medical Council (GMC) [30]. Following consultation, the UK government decided not to progress with distinct professional regulation of surgical care practitioners [31] and the healthcare professionals undertaking this advanced role will continue to be regulated by their qualifying professional regulator, such as the NMC or HCPC.

There are 10 regulatory bodies, including the NMC, HCPC, and GMC, responsible for the regulation of 33 health and social care professions in England. These bodies are established by statute but remain independent of government. They are overseen by the Professional Standards Authority, with the overarching purpose of ensuring public safety (see [32], section 5). To fulfil this purpose, each of the regulatory bodies has the following functions:

- setting and overseeing standards of education, competence and conduct;
- maintaining a register of professionals who are fit to practise and setting the requirements for renewing registration, including the upkeep of professional competence through continuing professional development; and
- investigating the fitness to practise of professionals due to concerns raised about their competence, character, or health that pose a risk to public safety.

The titles of regulated professions are protected titles. This means that for a person to claim to be a registered nurse, nursing associate, or operating department practitioner, they must be registered with the relevant professional regulator. It is a criminal offence to use these titles without being registered (see [33], section 39; [34], section 44). This provides protection for the public by ensuring that individuals fulfilling these roles are sufficiently competent and safe to practise, maintaining integrity and public confidence in the profession.

Each of the regulatory bodies sets standards and provides guidance in relation to the performance, conduct, and ethics expected of members of the relevant profession. Professional ethical codes provide a framework designed to protect the welfare and rights of patients and a standard against which healthcare professionals may be held to account for their conduct.

Although the precise content of the standards varies across the professions, broad and commonly held ethical and moral values highlighted earlier in the chapter underpin professional codes. These include protecting and promoting the welfare and interests of the patient, respecting patient autonomy through the requirement for informed consent, a duty of confidentiality, requirements for effective record keeping, non-discriminatory practice, and being honest and trustworthy [35, 36]. Principles such as these underpin the relationship of trust between healthcare professionals and their patients.

Fitness to Practise

One of the ways in which regulatory bodies fulfil their role of protecting the public is through the maintenance of a publicly available register of professionals who have successfully completed prerequisite training and qualifications and are considered fit to practise. This means that the individual is considered suitable and safe to practise. To remain on the professional register, healthcare professionals must continue to demonstrate that they have the requisite knowledge, skills, health, and good character to practise safely. Each regulatory body has its own registration and fitness-to-practise policies and processes, with variances in language and practices between regulators. The aim here is to provide a general overview of the common features of these processes.

For example, in the UK, registered nurses and nursing associates are required to revalidate with the NMC every three years and the HCPC requires operating department practitioners to renew their registration every two years. Registration renewal and revalidation usually entail the payment of a fee and requires the healthcare professional to provide evidence that they have met the relevant professional standards for continuing professional development and that they continue to be fit to practise [37, 38].

Professional regulators deal with complaints and concerns about healthcare professionals and may hold a registrant to account where a concern is raised that their fitness to practise is impaired. Fitness to practise may be impaired due to any of the following reasons (see [33], section 22; [34], section 21):

- misconduct;
- lack of competence;
- conviction or caution for a criminal offence;
- the physical or mental health of a healthcare professional that compromises patient safety or risks public trust in the profession;
- a determination by another health or social care regulatory or licensing body; and
- an entry in the register relating the healthcare professional that has been fraudulently procured or incorrectly made.

Fitness-to-practise procedures usually begin with an initial screen or triage of the concern by the professional regulator. The objective of professional regulation is public protection, which involves protecting patient safety, maintaining public confidence in the profession, and upholding professional standards. As such, the regulator will usually only proceed with a case where the nature of the impairment is one that relates to a concern in respect of these matters [39, 40].

If the threshold for investigation is met, then the professional regulator will proceed to investigate and where the matter is considered sufficiently serious and there is a realistic prospect of a finding that an individual's fitness to practise is impaired, the regulator may refer the matter to a fitness-to-practise panel for a public hearing of the case [41]. The healthcare professional will be judged according to the regulatory body's standards of competence, ethics, and conduct and any accompanying guidance [40, 42, 43]. For registered nurses and nursing associates, the relevant standards are those contained in the NMC Code [36]. In the case of operating department practitioners, these will be the HCPC's relevant standards of proficiency [44] and the standards of conduct, performance, and ethics [35]. If the panel finds that a healthcare professional's fitness to practise is impaired, there are a range of sanctions that may be applied which can include a warning, conditions being placed on an individual's practice, temporary suspension from the register, or, in the most serious of cases, permanent removal from the register. Sanctions will be recorded against the individual's entry on the professional register.

It is important to note, that the focus of a fitness-to-practise process is whether there is an ongoing risk to the public if the healthcare professional continues to practise or whether their conduct has been sufficiently serious as to jeopardise public confidence in the profession [41]. This focus on risk means that there is no specific requirement of harm to a patient or deliberate wrongdoing on the part of the healthcare professional. The process is not aimed at punishment of the healthcare professional or redress for previous misconduct or mistakes [45]. Rather, it is designed to ensure that where there is a finding of impairment of fitness to practise, sufficient measures are taken to protect the public.

Conscientious Objection in Healthcare

Within healthcare, there are interventions and services that are subject to long-standing ethical debate and controversy. Reproductive services such as abortion, contraception, and assisted reproduction all raise moral issues as to when life starts and when value should be placed on that life. In relation to end-of-life care, withdrawal of life-sustaining treatment also gives rise to moral disagreement. While euthanasia and physician-assisted dying are illegal in the UK, there is an active debate about their moral status and whether they should be legalised. Beyond the long-standing issues highlighted here, there are many ways in which surgical care can cause moral controversy. For example, the use of animal products in human surgery or whether cosmetic or aesthetic surgery is a legitimate medical intervention.

Healthcare professionals will have different views on these issues and in some cases a healthcare professional may not want to take part in a particular procedure or service where they feel to do so would violate their deeply held beliefs. This is known as a conscientious objection and it arises where an individual's personal morality is in opposition to expectations or duties arising from their professional or contracted role [46]. There are of course several reasons why a healthcare professional might refuse to perform a procedure; for example, they might lack the necessary competence, or the patient might request treatment that is not clinically appropriate. However, a conscientious objection differs from these types of objections because it is an objection based on one's core moral values [10].

There is much debate about whether healthcare professionals should have a right to conscientiously object to taking part in procedures (see, for example, [47–49]). We do not intend here to address these debates in depth but offer a brief summary of some of the more prominent and established positions.

Some ethicists argue that conscientious objection is incompatible with the professional role of healthcare professionals and their duty to provide care to their patients [50]; see discussion of the 'incompatibility thesis' in [49]. In contrast, there are those who dispute this position and emphasise the importance of preserving the healthcare professional's moral agency [51]. Other reasons invoked in support of a healthcare professional's right to conscientiously object include respect for autonomy and protection of the individual's moral integrity (see discussion in [52]). It can be argued that it is wrong to compel somebody to do something that they sincerely believe is immoral because it will cause them distress or may prevent them from taking up certain jobs or professions because of their beliefs.

However, there are also various arguments that point to the potential harms and risks that can arise from accommodating conscientious objection in healthcare. For example, that conscientious objection by healthcare professionals can contribute to a stigma around particular services; can place an undue burden on other colleagues and employers; and can deny or disrupt patient access to timely, effective care to which they are entitled (see discussions in [53–55]).

Where the right of healthcare professionals to conscientiously object is accepted in principle, there is debate about the scope of the right and how it should be exercised in practice. Although there are immediate professional issues that arise in relation to the responsibilities and duties of the healthcare professional who conscientiously objects (46, 56). There are other considerations, such as how a healthcare professional can or should prove a deeply held moral belief (see for example, discussions in [57]). The basis of the conscientious objection can also be important, such as whether it is based on a moral objection to the intervention itself or instead on a characteristic or lifestyle choice of the patient?[1]

Abortion and Conscientious Objection in Law

In England and Wales, the law provides explicit protection to healthcare professionals who wish to conscientiously object to participation in abortion and procedures under the Human Fertilisation and Embryology Act 1990 (see [58], section 38). These are referred to as 'statutory exemptions'. Section 4 of the Abortion Act 1967 [59] states that:

> no person shall be under any duty, whether by contract or by any statutory or other legal requirement, to participate in any treatment authorised by this Act to which he has a conscientious objection.

---

[1] In the provision of services, the Equality Act 2010 prohibits discrimination based on a protected characteristic and public organisations such as the NHS in the UK have a positive duty to promote equality. See also *Ladele* v. *London Borough of Islington* [2009] EWCA Civ 1357; and *McFarlane* v. *Relate Avon Ltd* [2010] EWCA Civ 880.

This is not an unlimited protection and, importantly, a healthcare professional is still under a duty to participate in an abortion where it is 'necessary to save the life or to prevent grave permanent injury to the physical or mental health of a pregnant woman' (see [59], section 4(2)).

The statutory exemption only applies to 'hands-on' activity in the procedure. In other words, it only applies to the procedure itself and not to ancillary or administrative tasks related to the procedure, such as typing a letter of referral for abortion services, booking in the patient; treatment relating to postoperative complications; or pre- and postoperative care [60, 61].

In law, the freedom to manifest one's belief, which may include exercising a conscientious objection, is a limited right under the European Convention on Human Rights. When deciding cases involving conscientious objections by healthcare professionals, the European Court of Human Rights has tended to leave a broad discretion to individual member states to decide on the extent of the limits placed on a healthcare professional's right to conscientiously object [62].

Conscientious Objection and Professional Standards

Professional and regulatory bodies differ in the degree to which they comment on conscientious objection. In the UK, the GMC provides specific and perhaps the most extensive treatment of the issue. The GMC's guidance on personal beliefs and medical practice is clear in its approach to enable doctors to practice in line with their beliefs, provided they act in accordance with relevant legislation, do not deny patients access to appropriate medical treatment or services, and do not discriminate or cause patients distress (see [63], sections 8–16). The guidance does not prescribe the types of procedures, treatment or care doctors may or may not object to, stating '[y]ou may choose to opt out of providing a particular procedure because of your personal beliefs and values' (see [63], sections 8–16). Importantly, objecting doctors must provide the patient with sufficient information and assistance to arrange for them to be seen by another doctor in a timely manner. Doctors must not leave their patient with nowhere to turn. The guidance notes that the employer can require doctors to fulfil contractual obligations provided they are not exempted by law, even where this would contravene their moral convictions (see [63], sections 8–16).

Both the NMC and the HCPC in the UK offer a more restrained approach to conscientious objection. The NMC Code, governing the conduct and behaviour of registrants, states that conscientious objection is only available to nurses, midwives, and nursing associates in limited circumstances, specifically, those subject to the statutory exemption clauses [36]. Nurses, midwives, and nursing associates are required to tell their colleagues, manager, and patient of their conscientious objection and arrange for a suitably qualified colleague to take over responsibility for the patient's care [36]. The NMC's accompanying guidance on conscientious objection does not go beyond an outline of the statutory clauses [64]. The HCPC provide no specific reference or guidance in relation the exercise of conscientious objection other than to state that registrants must not allow their personal views to affect their professional relationships or the care, treatment, or other services they provide [35].

References

1. J. Harris. The scope and importance of bioethics. In *Bioethics*, ed. J. Harris. Oxford: Oxford University Press, 2001, pp. 1–24.

2. R. Gillon. *Philosophical Medical Ethics*. Chichester: Wiley, 1986.

3. T. L. Beauchamp and J. F. Childress. *Principles of Biomedical Ethics*, 7th ed. Oxford: Oxford University Press, 2013.

4. M. Dunn and T. Hope. *Medical Ethics: A Very Short Introduction*, 2nd ed. Oxford: Oxford University Press, 2018.

5. M. Benjamin and J. Curtis. *Ethics in Nursing*, 3rd ed. Oxford: Oxford University Press, 1992.

6. G. T. Laurie, S. H. E. Harmon, and G. Porter. *Mason and McCall Smith's Law and Medical Ethics*, 10th ed. Oxford: Oxford University Press, 2016.

7. J. Rachels. Ethical theory and bioethics. In H. Kuhse and P. Singer (eds.), *A Companion to Bioethics*, 2nd ed. Chichester: Wiley Blackwell, 2009, pp. 15–23.

8. S. D. Pattinson. *Medical Law and Ethics*, 6th ed. London: Sweet & Maxwell, 2020.

9. M. Häyry. Utilitarianism and bioethics. In R. E. Ashcroft, A. Dawson, H. Draper, and J. McMillan (eds.), *Principles of Health Care Ethics*. Chichester: John Wiley & Sons, Ltd., 2007, pp. 303–336.

10. J. Herring. *Medical Law and Ethics*, 8th ed. Oxford: Oxford University Press, 2020.

11. J. J. C. Smart and B. Williams. *Utilitarianism: For and Against*. Cambridge: Cambridge University Press, 1973.

12. P. Singer. *Practical Ethics*, 3rd ed. Cambridge: Cambridge University Press, 2011.

13. N. Davis. Contemporary deontology. In P. A Singer (ed.), *A Companion to Ethics*. Oxford: John Wiley & Sons, Ltd., 1993, pp. 305–323.

14. D. McNaughton and J. P. Rawling. Deontology. In R. E. Ashcroft, A. Dawson, H. Draper, and J. McMillan (eds.),

Principles of Health Care Ethics. Chichester: John Wiley & Sons, Ltd., 2007, pp. 337–364.

15. T. Hill Jr. Kantianism. In H. LaFollette and I. Persson (eds.), *The Blackwell Guide to Ethical Theory*, 2nd ed. Hoboken, NJ: Wiley–Blackwell, 2013, pp. 311–331.

16. O. O'Neill. Kantian ethics. In P. A. Singer (ed.), *A Companion to Ethics*. Oxford: John Wiley & Sons, Ltd., 1993, pp. 263–277.

17. G. Trianosky. What is virtue ethics all about? *American Philosophical Quarterly* 1990; **27**: 335–344.

18. J. Oakley. A virtue ethics approach. In H. Kuhse and P. Singer (eds.), *A Companion to Bioethics*, 2nd ed. Chichester: Wiley Blackwell, 2009, pp. 91–104.

19. S. Holland. The virtue ethics approach to bioethics. *Bioethics* 2011; **25**: 192–201.

20. J. S. Gordon, O. Rauprich, and J. Vollmann. Applying the four-principle approach. *Bioethics* 2011; **25**: 293–300.

21. J. M. Harris. In praise of unprincipled ethics. *Journal of Medical Ethics* 2003; **29**: 303–306.

22. R. Gillon Defending the four principles approach as a good basis for good medical practice and therefore for good medical ethics. *Journal of Medical Ethics* 2015; **41**: 111–116.

23. G. Dworkin. Paternalism. In E. N. Zalta (ed.), *The Stanford Encyclopedia of Philosophy*, 2006; Available from: http://plato.stanford.edu/entries/paternalism/.

24. N. Harrison. Regressing or progressing: what next for the doctor–patient relationship? *The Lancet Respiratory Medicine* 2018; **6**: 178–80.

25. D. Rodger and B. P. Blackshaw. Using animal-derived constituents in anaesthesia and surgery: the case for disclosing to patients. *BMC Medical Ethics* 2019; **20**: 14.

26. G. Cullity. Beneficence. In R. E. Ashcroft, A. Dawson, H. Draper, and J. McMillan (eds.), *Principles of Health Care Ethics*.

Chichester: John Wiley & Sons, Ltd., 2007, pp. 159–190.

27. I. Goold and J. Herring. *Great Debates in Medical Law and Ethics*. London: Macmillan International Higher Education, 2018.

28. S. R. Cruess, S. Johnston, and R. L. Cruess. 'Profession': a working definition for medical educators. *Teaching and Learning in Medicine* 2004; **16**: 74–76.

29. E. D. Pellegrino. Professionalism, profession and the virtues of the good physician. *The Mount Sinai Journal of Medicine* 2002; **69**: 378–389.

30. Department of Health and Social Care. The regulation of physician associates (PAs) and anaesthesia associates (AAs). Available from: www.parliament.uk/business/publications/written-questions-answers-statements/written-statement/Commons/2019-07-18/HCWS1741/.

31. Department of Health and Social Care. The regulation of medical associate professionals in the UK, consultation response. Available from: www.gov.uk/government/consultations/regulating-medical-associate-professions-in-the-uk.

32. Health and Social Care (Safety and Quality) Act 2015. Available from: https://www.legislation.gov.uk/ukpga/2015/28/contents/enacted.

33. The Health Professions Order 2001. Available from: www.legislation.gov.uk/uksi/2002/254/article/39/made

34. Nursing and Midwifery Order 2001. Available from: www.legislation.gov.uk/uksi/2002/253/contents/made.

35. Health and Care Professions Council. Standards of conduct performance and ethics. Available from: www.hcpc-uk.org/standards/standards-of-conduct-performance-and-ethics/.

36. Nursing and Midwifery Council. The Code: professional standards of practice and behaviour for nurses, midwives and nursing associates. Available from: www.nmc.org.uk/standards/code/.

37. Nursing and Midwifery Council. Staying on the register. Available from: www.nmc.org.uk/registration/staying-on-the-register/.

38. Health and Care Professions Council. Registration renewals. Available from: www.hcpc-uk.org/registration/registration-renewals/.

39. Health and Care Professions Council. Threshold policy for fitness to practise investigations. Available from: www.hcpc-uk.org/globalassets/resources/policy/threshold-policy-for-fitness-to-practise-investigations.pdf.

40. Nursing and Midwifery Council. Fitness to practise library. Available from: www.nmc.org.uk/ftp-library/.

41. D. Blench. How regulators deal with poor registrant behaviour: the fitness to practise process explored. Professional Standards Authority Blog, 1 August 2018. Available from: www.professionalstandards.org.uk/news-and-blog/blog/detail/blog/2018/08/01/how-regulators-deal-with-poor-registrant-behaviour-the-fitness-to-practise-process-explored.

42. Health and Care Professions Council. Fitness to practise. Available from: www.hcpc-uk.org/concerns/what-we-investigate/fitness-to-practise/.

43. General Medical Council. Information for doctors under investigation. Available from: www.gmc-uk.org/concerns/information-for-doctors-under-investigation.

44. Health and Care Professions Council. Standards of proficiency: operating department practitioners. Available from: www.hcpc-uk.org/resources/standards/standards-of-proficiency-operating-department-practitioners/.

45. Nursing and Midwifery Council. Aims and principles for fitness to practice, No 2. NMC fitness to practise library. Available from: www.nmc.org.uk/ftp-library/understanding-fitness-to-practise/using-fitness-to-practise/.

46. M. Wicclair. *Conscientious Objection in Healthcare: An Ethical Analysis*. Cambridge: Cambridge University Press, 2011.

47. A. Giubilini and J. Savulescu. Conscientious objection in healthcare: problems and perspectives. *Cambridge Quarterly of Healthcare Ethics* 2017; **26**: 3–5.

48. S. Fovargue, S. McGuinnes, A. Mullock, and S. Smith. Conscience and proper medical treatment. *Medical Law Review* 2015, 23: 173–176.

49. M. Wicclair. Is conscientious objection incompatible with a physician's professional obligations? *Theoretical Medicine and Bioethics* 2008; **29**: 171–185.

50. J. Savulescu and U. Schuklenk. Doctors have no right to refuse medical assistance in dying, abortion or contraception. *Bioethics* 2017; **31**: 162–170.

51. M. Neal and S. Fovargue. Is conscientious objection incompatible with healthcare professionalism? *The New Bioethics* 2019; **25**: 221–235.

52. M. Wicclair. Conscientious objection in healthcare and moral integrity. *Cambridge Quarterly of Healthcare Ethics* 2017; **26**: 7–17.

53. U. Schuklenk. Conscience-based refusal of patient care in medicine: a consequentialist analysis. *Theoretical Medicine and Bioethics* 2019; **40**: 523–538.

54. P. West-Oram and A. Buyx. Conscientious objection in healthcare provision: a new dimension. *Bioethics* 2016; **30**: 336–343.

55. J. Savulescu. Conscientious objection in medicine. *British Medical Journal* 2006; 332: 294–297.

56. R. Trigg. Conscientious objection and 'effective referral'. *Cambridge Quarterly of Healthcare Ethics* 2017; **26**: 32–43.

57. A. Giubilini. Conscientious objection and medical tribunals. *Journal of Medical Ethics.* 2016; 42: 78–79.

58. Human Fertilisation and Embryology Act 1990. Available from: www .legislation.gov.uk/ukpga/1990/37/ introduction.

59. Abortion Act 1967. Available from: www .legislation.gov.uk/ukpga/1967/87/ contents.

60. *Doogan* v. *Greater Glasgow and Clyde Health Board* [2013] SCIH 36.

61. *Janaway* v. *Salford Area General Authority* [1989] AC 537 (HL).

62. M. Campbell. Conscientious objection, health care and Article 9 of the European Convention on Human Rights. *Medical Law International* 2011; **11**: 284–304.

63. General Medical Council. Guidance on personal beliefs and medical practice. Available from: www.gmc-uk.org/ ethical-guidance/ethical-guidance-for-doctors/personal-beliefs-and-medical-practice.

64. Nursing and Midwifery Council. Conscientious objection by nurses, midwives and nursing associates. Available from: www.nmc.org.uk/standards/code/ conscientious-objection-by-nurses-and-midwives/.

Operating Department Practice and the Law

Edmund Horowicz and Amy Williams

Introduction

Healthcare law is concerned with how different areas of law apply specifically to the provision and practice of healthcare. It focuses on the relationships that arise between the State, healthcare professionals, healthcare institutions, and individuals. It encompasses patient safety, access to services, medical research, and the management of public health. Ultimately, healthcare law is about people, their bodies, and those entrusted to care for them. Fast-paced, continuing advances in technology and healthcare practice make this a dynamic and complex area of law that must address long-standing, new, and evolving professional and ethical considerations.

Healthcare policy is largely a devolved matter in the UK, with the four nations of the UK adopting differing approaches to governance and spending. In addition, Scotland and Northern Ireland have separate legal systems to that of England and Wales. This chapter focuses on healthcare law and policy in England.

Criminal and Civil Law

The law can be categorised in several ways and one helpful distinction is that between criminal law and civil law. Criminal law is a type of public law through which the State, on behalf of society, circumscribes and punishes conduct by individuals that is considered unacceptable by the State [1]. Civil law regulates the relationships between individuals, such as employers and their employees or retailers and their customers. Each has a separate court system and legal processes. The highest court in both areas of law is the UK Supreme Court [1].

Sources of Law

English law is found in a variety of sources:

- **Primary legislation**: Acts of Parliament, for example, the Mental Capacity Act 2005 [2], the Mental Health Act 1983 [3], and the Children Act 1989 [4].
- **Secondary or delegated legislation** made by nominated authorities to implement or give practical effect to requirements under Acts of Parliament (see, for example, [5, 6]).
- **Common or case law**: Principles of law or rules contained in legal cases.

Courts develop common law in two ways:

(1) they interpret the meaning of legislation and how it applies in individual cases;[1] and

---

[1] See, for example: *Aintree University Hospitals NHS Foundation Trust (Respondent)* v. *James (Appellant)* [2013] UKSC 67, where the Supreme Court detailed how the best-interests checklist contained in the Mental Capacity Act 2005 should be interpreted.

(2) they develop legal rules and principles through case law in areas where the issue is not explicitly dealt with by statute.[2]

To ensure consistency and fairness, the courts apply the doctrine of judicial precedent or *stare decisis*, which requires that lower courts follow the decisions of the higher courts and the decisions made in previous cases with similar facts (see [1], pp. 137–181).

- **European Union (EU) law:** When the UK was as member of the EU, principles of EU law were reproduced in UK legislation and case law. EU law encompasses a wide range of areas relevant to healthcare including the processing of patient data, the storage and transport of medicines, and access to healthcare by EU citizens travelling between member states. Following the UK's withdrawal from the EU in January 2020, the European Union (Withdrawal) Act 2018 allowed for directly applicable EU law existing at the date of exit to be brought into UK law (see [7], section 3).
- **European Convention on Human Rights:** The Human Rights Act 1998 [8] came into force in 2000 and enabled UK citizens to have cases involving their Convention rights heard by UK courts. There are two ways in which the Human Rights Act 1998 gives effect to Convention rights in the UK (see [9], pp. 75–78):

  (1) '[S]o far as is it is possible to do so' all legislation 'must be read and given effect in a way which is compatible with the Convention rights' (see [8], section 3(1)).
  (2) Decisions and actions taken by a 'public authority', such as the NHS [National Health Service in the UK] trusts and a court or tribunal, or an organisation acting in a public function, must comply with the Act (see [8] section 6(1)).

Some rights are unqualified rights such as the right to freedom from torture and inhuman or degrading treatment (Article 3) and there can be no justification for infringing an individual's enjoyment of these rights. Most rights, however, are known as qualified or limited rights including the right to life (Article 2), the right to liberty and security (Article 5), and the right to respect for private and family life (Article 8). They may be lawfully restricted where it is necessary to protect the rights of others or to protect the wider interests of the community; for example, in the interests of public health or security, provided the restriction is proportionate [8].

Many of the rights protected by the Act are particularly relevant to healthcare practice and have been considered in the interpretation and application of law, policy, and practice within health and social care across a wide range of issues including assisted dying [10], confidentiality [11], bodily integrity [12], and fertility treatment [13].

Equality and Non-discriminatory Practice

The requirement to treat all service users and carers with respect, and in a way that does not discriminate against them, is a core value of professional ethics (see [14], standard 20.2; [15], standards 1.5 and 1.6). The obligation to not only practice in a way that does not discriminate against patients with particular characteristics, lifestyles, or backgrounds is further enhanced by requirements to challenge discrimination and promote equality in both healthcare practice and the workplace (see [16], section 29(7) and section 149). A key part of the legal framework in this respect is the Equality Act 2010, which protects individuals

---

[2] See, for example: *Gillick* v. *West Norfolk and Wisbech Area Health Authority* [1986] AC 112, where the court laid down the principles of consent in the case of adolescents.

from unlawful discrimination. The Act applies in several areas including employment, education, and access to goods and services, which includes the provision of healthcare. There are nine 'protected characteristics' upon which unlawful discrimination may be based:

(1) age;

(2) disability;

(3) gender reassignment;

(4) marriage and civil partnership;

(5) pregnancy and maternity;

(6) race;

(7) religion or belief;

(8) sex; and

(9) sexual orientation.

Discrimination may be direct or indirect. Direct discrimination occurs if, because of a protected characteristic, person A treats person B less favourably than person A treats or would treat others (see [16], section 13(1)). Indirect discrimination occurs where an apparently neutral provision, criterion, or practice would put persons with a protected characteristic at a disadvantage compared with other persons (see [16], section 19).

The Public Sector Equality Duty contained in section 149 of the Act, requires public bodies to have due regard to the need to eliminate discrimination, advance equality of opportunity, and foster good relations between persons who share a relevant protected characteristic and persons who do not share it, which involves tackling prejudice and promoting understanding. (For further information, see [17].)

More broadly, there is evidence that social and economic inequalities lead to poorer health outcomes for many patients [18]. Alongside the Equality Act 2010, the Health and Social Care Act 2012 also provides legal mechanisms to reduce inequalities, to promote better outcomes for all patients (see [19], sections 4 and 26). The Act places a duty on the Secretary of State (see [19], section 4) and public health bodies to reduce inequalities between people in respect of the benefits they receive from healthcare.

The perioperative practitioner must work within this framework and understand both the ethical and legal significance of respecting and promoting the rights and dignity of each patient. This includes the need for personalised care, which involves identifying and appropriately adapting care and treatment to meet the diverse and individual needs of patients, challenging discriminatory practices, and effectively promoting equality for all patients.

Responsibility and Accountability

The UK's Department of Health and Social Care have noted that the terms responsibility and accountability are used interchangeably but their meanings should be distinguished [20]:

Responsibility (for): A set of tasks or functions that an employer, professional body, court of law, or some other recognised body can legitimately demand.

Accountability (to): The mechanism by which failure to exercise responsibility may produce sanctions such as warnings, disciplining, suspension, criminal prosecution, or removal from the professional register. It can be called 'answerability'.

Healthcare professionals can be held accountable for those aspects of care and treatment for which they are responsible.

In What Ways Is a Healthcare Professional Accountable?

A healthcare professional is accountable in the following ways:

- **Professional regulation**
  In Chapter 3, we explained that, through the fitness-to-practise process, healthcare professionals can be held to account by their professional regulator for breaching the professional standards of conduct or proficiency.

- **Employment law**
  An individual is also accountable to their employer and can face disciplinary proceedings for not exercising their contractual responsibilities to the required standard.

- **Criminal law**
  Prosecutions can be brought against those whose behaviour amounts to criminal conduct: for example, gross negligence manslaughter, wilful neglect, murder, or fraud.

- **Civil law** – tort (wrongful action): negligence, battery, etc.
  A healthcare professional can be held accountable in civil law through the tort of negligence where the care they provide falls below the required standard and causes harm to a patient [21]. A healthcare professional can also be held accountable in the tort of battery for making physical contact with a patient to provide treatment or care without their consent or other legal authority [22].

The extreme case of the former consultant breast surgeon Ian Paterson demonstrates how a healthcare professional may be held accountable in several ways for the same instance of conduct. Over two decades, Paterson performed unnecessary or inappropriate breast surgery on potentially hundreds of women. He was found guilty of the crime of wounding with intent, and was imprisoned. He was also struck off the register of the UK's General Medical Council, dismissed by his employer for gross misconduct, and, collectively, many of Paterson's victims were successful in civil legal action against him [23]. In February 2020, the 'Report of the independent inquiry into the issues raised by Paterson' was published and in it the significance of accountability was emphasised; but it was also noted that being accountable did not in itself necessarily prevent continued malpractice [24].

Accountability and Negligence

When a patient claims to have been harmed, a key issue is whether that harm was an accepted risk of a procedure carried out correctly and with due care, or whether the harm resulted from care that had fallen below the standard expected in law. Negligence in healthcare has been subject to increasing public and political scrutiny because of the significant costs resulting from monetary damages paid to claimants (see, for example, [25], [26], and [27]). However, harm caused by negligent healthcare can be catastrophic and life changing for the patient and their loved ones. NHS Resolution, the body that deals with negligence claims and compensation in the NHS in England, explain that negligence claims are not only important to the individual affected but also allow lessons to be learned by healthcare providers to prevent similar harm occurring again [28]. Although unintentional, healthcare professionals can make mistakes that may cause harm to a patient in their care. The law of negligence provides a form of redress for those harmed and holds the healthcare professional accountable for careless, negligent acts and omissions that result in harm.

For a claimant to succeed in a negligence action they must satisfy all three of the following elements established in the case of *Donoghue* v. *Stevenson* [29]:

(1) that the defendant owed the claimant a duty of care;

(2) that there was a breach of that duty; and

(3) that because of this breach, harm occurred to the claimant.

Duty of Care

In law, a duty of care is imposed where a person has responsibility for a task or function that, if not carried out with the required standard of care, may cause reasonably foreseeable harm to another person (see [25]; see also [29]). It is likely to be a straightforward task to demonstrate that a healthcare professional owes a duty of care to the patients to which they are responsible for providing care and treatment. It is less obvious whether a perioperative practitioner also owes a legal duty of care to a patient's relatives, the public, or the patient's employer.

The courts have held that for a duty of care to arise, there must be some form of sufficiently close or proximate relationship between the claimant and the defendant and it must be fair, just, and reasonable to impose a legal duty of care in the circumstances [30]. In the case of *West Bromwich Albion* v. *El Safty* [31], the court held that while the surgeon had a duty of care to their patient (a footballer employed by the defendant); they did not owe a duty of care to his club for negligent advice regarding treatment, which resulted in an end to his playing career. It was held that there was insufficient proximity between the defendant and the club and it would not be fair to impose a duty of care in the circumstances which could potentially expose healthcare professionals to huge liabilities owed to employers (see [32], appendix one).

Another consideration is whether a student in the operating department owes a duty of care to the patients they provide treatment to? The simple answer is, 'yes'. Professional bodies produce education standards for the supervision of students training in theatre, and guidance on conduct outlining the expectations placed on students (see, for example, [33–35]).

The Standard of Care

There will be a breach of the duty of care where the conduct of the healthcare professional falls below the standard of care expected in law. Judges and lawyers are generally not medically qualified, so how can a court determine the proper standard of care in a case? This problem was addressed in the famous case of *Bolam* v. *Friern Hospital Management Committee* [21]. The case established what is known as the 'Bolam test' for assessing the standard of care: A doctor 'is not guilty of negligence if he has acted in accordance with a practice accepted as proper by a responsible body of men skilled in that particular art' (see [21], at 587).

The test applies what can be referred to as a 'professional standard'. That is, if a healthcare professional can show that their professional peers would have acted in a similar way in the circumstances, then the healthcare professional will not be considered negligent. The court made clear that the standard is that of the ordinary level of competence of a person in the relevant profession and speciality, rather than an expert.

The test has been criticised for effectively allowing doctors to set the legal standard of care regardless of the reasonableness of the accepted practice [36]. The case of *Bolitho* v. *City and Hackney Health Authority* [37] went some way to address this by stating that where a professional expert witness reported that the actions of the defendant were proper medical practice, judges were entitled to scrutinise the logical basis and reasonability of that conclusion [37].

The Courts have further held that inexperience will not be a defence to negligence so, newly qualified or less experienced perioperative practitioners are held to the standard of a reasonably competent practitioner in that particular skill [38]. In the case of *Wilsher* v. *Essex Area Health Authority* [38], the court recognised the importance in healthcare of training on the job and with patients. The case suggests that inexperienced healthcare professionals may not be negligent where they refer to and seek the advice of senior colleagues when appropriate (see [38], [39], pp. 155–156).

Perioperative practitioners must recognise the scope of their practice and competency when developing new skills. The standard of care focuses on how the skill ought to be carried out, rather than who is carrying it out, which is particularly important for students and those undertaking roles traditionally carried out by doctors such as surgical first assistants or surgical care practitioners. In this respect, evidence of compliance with recognised clinical guidelines [40], such as those developed by the Perioperative Care Collaborative [41] or the Royal College of Surgeons [42], can provide evidence that an individual's conduct was in accordance with a body of medical opinion. Standards for undertaking the 'dual role', assisting and acting as the scrub practitioner, are also outlined in these documents.

Causation

If a breach is proved, the claimant must show that it is more likely than not that the harm they suffered was caused by the breach. This is known as causation. The traditional approach of the courts has been to apply the 'but-for' test: but for the breach, the harm would not have occurred [43].

In some cases, there may be more than one potential cause of the harm the claimant has suffered; or there could have been a series of factors that together resulted in the harm. In the Wilsher case, an infant suffered retinal damage and limited sight for which there were five potential causes identified. One was administration of excess oxygen following a trainee doctor's error, and the others were linked to the infant's prematurity and health. It was not possible on the evidence to know which one was responsible for the infant's loss of sight. The court dismissed the notion that causation could be found just by materially contributing to the risk of the harm suffered; therefore, in order for a claim in negligence to succeed, the claimant must show that of all the potential causes it was the defendant's breach that caused the harm [38].

In serious cases of negligence, which result in the death of a patient, the healthcare professional may be prosecuted for the criminal offence of gross negligence manslaughter. In *R* v. *Adomako* [44], an anaesthetist negligently failed to notice or respond to obvious signs that the oxygen had become disconnected and the patient had stopped breathing, resulting in their death. On appeal, Lord Mackay LC stated that the question for the jury in deciding whether the negligence amounted to gross negligence 'is whether having regard to the risk of death involved, the conduct of the defendant was so bad in all the circumstances as to amount in their judgment to a criminal act or omission' [44].

In a more recent, highly publicised case, the court found that Dr Hadiza Bawa-Garba was responsible for errors that led to the death of a 6-year-old boy in her care and she was convicted of gross-negligence manslaughter. The case highlighted concerns about the criminal prosecution of healthcare professionals for negligence that occurs within a context of broader systemic issues carrying increased risk of errors such as staffing shortages, problems with policies and processes, and inadequate support for less-experienced healthcare professionals [45, 46].

In 2013, Sir Robert Francis published his report into the catastrophic failings in care at the Mid-Staffordshire General Hospital Trust in England between 2005 and 2008, and its recommendations had wide-reaching consequences for the NHS. Following the report, an offence of wilful neglect was created which allowed for the prosecution of individuals who deliberately or recklessly mistreated or neglected patients, whether or not it resulted in the harm or threat of harm to a patient's health (see [47], sections 20 and 21).

The report also highlighted a need for a culture in which healthcare staff could feel able to raise concerns about patient care and safety and have them taken seriously. The report emphasised a need to be open and honest when things go wrong and recommended the introduction of a duty of candour. A duty of candour is defined in the report as the requirement that [48]:

> Any patient harmed by the provision of a healthcare service is informed of the fact and an appropriate remedy offered, regardless of whether a complaint has been made or a question asked about it.

In response to the report, the UK government introduced a statutory duty of candour which applies to all Care and Quality Commission regulated providers (see [49], regulation 20). A professional duty of candour was also incorporated into all professional codes of conduct. The General Medical Council and the Nursing and Midwifery Council explained these professional obligations in a jointly authored guidance document [50].

Autonomy and Consent

The principle of respect for autonomy finds legal and professional expression through the requirement for patient consent to medical treatment. Brazier explains that [51]:

> [a] patient who is sufficiently mature and intellectually competent to understand what is entailed in a treatment is entitled to make up his or her own mind as to whether to accept or reject proposed medical treatment. This right is part and parcel of his or her autonomy, of sovereignty over one's own body.

Within the NHS in the UK, it is customary practice for a standard pro forma to be used to record the consent of a patient to surgery. While obtaining written consent of this type is advisable and may be a compulsory requirement in practice, a signed consent form is only *evidence* that consent has been provided and does not necessarily constitute a valid consent to treatment. Consent may be communicated verbally and might also be implied by the conduct of the patient [52]. Whatever form consent takes, to be valid the patient must have capacity to make the decision and be sufficiently informed about the procedure [53].

Treatment without Consent

The consequences for the perioperative practitioner in performing treatment on a patient without valid consent are serious and can give rise to liability in both criminal and civil law [54]. The general position is that a healthcare professional commits the crime of assault (see [55], section 39) and the tort of trespass to the person (battery) [56] where they intentionally or recklessly touch a patient without their consent.[3]

To lawfully provide treatment to a patient, the perioperative practitioner must therefore have what has been called a 'flak jacket' [57]: protection from liability in the form of legal authority to provide the treatment. In the case of a competent patient, their valid, informed consent will provide such protection. Otherwise, the consent of a person authorised to consent on behalf of a person without capacity is required; or specific defences within common law and statutes such as the Mental Capacity Act 2005 [2]. We will consider each of these in this section but firstly we must understand what is meant by obtaining informed consent.

Informed Consent

For a patient to be able to make the decision that is best for them, it is important that the perioperative practitioner supports their patient through the provision of accurate, relevant, and tailored information. The perioperative practitioner must provide adjustments and support to enable the patient to understand the information and communicate their decision. Finally, they must take reasonable steps to ensure the patient's understanding and allow time for them to ask questions. In this respect, it is important for the perioperative practitioner to consider where and when consent should be obtained. For example, obtaining consent for surgery in the anaesthetic room may not allow the patient sufficient time to think and ask questions and the patient may feel pressure to consent to surgery so as not to cause any inconvenience to the surgical team. Ultimately, the perioperative practitioner must act as the patient's advocate, supporting their right to consent to or refuse treatment where they are able.

Where the patient in providing consent, understands in broad terms the nature of the treatment but there are deficiencies in the information provided by the healthcare professional, then liability will not arise in battery but in the tort of negligence [58]. Traditionally, the law had applied the 'professional standard' in the *Bolam* test to both the standard of care in the provision of clinical treatment and the practice of informed consent. However, in the leading case of *Montgomery* v. *Lanarkshire Health Board* [53], the Supreme Court reviewed the law relating to consent and endorsed the more patient-focused approach contained in General Medical Council guidelines [59], known as the 'reasonable patient standard'. The case establishes that the perioperative practitioner seeking a patient's consent will be under a duty (see [53], at 87):

> ... to take reasonable care to ensure that the patient is aware of any material risks involved in the recommended treatment and of any reasonable alternatives or variant treatments.

---

[3] For example, in the case of *Devi* v. *West Midlands Area Health Authority* [1980] the patient provided consent for a minor gynaecological procedure but during surgery it was discovered that her womb was ruptured so a sterilisation was performed. Mrs Devi was successful in her claim for battery because she had not consented at any point to the sterilisation; see also *Re B (Adult: Refusal of Medical Treatment)* [2002] 2 All England Reports 449, [2002] EWHC 429, (2002) 65 BMLR.

The Court explained the meaning of 'material risks' (see [53], at 87):

'in the circumstances of the particular case, a reasonable person in the patient's position would be likely to attach significance to the risk, or the doctor is or should reasonably be aware that the particular patient would be likely to attach significance to it.'

Here, the focus is not on the percentages of probabilities, but rather on the individual information needs of the patient. Consideration needs to be given to the likely impact on the patient of the actualisation of any particular risk, and the patient's motivation and expectations of treatment. The Royal College of Surgeons' guidance for information provision is likely to be helpful to the perioperative practitioner and recommends that in providing information about the procedure and its possible implications, discussion should include the following [60]:

- the patient's diagnosis and prognosis;
- options for treatment, including non-operative care and no treatment;
- the purpose and expected benefit of the treatment;
- the likelihood of success;
- the clinicians involved in their treatment;
- the risks inherent in the procedure, however small the possibility of their occurrence, side effects, and complications – the consequences of non-operative alternatives should also be explained; and
- potential follow-up treatment.

The court in the Montgomery case emphasised the importance of dialogue in the consent process. It is important that sufficient time and space is afforded to the consent discussion in a way that considers the seriousness or complexity of the particular procedure and enables the practitioner to build a good understanding of their patient's wishes and information needs. The court was clear that bombarding the patient with information and technical jargon was not acceptable, and that information should be provided in an accessible way for the patient to be able make their own decision [53]. The importance of warning patients about postoperative risks was highlighted in *Spencer* v. *Hillingdon NHS Trust* [61], a case that involved a failure to warn a patient of the postoperative risk of deep vein thrombosis.

The court in the Montgomery case also discussed the 'therapeutic exception' which permits the healthcare practitioner, in rare and only the most exceptional circumstances, to withhold information if disclosing it to the patient would cause them serious harm [53].

Refusal of Treatment

The law not only protects the patient's decision-making rights in relation to consent but also the refusal of treatment. In the case of *Re B (Adult: Refusal of Medical Treatment)* [22], a tetraplegic patient refused continuation of life-sustaining treatment. Doctors treating her wanted to continue ventilation and considered that, with rehabilitative treatment to help improve the quality of her life, Ms B may in time feel better about her situation. They felt that to remove ventilation at this stage would be akin to killing their patient. The court held that Ms B had the necessary capacity and understanding to make the decision and she was entitled to refuse ongoing treatment. Her continued ventilation in the face of her refusal amounted to battery and she was awarded nominal damages of £100 in recognition of this infringement of her rights. The court's concern in the case was not whether the patient was right to consent or refuse the treatment but rather whether they had the necessary mental capacity to consent or refuse the treatment [22].

Capacity

Capacity is key to autonomous decision making and, once a patient is found to have the necessary capacity and is sufficiently informed, their decision about whether to consent or refuse the treatment being offered must be respected [62].

The legal test for capacity is set out in the Mental Capacity Act 2005 (MCA) [2] and the accompanying code of practice [63]. When assessing whether a patient has the capacity to decide about their treatment, the perioperative practitioner must have regard to fundamental principles underpinned by the MCA. All adult patients and children aged 16 and 17 years are presumed to have capacity (see [64], section 8). The MCA states that no assumptions should be made about a patient's capacity based on age, appearance or behaviour, disability, or the existence of a mental disorder (see [2], section 2).

The test is focused on the ability to make a particular decision, rather than a more universal ability to make decisions. Some patients may be able to make simple decisions, such as what to have for breakfast, but may lack the necessary understanding to make complex decisions about their long-term treatment or care. As far as a person is able to make decisions for themselves, they must be permitted to do so, and the MCA requires that all reasonable steps are taken to enable them to make a decision before they can be found to lack capacity (see [2], section 1(3)).

A person may make decisions that are seemingly irrational or refuse treatment that might generally be in their best interests. This is not in itself sufficient grounds for a finding that they lack capacity (see [2], section 1(4); [63], pp. 24–26). A patient's decision making may not be based solely on their medical interests. They are also often likely to be influenced by personal values, beliefs, practical considerations, and priorities. However, seemingly harmful or irrational decisions, particularly where they are out of character, may give rise to a legitimate suspicion that the patient lacks either capacity or all the relevant information to make the decision. This may require further investigation of the patient's capacity (see [63], p. 25). Ultimately, however, where a patient has capacity, they are entitled to make the decision that they consider best for them overall, even where the perioperative practitioner may think they should have decided otherwise (see [63], pp. 24–26).

The Test for Capacity

To assess a patient's capacity, the perioperative practitioner is therefore concerned with whether the patient can decide about their treatment at the time that they need to make the decision. The MCA stipulates a two-stage test. The perioperative practitioner must consider:

(1) Does the person have 'an impairment of, or a disturbance in the functioning of, the mind or brain?' (see [2], section 2).

(2) If so, does the impairment or disturbance mean they are unable to make the particular decision?

The impairment may be temporary or permanent (see [2], section 2). The MCA states that a person is unable to decide for the purpose of the test if, at the material time, they are unable to:

(a) understand the information relevant to the decision;

(b) retain that information;

(c) use or weigh that information as part of the process of making the decision; and

(d) communicate their decision (whether by talking, using sign language or any other means) (see [2], section 3; [65], pp. 175–188).

It is important for those involved in a patient's care to make a comprehensive record of the test, the outcome, and the reasons for their conclusions. If a practitioner is uncertain about the patient's capacity then it is advisable to consult with the wider healthcare team and, if appropriate, the patient's family and carers. In case of a disagreement about capacity, it may be necessary to consider an application to the Court of Protection for an order relating to the patient's capacity (see [63], p. 63).

Best-Interests Decision-Making

Where a patient lacks capacity, decisions in relation to their care and treatment must be made in their best interests (see [2], section 1(5)) In determining the best interests of the patient, the following must be considered:

- all the relevant circumstances;
- whether it is likely the patient will regain capacity and, if so, when;
- the person's past and present wishes and feelings, in particular, any written statement made when the person had capacity;
- the beliefs and values that may have influenced the person's decision if they were able to decide for themselves; and
- decisions relating to life-sustaining treatment should not be motivated by a desire to bring about the person's death (see [2], section 4).

As far as reasonably practical, the patient themselves should be permitted, encouraged, and enabled to take part in the decision-making process (see discussion in [65], pp. 175–188). Where possible, best-interests decisions should be informed by consultation with family members, carers, and/or those named or appointed by the patient as someone to be consulted (see [63], pp. 80–86). To support the courts in establishing what is in a person's best interests, a balance sheet approach has been adopted from the case of *Re A* [2000], to better highlight the risks and potential benefits for the decision in question [66].

The MCA is designed to empower those who may face barriers to exercising their decision-making capacity. (For further discussion on this point see [67, 68].) The MCA confers obligations on those involved in the care and treatment of individuals to support autonomous decision making and protects a person's right to meaningful involvement in decisions about their own care and treatment. It also provides several mechanisms for those who have capacity to undertake advance planning about their care and treatment for such a time when they lack the necessary capacity to make such decisions.

Advance Decisions

A valid advance decision enables a person to refuse a particular treatment should they lack capacity in the future (see [2], section 24). They can be distinguished from advanced statements which may include the patient's preferences or request for particular treatments in the event they lose capacity (see [63], p. 82). Valid advanced refusals of treatment by a person with capacity are legally binding on healthcare professionals. Conversely, while advanced requests for treatment may be useful in informing a best-interests decision, they are not legally binding, and healthcare professionals cannot be compelled to provide treatments contrary to their clinical judgment [69].

To be valid, the person making the advance decision must be over 18 and have capacity. The decision needs to be voluntary and the advance decision must detail specifically the treatment and circumstances of the refusal. The decision will only be valid if it specifically applies to the situation in question and circumstances have not changed in such a way as to suggest the person has changed their mind (see [2], section 25; [63], pp. 171–172).

In circumstances where a person wishes to refuse life-sustaining treatments, the refusal will only be valid if it is in writing and signed by the patient and two witnesses (see [2], section 25(5)–(6); [65], pp. 195–198).

Lasting Power of Attorney

The MCA also allows a person over 18 with capacity to appoint one or more people to make decisions about their welfare, care, and treatment on their behalf when they no longer have capacity. This is known as a lasting power of attorney (LPA). To be valid, an LPA must be in writing, comply with certain legal formalities, and be registered with the Office of the Public Guardian (see [2], section 9 and Schedule 1). The decisions that an appointed person (a donee) can make are limited to what is provided for in the LPA (see [2], section 9(4b)). A person may only make decisions relating to life-sustaining treatment where this has been explicitly provided for in the LPA. Donees must make decisions in the best interests of the patient (see [2], section 9(4a)).

In the absence of an advance decision or LPA relating to the decision to be made, the decision will fall to the carers or healthcare professionals providing the relevant care or treatment to the patient. In the healthcare setting, best-interests decisions are usually made by a team of professionals involved with the care of the patient, in consultation with family members and carers. Where there is disagreement, the matter can be bought to court for a decision as to the patient's best interests (see, for example, [70]).

Decision making is, as we have seen, one of the fundamental legal issues within operating department practice. We have seen that perioperative practitioners must support patients to obtain lawful and valid informed consent. Where a person over the age of 16 years is unable to provide consent, the law ensures that decisions must be made in their best interests but focus on the needs of the person. While decision making for adults presents challenges for the perioperative practitioner, they must understand the requirements to act as an effective advocate for their patient.

Emergencies

In emergency situations, it may not always be possible to seek consent from the patient. In some cases, they may require urgent, life-saving surgery but be unable to consent because they are unconscious or otherwise incapacitated. In other circumstances, during an operation, a person may need an additional emergency procedure to save their life or prevent a serious deterioration in their health. In these circumstances, treatment may proceed without consent provided it is immediately necessary and, in the patient's best interests on the basis of medical necessity [2, 25]; see also [63], p. 31 and p. 104. There must be good medical reasons why the procedure cannot be delayed allowing time to seek the patient's consent. Also, as discussed above, if the patient, at a time when they had capacity, made a valid advanced decision, refusing the life-saving procedure in the circumstances, then that decision must be respected [2] (see also [63], p. 174).

Children, Healthcare, and the Law

Within healthcare, children present specific issues in relation to decision making because they have not yet achieved the full set of legal rights conferred to adults. Children occupy a complex area of healthcare law because a tripartite relationship exists between the child, their parents or carers, and healthcare professionals.

A child is any person under the age of 18 years (see [64], section 8) and, generally, there is no presumption that children under 16 years have capacity to consent for themselves. However, the law recognises that children are not a homogenous group. Childhood is a marked period of growth and development in a person's life. Levels of understanding and maturity develop as a child grows but can differ even in children of the same age. The law has evolved to recognise the emerging autonomy of children as they mature into adulthood.

Generally, those with parental responsibility for a child may provide consent for their treatment and parents are usually expected to make decisions that are in the interests of the child's welfare. Usually, the consent of any person with parental responsibility will be sufficient for treatment to be provided lawfully. In the case of serious or irreversible procedures, such as non-therapeutic male circumcision, the courts have indicated that the consent of all those with parental responsibility will be required (see [71]; for an ethical discussion on this point, see [72]). Where parents disagree, the courts have been called upon to determine the best interests of children, for example, in disputes concerning vaccination (for a recent example, see [73]).

16- and 17-Year-Olds

As discussed above, 16- and 17-year-olds are presumed to have capacity and can provide effective consent to surgical, medical, and dental treatment without the need for parental consent (see [64], section 8). Case law suggests, however, that while they may consent to treatment, refusals, particularly of life-saving treatment, can be overridden by the courts. In the case of *Re P (Medical treatment: best interests)* [74], the court held that a 17-year-old was not able to refuse a blood transfusion on the basis that he was unable to contemplate his own mortality. The _Re P_ case highlights that had the young person been 18 (just a few months older) the court would have to respect their decision as an adult. The law in this area has been subject to criticism because of the reliance on chronological age rather than maturity [75].

Children Under 16

Very young children will not usually have capacity to consent to treatment but in the case of older children, particularly adolescents, the situation is less clear and it is necessary to consider whether the child is themselves sufficiently competent to consent to treatment without the need for parental consent. The English legal principle that a competent minor could provide lawful consent was established in *Gillick v. West Norfolk and Wisbech Area Health Authority* [76]. Lord Scarman stated that the minor must have 'sufficient understanding and intelligence to enable him or her to understand fully what is proposed'. This principle, known as 'Gillick competence', reflects the stance of the United Nations Convention on the Rights of the Child, which asserts that, as a child matures into adolescence, gaining maturity and intelligence, the increased ability to make informed autonomous treatment choices must be recognised by the State [77]. The considerations for the healthcare professionals and the courts to assess competence are:

- Does the child understand the nature of their medical condition and the proposed treatment?
- Does the child understand the moral and family issues involved?
- Does the child have sufficient life experience and maturity?
- Is the child capable of weighing up the information appropriately?
- If the child's competence is fluctuating, they will be treated as incompetent.
- The court will be concerned that the child is making their own decision and not merely repeating the views of their parents.

As with 16- and 17-year-olds, the ability to consent to treatment does not necessarily mean the court will find a child has capacity to refuse treatment. In this respect, Cave states that 'the ambiguous definition of competence enabled judges to raise the threshold to arguably unattainable levels' [78].

The Child's Welfare

Where disagreements arise between healthcare professionals and those with parental responsibility and/or older children about the best way to proceed with care or treatment, the court can be asked to decide the matter. In doing so, the court will apply the paramountcy principle which requires that 'the welfare of the child shall be the court's paramount consideration' (see [4], section 1(1)).

In determining the child's welfare, the court must consider the range of factors in the 'welfare checklist' contained in the Children Act (see [4], section 1(3)). The checklist includes consideration of any harm the child has already suffered or is likely to suffer. Harm is defined as 'ill-treatment or the impairment of health or development; health includes physical and mental health' (see [4], section 1(3)).

Determining the best interests of a child is not always straightforward. Recent cases around withdrawal of treatment from infants, such as *Great Ormond Street Hospital* v. *Yates and Gard* [79], have highlighted the tension that can arise where parents and or healthcare professionals disagree as to the child's best interests.

Although we have focused on children and decision making in this section, in the next section we will return to confidentiality in relation to children. In all cases, the focus of the perioperative practitioner must be the best interests of the child.

Confidentiality

Trust is of fundamental importance to the professional–patient relationship and is underpinned by an understanding that the information shared by a patient will be treated discreetly and in confidence. To understand how the law protects patient confidentiality it is necessary to consider the common law, the influence of the Human Rights Act 1998, and the EU General Data Protection Regulation.

The Common Law Duty of Confidentiality and the Right to Privacy

The common law has long recognised a duty of confidentiality arising from a confidential relationship such as that between a doctor and their patient [80] and is usually considered to continue after the death of the patient [81]. A duty of confidentiality may also arise in circumstances 'whenever a person receives information he knows or ought to know is fairly and reasonably to be regarded as confidential' [11]. Medical information has been held to be 'obviously private' and therefore subject to a duty of confidentiality [11]. While it is indisputable that healthcare professionals are under a duty not to disclose medical and other personal information about their patients, issues arise where the failure to share such information might risk harm to the welfare, rights, or interests of others.

Disclosure and Breach of Confidentiality

Public Interest

Case law demonstrates that the duty of confidentiality is not an absolute duty and that in certain circumstances healthcare professionals may be permitted to disclose confidential information where it is necessary in the public interest to do so [82].

In *W* v. *Edgell* [82], the Court of Appeal held that while Dr Edgell owed W a duty of confidentiality, the public interest in the safety of others outweighed the public interest in maintaining W's confidentiality. Disclosure of a psychiatric report to those responsible for decisions about W's detention and treatment in a secure hospital was a proportionate means to protect the public and thereby lawful. The case provides important guidance about the duty of confidentiality and disclosure. For a breach of confidentiality to be justified there must be an ongoing, real, and serious risk of harm to others. Disclosure must only be made to those with a legitimate interest in the information and must be confined to the minimum necessary to prevent the harm in question [82].

The case of *Campbell* v. *MGN* [11] established that the duty of confidentiality incorporates a person's right to respect for their privacy under Article 8 in the Human Rights Act 1998. The right to privacy under Article 8 is a qualified right and interference may be limited where it is necessary to achieve a legitimate aim under Article 8 [8]. Namely, national security, public safety, or the economic well-being of the country, for the prevention of disorder or crime, for the protection of morals, or for the protection of freedom and rights of others [see [8], Article 8). Any breach of confidence must be the minimum necessary to protect the relevant public interest.

Consent to Disclosure

There will be no breach of confidentiality if the patient provides valid consent to information being disclosed and, wherever possible, consent to a disclosure of their personal information should be obtained. (For further discussion on confidentiality and consent, see [9], pp. 245–247.) Where consent is not required or being sought, the patient should be informed of the intention to breach confidence, provided it does not place the healthcare professional or others at risk of harm or undermine the purpose for disclosing the information. (For further discussion, see [25], pp. 245–256; [83], section 9.)

Healthcare is generally provided by a team of professionals and usually a patient, in accessing these services, is considered to have impliedly consented to their medical information being shared between those responsible for their care (see [84], paragraph 15). This is subject to the limitation that only the information necessary for providing care should be shared between healthcare colleagues and strictly for the purposes of providing such care and treatment. If a competent patient requests that information is not shared in this way, they should be advised of the consequences this could have for their care [25] (see also [84], paragraph 14).

In limited circumstances, there is a mandatory legal requirement for healthcare professionals to disclose information about their patients, for example, reporting notifiable infectious disease. (See, for example, [39], pp. 209–213; [85], section 5B; [86, 87].)

Disclosure under the MCA

Where an adult lacks capacity to consent to disclosure of their medical information, disclosure must only be made to the extent it is considered to be in their best interests (see [2], section 1(5)). It may be permissible to provide a close relative or friend with limited information about a patient's condition and what they can expect, provided there is nothing to suggest that the patient would be opposed to this or that it would cause harm to the patient or others. The particular disclosure and the reason for it should be recorded (see [84], paragraphs 13–15).

Children and Confidentiality

Children enjoy the same rights as adults to respect for their confidentiality and their rights to privacy under Article 8, and consent to disclose their medical information should be sought from a competent child or those with parental responsibility. All decisions relating to the disclosure of a child's confidential information should be made in their best interests. In the case of children who are not able to provide consent, those with parental responsibility can provide consent for disclosure of the child's medical information (see [84], paragraphs 9 and 10).

In the case of older children, the previously mentioned case of *Gillick* v. *West Norfolk and Wisbech Area Health Authority* [76] suggests that the capacity to consent or refuse the disclosure of confidential information aligns with the child's capacity to consent to treatment. However, the court has made clear that where a child was seeking contraceptive advice or abortion services, the healthcare professional is under a duty to persuade them to discuss the matter with their parents [76, 88]. (For a more detailed discussion see [39], pp. 198–204.)

Healthcare professionals are under a professional and legal obligation to take reasonable steps to protect a vulnerable adult or child that they are concerned is at risk of harm, abuse, or negligence, which may include the disclosure of confidential information where necessary [89]. (For further discussion, see [90].)

Data Protection Law

The General Data Protection Regulation (GDPR) provides a further dimension of protection for patient confidentiality (see [91]; for further discussion see [9], pp. 241–243). The GDPR has been kept in UK law as the 'UK GDPR' following Britain's departure from the EU and is to be read alongside the Data Protection Act 2018. Together, they regulate the collection, storage, and processing of personally identifiable information. Organisations must ensure that any processing of information is subject to the principles contained in the Data Protection Act, including that:

- processing must be lawful and fair;
- information must only be used for the specific, explicit, and legitimate purpose for which it was collected;
- data must be adequate, relevant, and not excessive in relation to the stated purpose for which they are processed;
- all reasonable steps should be taken to ensure the data are accurate and kept up to date;
- information should be kept no longer than is necessary; and
- data should be handled in a way that ensures proper security of the information (see [92], sections 34–41; see also [93]).

Added safeguards apply to more sensitive information including health data, and patients have the right to request access to data held about them. There are significant fines for breach of the regulations and any breach should be reported swiftly [94].

Professional standards and guidance informed by this complex area of law provide a practical framework for following both legal and ethical requirements relating to confidentiality (see [14], standard 5); see also [83] and [95]). Within NHS trusts in the UK, all NHS staff, students, trainees, authorised agencies, and the trust itself are considered to have a duty of confidentiality and each trust must appoint a 'Caldicott guardian' who is responsible for ensuring that personal information is only shared for justified purposes and only to the extent necessary to achieve a justifiable purpose (see [96] and [89]; see also [25], pp. 238–239).

Summary

While the focus of this textbook is operating department practice, it is important to appreciate that healthcare law is broad and, as such, must be applied rather than be specific to operating department practice. Healthcare law is also complex, but we have seen that in part this is because it highlights and aims to address the issues that arise in the provision of healthcare and the rights of patients. Importantly, the standards set by healthcare law must be met by perioperative practitioners alongside the professional obligations set by their regulating body and in consideration of ethical reasoning about issues that arise. Perhaps one way to think of healthcare law specifically relating to operating department practice is to consider the way in which treatment and interventions are provided. Every aspect of perioperative care therefore requires the practitioner to recognise, understand, and uphold the legal standard expected.

References

1. G. Slapper and D. Kelly. *The English Legal System*, 18th ed. London: Routledge, 2017.

2. Mental Capacity Act 2005. Available from: www.legislation.gov.uk/ukpga/2005/9/contents.

3. The Mental Health Act 1993. Available from: www.legislation.gov.uk/ukpga/1983/20/contents.

4. Children Act 1989. Available from: www.legislation.gov.uk/ukpga/1989/41/section/1.

5. The Controlled Drugs (Supervision of Management and Use) Regulations 2013 (created by the Secretary of State for Health under powers conferred by the Health Act 2006). Available from:

www.legislation.gov.uk/uksi/2013/373/contents/made.

6. The Nursing and Midwifery Order 2001. Available from: www.legislation.gov.uk/uksi/2002/253/contents/made.

7. European Union (Withdrawal) Act 2018. Available from: www.legislation.gov.uk/ukpga/2018/16/section/3/enacted.

8. Human Rights Act 1998. Available from: www.legislation.gov.uk/ukpga/1998/42/contents.

9. S. D. Pattinson. *Medical Law and Ethics*, 6th ed. London: Sweet & Maxwell, 2020.

10. *Pretty* v. *United Kingdom* no. 2346/02 [2002] ECHR 423 (29 April 2002).

11. *Campbell* v. *Mirror Group Newspapers Ltd* [2004] UKHL 22.

12. *Glass* v. *United Kingdom* [2004] 1 FCR 553.

13. *Evans* v. *United Kingdom* [2007] ECHR 264.

14. Nursing and Midwifery Council. The Code. : professional standards of practice and behaviour for nurses, midwives and nursing associates. Available from: www.nmc.org.uk/standards/code/.

15. Health and Care Professions Council. Standards of conduct, performance and ethics. Available from: www.hcpc-uk.org/standards/standards-of-conduct-performance-and-ethics/.

16. Equality Act 2010. Available from: www.legislation.gov.uk/ukpga/2010/15/contents.

17. Government Equalities Office and Equality and Human Rights Commission. Equality Act 2010 guidance. Available from: www.gov.uk/guidance/equality-act-2010-guidance#public-sector-equality-duty.

18. J. N. Newton, A. D. M. Briggs, C. J. L. Murray, et al. Changes in health in England, with analysis by English regions and areas of deprivation, 1990–2013: a systematic analysis for the Global Burden of Disease Study 2013. *The Lancet* 2015; **386**: 2257–2274.

19. Health and Social Care Act 2012. Available from: www.legislation.gov.uk/ukpga/2012/7/contents/enacted.

20. Department of Health. *Responsibility and Accountability: Moving on from New Ways of Working to a Creative, Capable Workforce: Best Practice Guidance*. London: HMSO, 2010.

21. *Bolam* v. *Friern Hospital Management Committee* [1957] 2 All ER 118.

22. *Re B (Adult: Refusal of Medical Treatment)* [2002] 2 All ER 449.

23. L. Dearden. Ian Paterson: High Court approves £37 m compensation for 750 victims of jailed breast surgeon. *Independent*, September 27, 2017. Available from: www.independent.co.uk/news/uk/home-news/ian-paterson-victims-compensation-breast-surgeon-mutilate-wounding-patients-high-court-nhs-a7970666.html.

24. G. James. Report of the independent inquiry into the issues raised by Paterson. Available from: https://assets.publishing.service.gov.uk/government/uploads/system/uploads/attachment_data/file/863211/issues-raised-by-paterson-independent-inquiry-report-web-accessible.pdf.

25. J. Herring. *Medical Law and Ethics*, 8th ed. Oxford: Oxford University Press, 2020.

26. NHS Resolution. Report and accounts 2018/2019. Available from: https://resolution.nhs.uk/wp-content/uploads/2019/08/NHS-Resolution-Annual-Report-2018-19.pdf.

27. N. Slawson. NHS compensation pay-outs 'unsustainable', say health leaders. *Guardian*, February 2, 2018. Available from: www.theguardian.com/society/2018/feb/02/nhs-compensation-payouts-unsustainable-say-health-leaders.

28. NHS Resolution. About NHS Resolution. Available at: https://resolution.nhs.uk/about/.

29. *Donoghue* v. *Stevenson* [1932] UKHL 100.

30. *Caparo Industries PLC* v. *Dickman* [1990] UKHL 2.

31. *West Bromwich Albion Football Club Limited* v. *El Safty* [2005] EWHC 2866.

32. R. P. Mulheron. *Medical Negligence: Non-Patient and Third-Party Claims*. Farnham: Ashgate Publishing, 2010.

33. Health and Care Professions Council. Education standards. Available from: www .hcpc-uk.org/education/resources/ education-standards/.

34. Nursing and Midwifery Council. Standards for education. Available from: www .nmc.org.uk/education/standards-for-education2/.

35. Health and Care Professions Council. Guidance on conduct and ethics for students. Available from: www.hcpc-uk.org/globalassets/resources/guidance/ guidance-on-conduct-and-ethics-for-students.pdf.

36. M. Brazier and J. Miola. Bye-Bye Bolam: a medical litigation revolution? *Medical Law Review* 2000; **8**: 85–114.

37. *Bolitho* v. *City and Hackney Health Authority* [1997] 4 All ER 771.

38. *Wilsher* v. *Essex Area Health Authority* [1986] 3 BMLR 37.

39. G. T. Laurie, S. H. E. Harmon, and G. Porter. *Mason and McCall Smith's Law and Medical Ethics*, 10th ed. Oxford: Oxford University Press, 2016.

40. *Penney and others* v. *East Kent Health Authority* [1999] All ER (D) 1271.

41. Perioperative Care Collaborative. The perioperative care collaborative position statement: surgical first assistant. Available from: www.afpp.org.uk.

42. Royal College of Surgeons. Surgical care team guidance framework. Available from: www.rcseng.ac.uk.

43. *Barnett* v. *Chelsea and Kensington Hospital Management Committee* [1968] 2 WLR 422.

44. *R* v. *Adomako* [1995] 1 A.C. 171.

45. J. Vaughan Post Bawa-Garba: how do we detoxify the climate of fear? *The Bulletin of the Royal College of Surgeons of England* 2018; **100**: 325.

46. C. Dyer Bawa-Garba case has left profession shaken and stirred. *British Medical Journal* 2018; **360**: DOI https://doi .org/10.1136/bmj.k456.

47. Criminal Justice and Courts Act 2015. Available from: www.legislation.gov.uk/ ukpga/2015/2/contents

48. R. Francis QC (Chair). Report of the Mid Staffordshire NHS Foundation Trust public inquiry. Available from: https:// assets.publishing.service.gov.uk/ government/uploads/system/uploads/ attachment_data/file/279124/0947.pdf.

49. Health and Social Care Act 2008 (Regulated Activities) Regulations 2014. Available from: www.legislation.gov.uk/ ukdsi/2014/9780111117613/contents.

50. General Medical Council and the Nursing and Midwifery Council. Openness and honesty when things go wrong: the professional duty of candour. Available from: www.gmc-uk.org/ethical-guidance/ ethical-guidance-for-doctors/candour---openness-and-honesty-when-things-go-wrong.

51. M. Brazier. Patient autonomy and consent to treatment: the role of the law. *Legal Studies* 1987; **7**: 169–179.

52. *O'Brien* v. *Cunard SS Co.* (Mass. 1891) 28 NC266.

53. *Montgomery* v. *Lanarkshire Health Board* [2015] UKSC 11.

54. *Lord Goff of Chieveley in F* v. *West Berkshire HA* [1991] UKHL 1.

55. Criminal Justice Act 1988. Available from: www.legislation.gov.uk/ukpga/1988/33/ contents.

56. C. Elliott and F. Quinn. *Tort Law*. Harlow: Pearson Education, 2013.

57. *Re W (A Minor) (Medical Treatment)* [1992] 4 All ER 627.

58. *Chatterton* v. *Gerson* [1981] QB 432, [1981] 1 All ER 257.

59. General Medical Council. Good medical practice: working with doctors working for patients. Available from: www.gmc-uk .org/-/media/documents/good-medical-practice---english-20200128_pdf-51527 435.pdf.

60. Royal College of Surgeons. Good surgical practice, a guide to good practice: consent. Available from: www.rcseng.ac.uk/

standards-and-research/gsp/domain-3/
3-5-1-consent/.

61. *Spencer* v. *Hillingdon NHS Trust* [2015]
    EWHC 1058.

62. M. Brazier and E. Cave. *Medicine, Patients
    and the Law*, 6th ed. Manchester:
    Manchester University Press, 2016.

63. Department for Constitutional Affairs.
    Mental capacity act code of practice.
    Available from: www.gov.uk/government/
    publications/mental-capacity-act-code-of-
    practice.

64. Family Law Reform Act 1969. Available
    from: www.legislation.gov.uk/ukpga/1969/
    46/section/8.

65. P. Bartlett and R. Sandland. *Mental Health
    Law: Policy and Practice*. Oxford: Oxford
    University Press, 2014.

66. L. J. Thorpe in *Re A* [2000] 1 FLR 549
    at 560.

67. C. S. Johnston. Lack of capacity is not an
    'off switch' for rights and freedoms: Wye
    Valley NHS Trust v. Mr B (By His
    Litigation Friend, the Official Solicitor)
    2015 EWCOP 60. *Medical Law Review*
    2017, 25: 662–671.

68. E. Cave. Determining capacity to make
    medical treatment decisions: problems
    implementing the Mental Capacity Act
    2005. *Statute Law Review* 2015; 36: 86–106.

69. *Re J* [1993] Fam 15, at 29; [1992] 4 All ER
    614 at 625.

70. *Aintree University Hospitals NHS
    Foundation Trust* v. *James* [2013].

71. British Medical Association. Guidance for
    non-therapeutic male circumcision:
    practical guidance for doctors. Available
    from: www.bma.org.uk/media/1847/
    bma-non-therapeutic-male-circumcision-
    of-children-guidance-2019.pdf.

72. B. D. Earp and R. Darby. Circumcision,
    autonomy and public health. *Public Health
    Ethics* 2019; 12: 64-81.

73. *B (A Child: Immunisation)* [2018]
    EWFC 56.

74. *Re P (Medical Treatment: Best Interests)*
    [2003] EWHC 2327 (Fam).

75. E. Horowicz. Transgender adolescents and
    genital-alignment surgery: is age restriction
    justified? *Clinical Ethics* 2019; 14: 94–103.

76. *Gillick* v. *West Norfolk and Wisbech Area
    Health Authority* [1986] A.C. 112.

77. United Nations. Convention on the rights
    of the child. Available from: www
    .ohchr.org/en/professionalinterest/pages/
    crc.aspx.

78. E. Cave Goodbye Gillick? Identifying and
    resolving problems with the concept of
    child competence. *Legal Studies* 2014; 34:
    103–122.

79. *Great Ormand Street Hospital* v. *Yates and
    Gard* [2017] EWHC 972 (Fam).

80. *Hunter* v. *Mann* [1974] QB 7674.

81. *Lewis* v. *Secretary of State for Health* [2008]
    EWHC 2196.

82. *W* v. *Egdell* [1990] 1 All ER 835.

83. Health and Care Professions Council.
    Guidance on confidentiality. Available
    from: www.hcpc-uk.org/registration/
    meeting-our-standards/guidance-on-
    confidentiality/.

84. Department of Health. Confidentiality:
    NHS code of practice. Available from:
    https://assets.publishing.service.gov.uk/
    government/uploads/system/uploads/
    attachment_data/file/200146/
    Confidentiality-NHS_Code_of_Practice.pdf.

85. Female Genital Mutilation Act 2003.
    Available from: https://www
    .legislation.gov.uk/ukpga/2003/31/
    contents.

86. Health Protection (Notification)
    Regulations (SI 2010/659), as amended.
    Available from: www.legislation.gov.uk/
    uksi/2010/659/regulation/2/made.

87. Regulation (EU) 2016/679 on the
    protection of natural persons with
    regard to the processing of personal
    data and on the free movement of
    such data, and repealing Directive
    95/46/EC (General Data Protection
    Regulation). Available from: https://
    eur-lex.europa.eu/legal-content/
    EN/TXT/PDF/?uri=CELEX:32016R0679&
    from=EN.

88. *R (on the application of Axon)* v. *Secretary of State for Health* [2006] 2 WLR 1130.

89. Department of Health. Confidentiality: NHS code of practice supplementary guidance – public interest disclosures. Available from: https://assets .publishing.service.gov.uk/government/ uploads/system/uploads/attachment_data/ file/216476/dh_122031.pdf;

90. E. Cave Disclosure of confidential information to protect the patient: the role of legal capacity in the evolution of professional guidance. *Journal of Medical Law and Ethics* 2015; 3: DOI 10.7590/ 221354015X14319325749982.

92. Data Protection Act 2018. Available from: www.legislation.gov.uk/ukpga/2018/12/ contents/enacted.

93. Information Commissioner's Office. Guide to data protection. Available from: https:// ico.org.uk/for-organisations/guide-to-data-protection/.

94. Information Commissioners Office. Personal data breaches. [Available from: https://ico.org.uk/for-organisations/guide-to-data-protection/guide-to-the-general-data-protection-regulation-gdpr/personal-data-breaches/.

95. General Medical Council. Confidentiality: good practice in handling patient information. Available from: www.gmc-uk.org/ethical-guidance/ethical-guidance-for-doctors/confidentiality.

96. Department of Health. The Caldicott Committee Report on the review of patient-identifiable information. Available from: https://webarchive .nationalarchives.gov.uk/20130124064947/ http://www.dh.gov.uk/prod_consum_dh/ groups/dh_digitalassets/@dh/@en/ documents/digitalasset/dh_4068404.pdf.

Health and Safety in the Perioperative Environment

Kevin Henshaw

Introduction

The Health and Safety at Work Act 1974 [1] (often referred to as the HSWA) is a fundamental piece of UK legislation that specifies the obligations and responsibilities of employers regarding the health and safety of employees – as well as temporary workers and visitors – within the workplace.

The HSWA is huge in its remit and includes all places of work – including healthcare providers in both independent and public sectors. It is part of statute law (as opposed to civil or common law), which means that it has been approved by the UK parliament and can result in both criminal and civil prosecutions. Fines, prison sentences, or both, can be imposed on those convicted of breaches of the HSWA. The Health and Safety Executive (HSE) [2] are the regulatory body in the UK who can inspect, investigate, and enforce practices that may be harmful within organisations. This chapter focuses on some of the fundamental areas of perioperative care in relation to health and safety with an onus on the responsibilities of both employers and employees.

Rationale for Health and Safety

It is useful to consider the health and safety process as an enabling feature of perioperative practice. This is because the rationale for all health and safety legislation is to enable individuals to safely carry out their duties without fear of injury and harm. From an individual practitioner's perspective, there are both professional and moral obligations to ensure a safe working environment.

In the UK, the Health and Care Professions Council (HCPC) and Nursing and Midwifery Council (NMC) registrants are required to consider their own personal safety and those in their care [3, 4]. The HCPC and NMC set standards of proficiency for each of the professional groups on their register and these outline the threshold standards that are necessary to protect the public from harm. Any registrant must possess the relevant knowledge and abilities detailed in the standards of proficiency when they start practicing and must continue to for as long as they remain on the register.

The standards of proficiency for operating department practitioners state the following with respect to health and safety (see [4], standards 15.3–15.7):

- be aware of applicable health and safety legislation, and any relevant safety policies and procedures in force at the workplace, such as incident reporting, and be able to act in accordance with these;

- be able to work safely, including being able to select appropriate hazard control and risk management, reduction or elimination techniques in a safe manner and in accordance with health and safety legislation;
- be able to select appropriate personal protective equipment and use it correctly; and
- be able to establish safe environments for practice, which minimise risks to service users, those treating them, and others, including the use of hazard control and particularly infection control.

From a legal point of view, all employers and employees have a duty to comply with the HSWA within their day-to-day activities. Employers have a responsibility to ensure that their employees' health, safety, and well-being are addressed during their time at work. The focus of any normal activity is to reduce the chances of occupational harm, injury, or ill health which may occur as a result of any work-related activities. This is partly achieved by the implementation of a risk-management process. Risk management is contained within the overall clinical governance framework and is reported back to trust boards via health and safety committees and clinical risk management groups. Any 'near misses', 'critical incidents', or 'never events' (see Table 5.1) should be recorded and fed back to the appropriate group by use of whatever local reporting system is in place. This reporting helps to build up a database of health and safety issues and identify trends. This system can only work if all staff are prepared to report any incident, however insignificant or minor they appear to be.

Risk management is one of the key principles of clinical governance and is directly associated with the HSWA. Risk management, and the reporting of incidents, is one of the metrics used to measure the effectiveness of health and safety strategies.

HSWA Overview

Employees have a legal duty to take care of their own health and safety and that of others who may be affected by their actions at work. They must cooperate with employers and co-workers to help everyone meet their legal requirements. If an employee has a specific query or concern relating to health and safety in their workplace they should talk to their employer, manager/supervisor, or a health and safety representative.

Employers have a legal duty to protect the health, safety, and welfare of their employees and other people who might be affected by their business. Employers must do whatever is reasonably practicable to achieve this. This means making sure that their employees and others are protected from anything that may cause harm, effectively controlling any risks to injury or health that could arise in the workplace. They also have a duty to assess risks in the workplace; risk assessments should be carried out that address all risks that might cause

Table 5.1 Incident definitions

Near miss	Any event that could have resulted in an adverse outcome but did not
Critical incident	Any untoward medical occurrence in a patient that results in some degree of harm
Never event	Any wholly preventable event where national guidance or safety recommendations provide strong systemic protective barriers that should have been implemented by all healthcare providers [5]

harm in the workplace. Employers must provide their employees with information about the risks in their workplace and how they are protected; they should also instruct and train their employees on how to deal with the risks. They must also consult their employees on health and safety issues. Consultation must be either direct or carried out through a safety representative who is either elected by the workforce or appointed by a trade union.

What Is a Hazard?

A hazard is something that can *become* unsafe and, under the right circumstances, has the potential to do harm. For example, sharps become a risk when not managed or handled properly. It may be useful to consider hazards as something (or someone!) who has the potential to cause harm. Floors can become a hazard when they are wet and may cause harm if someone slips.

What Is a Risk?

A risk is something that has the *potential* to do harm because of a hazard being present. The level of risk is dependent on how the situation is managed. In our analogy, a wet floor presents a high risk of accidental slips unless warning signs are displayed and the risk is made obvious to anybody 'using' the floor. Conversely, the risk is increased if the floor becomes slippery and users are oblivious to the hazard. Used needles are hazardous but become a high risk if they are not safely discarded immediately after use or are 'hidden' on a surface or patient trolley.

All risks need to be identified, assessed, and managed wherever possible. Risk assessment (and the reduction of harm) is the essence of good health and safety management and is central to quality assurance and safe patient management, and it is one of the pillars of clinical governance. Rather than being seen as restrictive and bureaucratic, as already stated, health and safety should be perceived as enabling a process that allows practitioners to provide safe care in a safe environment.

Clinical governance is 'a system through which NHS [UK National Health Service] organisations are accountable for continuously improving the quality of their services and safeguarding high standards of care by creating an environment in which excellence in clinical care will flourish' [6]. It is an umbrella term that describes any activities that help sustain and improve high standards of patient-centred care. All the activities that intend to improve the quality and safety of healthcare are grouped together under 'clinical governance' so they can be more effective.

What Exactly Are Health and Safety Regulations?

The Workplace (Health, Safety and Welfare) Regulations 1992

The Workplace (Health, Safety and Welfare) Regulations 1992 [7] specifically refer to adequate lighting, heating, ventilation, facilities, and safe passageways. Care should be taken within the perioperative area when low lighting is required, such as in interventional radiology suites or during some endoscopy procedures. Trip hazards in low lighting, such as trailing electrical cables and tubing, pose a risk and may require specific risk assessment. Examples of the need to maintain 'safe passageways' can often be seen on common corridors where bulky equipment such as operating tables, image intensifiers, and patient trollies are stored. A lack of space often means that corridors are the only option for storage. Nevertheless, a risk assessment should be carried out, with the need to maintain access to fire exits and clear passages being highlighted. A clear communication strategy may be required to ensure that all staff are aware of the hazards of unsafe passageways. Similar risk-assessment principles can be applied to temperature control and the need to monitor anaesthetic gases and volatile agents within the perioperative area.

The Health and Safety (Display Screen Equipment) Regulations 1992

The Health and Safety (Display Screen Equipment) Regulations 1992 [8] place specific requirements on employers to protect their staff from the harm that can arise from using display screen equipment. This includes the use of computers and monitors within the clinical area.

The Personal Protection Equipment at Work Regulations 1992

The Personal Protection Equipment at Work Regulations 1992 [9] state that personal protective equipment (PPE) should be provided where necessary, including adequate training and instruction in its use. This includes 'fit testing' for respiratory protective equipment (RPE), such as the FFP3 disposable mask which relies on an airtight seal to protect the wearer against airborne contaminates. Like many health and safety procedures, fit testing (and risk assessment in general) should be thought of as a dynamic, ongoing process that may change during, or even after, an intervention. For example, users should carry out a fit test the first time an RPE is used. To preserve the integrity of the mask seal, a new fit test should be initiated following one of the following:

- sudden weight gain or weight loss;
- dental work which may change the shape of the face;
- aesthetic procedures or scars, surgery, or general changes to the face; and
- change of make or type of RPE.

Manual Handling Operations Regulations 1992

The Manual Handling Operations Regulations 1992, which were amended in 2002 [10], include: the removal, where possible, of the need for workers to undertake manual handling, which is associated with a risk of injury; a due assessment of the risks; and the provision of weight information regarding loads. Again, these regulations are generic and apply to all occupations throughout the UK. A common example from perioperative practice would be transferring an anaesthetised patient from a trolley to an operating table. An obvious risk will be that the patient will have no functioning protective reflexes or muscle tone. Therefore, they are at high risk of injury from what is generally considered a 'simple' manoeuvre. Each year, there are documented accounts of patients falling from the operating table during transfer to or from a patient trolley. In 2021, 70-year-old Jeannette Shields was 'dropped' from the operating table following hip surgery and died 6 weeks later from her injuries [11].

A risk assessment should be carried out before any moving and handling task. All risk assessments should be dynamic and can change within a short time period. They are not a one-off 'tick-box' exercise. For example, the manual handling risk may change intraoperatively (tilting the operating table) or postoperatively (transferring of the patient back to a trolley or bed). The risk may have increased because of additional hazards such wound drains, dressings, casts, splints, or even external metalwork such as fixators. Patients emerging from general anaesthesia while still on the operating table or trolley pose a particular problem as they are often disorientated and can be unpredictable when moving.

Where possible, all patients who are mobile and can move themselves should be encouraged to do so following a risk assessment of mobility. This may include transfer from the preoperative area to the anaesthetic room or directly into the operating theatre. Any independent patient mobility will reduce the chances of manual handling accidents but must be risk-assessed appropriately for each individual patient.

The Reporting of Injuries, Diseases and Dangerous Occurrences Regulations (RIDDOR) 1995

The Reporting of Injuries, Diseases and Dangerous Occurrences Regulations (RIDDOR) 1995 [12] outline the reporting of work-related injuries, accidents, incidents, and diseases to the HSE and their recording within the workplace. It is an essential (as well as a legal requirement) that any of the above incidents should be reported and recorded to help compile a database which will enable the HSE and employers to build up a profile of dangerous incidents or near misses. A simple example of the need to report an incident may be that the employer has decided to change the brand of sterile gloves. This may result in an increase of contact dermatitis for users which, if unreported and uncollated, will simply be considered as an issue for individual users. The reporting of multiple users 'reacting' to the new gloves will highlight that the common denominator is the gloves and that the change of supplier will therefore need to be reconsidered.

In the case of an accidental needlestick injury (where a sharp object pierces the skin), the incident is only reported to RIDDOR if the injury causes more than 7 days absence from work through an illness which is directly attributable to the needlestick puncture. If the needle is contaminated with a known blood-borne virus or if the source of the injury cannot be traced (if the sharp is among paper waste, for example) then prophylactic treatment should be commenced, and the injury reported and recorded as an incident which was dangerous. An investigation into how the incident occurred will follow, with recommendations for how to avoid similar incidents in the future – these recommendations are then disseminated via the HSE.

The Provision and Use of Work Equipment Regulations 1998

The Provision and Use of Work Equipment Regulations 1998 [13] require employers to ensure the safety and suitability of work equipment, including its maintenance, and relevant training. These regulations relate to any equipment or devices that are provided by an employer and require a level of training. For example, anyone taking part in the transfer of a patient using a lateral transfer device (e.g., PATSLIDE®) should be trained to an appropriate level and understand the principles of safe manual handling. All employees have a duty of care to the patient and should express any reservations or concerns they may have before taking part in any transfer procedure. This principle of safe 'usage' applies to any equipment or devices within the perioperative area, including any newly purchased items.

Management of Health and Safety at Work Regulations 1999

The Management of Health and Safety at Work Regulations 1999 [14] ensure that employers need to ensure that a delegated member of staff is appointed in the role (often additional) of overseeing health and safety in the workplace. This person is often referred to as the health and safety representative; they are independent of management and should represent the health and safety concerns and interests of their co-workers. A copy of the HSWA should be readily available and accessible in each department.

Control of Substances Hazardous to Health 2002 (COSHH)

All employers are obliged to comply with the Control of Substances Hazardous to Health 2002 (COSHH) regulations [15] (see also the COSHH 2004 (amendment) [16]). The perioperative environment contains many examples of substances that are harmful to health, which are beyond the remit of this chapter. Each employer must ensure that any hazardous materials such as chemical cleaning agents or specimen fixatives are assessed in accordance with local guidelines. These guidelines are designed to minimise employees' exposure to hazardous substances and, where possible, provide alternatives or provide safe systems of delivery.

Surgical smoke is the release of smoke into the atmosphere as a direct result of tissues being vaporised or destroyed by lasers, ultrasonic devices, or diathermy. Surgical smoke is primarily constituted of water vapour but also contains bacteria, viruses, and gases that are known carcinogens, mutagens, and teratogens [17, 18]. Surgical smoke evacuation devices should be used to reduce the levels of exposure to surgical smoke and are indicated any time that a surgical plume is generated. Under optimal conditions, surgical smoke evacuators can reduce smoke exposure by 99% [19]. Wall-mounted suction should not be used to remove surgical smoke because it was not designed for that purpose and there is no evidence to support its efficacy. The COSHH legislation requires an employer to conduct a risk assessment and put measures in place to limit or control exposure to hazardous substances; however, in practice, this remains uncommon.

A further example of the relevance of COSHH regulations is the storage of skin preparations. Some skin preparations are alcohol based, and are flammable, and so these solutions should always be stored as recommended by the manufacturer. Moreover, alcohol-based skin preparations can cause chemical burns and act as fuel for a surgical fire, and they should always be used according to the manufacturer's instructions. Care should be taken to ensure that the alcohol-based skin preparation is not allowed to pool on the skin's surface or be absorbed into the drapes, and that the recommended drying time is observed. Between January 2012 and December 2018 there were 37 reported surgical fires in England and Wales, and more than half resulted in some degree of patient harm – the actual number of surgical fires is likely to have been significantly higher than this [20].

A surgical fire requires three components to be present, which are known as the fire triad: fuel, ignition source, and an oxidiser. When these three are present there is always a risk of a surgical fire, and they are frequently present during surgery (see Table 5.2). However, this can be mitigated by understanding the risks and acting accordingly: for example, not applying drapes before the recommended drying time is observed; using a laser-resistant endotracheal tube when indicated; reducing the fraction of inspired oxygen to less than 30% when using supplemental oxygen; and using a skin preparation applicator to reduce excess solution.

Table 5.2 Fire triad

1. Fuel	2. Ignition source	3. Oxidiser
• Drapes	• Electrosurgical devices	• Oxygen
• Dressings	• Fibre-optic light sources	• Nitrous oxide
• Swabs	• Lasers	
• Alcohol-based skin preparations	• Surgical drills	
• Drains	• Defibrillators	
• Patient gowns		
• Smoke evacuator hoses		
• Endotracheal tubes		

References

1. Health and Safety at Work etc. Act 1974. Available from: www.legislation.gov.uk/ukpga/1974/37/contents.

2. Health and Safety Executive (HSE). Available from: www.gov.uk/health-and-safety-executive.

3. Nursing and Midwifery Council. The Code: professional standards of practice and behaviour for nurses, midwives and nursing associates. Available from: www.nmc.org.uk/globalassets/sitedocuments/nmc-publications/nmc-code.pdf.

4. Health and Care Professions Council. Standards of proficiency: operating department practitioners. Available from: www.hcpc-uk.org/standards/standards-of-proficiency/operating-department-practitioners/.

5. NHS England. Never events policy and framework. Available from: www.england.nhs.uk/wp-content/uploads/2020/11/Revised-Never-Events-policy-and-framework-FINAL.pdf.

6. G. Scally and L. J. Donaldson. Clinical governance and the drive for quality improvement in the new NHS in England. *British Medical Journal* 1998; **317**: 61–65.

7. The Workplace (Health, Safety and Welfare) Regulations 1992. Available from: www.legislation.gov.uk/uksi/1992/3004/contents/made.

8. The Health and Safety (Display Screen Equipment) Regulations 1992. Available from: www.legislation.gov.uk/uksi/1992/2792/contents/made.

9. The Personal Protective Equipment at Work Regulations 1992. Available from: www.legislation.gov.uk/uksi/1992/2966/contents/made.

10. The Manual Handling Operations Regulations 1992. Available from: www.legislation.gov.uk/uksi/1992/2793/contents/made.

11. F. Williams. Cumberland Infirmary patient 'dropped' from operating table dies within weeks. Available from: www.bbc.co.uk/news/uk-england-cumbria-57254855.

12. The Reporting of Injuries, Diseases and Dangerous Occurrences Regulations 1995. Available from: www.legislation.gov.uk/uksi/1995/3163/contents/made.

13. The Provision and Use of Work Equipment Regulations 1998. Available from: www.legislation.gov.uk/uksi/1998/2306/contents/made.

14. The Management of Health and Safety at Work Regulations 1999. Available from: www.legislation.gov.uk/uksi/1999/3242/contents/made.

15. The Control of Substances Hazardous to Health Regulations 2002. Available from: www.legislation.gov.uk/uksi/2002/2677/regulation/7/made.

16. The Control of Substances Hazardous to Health (Amendment) Regulations 2004.

Available from: www.legislation.gov.uk/uksi/2004/3386/contents/made.

17. T. Searle, F. R. Ali, and F. Al-Niaimi. Surgical plume in dermatology: an insidious and often overlooked hazard. *Clinical and Experimental Dermatology* 2020; **45**: 841–847.

18. R. Vortman, S. McPherson, and M. Cecilia Wendler. State of the science: a concept analysis of surgical smoke. *AORN Journal* 2021; **113**: 41–51.

19. H. M. Seipp, T. Steffens, and J. Weigold, et al. Efficiencies and noise levels of portable surgical smoke evacuation systems. *Journal of Occupational and Environmental Hygiene* 2018; **15**: 773–781.

20. D. Rodger. Surgical fires: still a burning issue in England and Wales. *Journal of Perioperative Practice* 2020: **30**: 135–140.

Chapter

6

Fundamentals of Operating Department Design

Shane Roadnight and Anne Followell

Introduction

Within the operating department, essential care is delivered to a vulnerable group of patients by a highly skilled multidisciplinary team, and surgical facilities should be designed to support and enable the smooth flow of patients from admission to discharge. Surgical activities are broad, ranging from scheduled to unscheduled, and from routine day procedures to complex major surgery. Theatre services are central to the hospital system and rely on interdependent relationships with other hospital departments. This presents organisational, planning, and design challenges, as healthcare providers seek to improve services and utilise existing infrastructure to offer facilities that meet demand in a fast-paced and progressive field. Patients are entitled to receive high-quality healthcare, provided safely and effectively, and theatre teams should expect to deliver those high standards of care in an appropriate workspace. All National Health Service (NHS) healthcare facilities must adhere to building regulations, and the Health Building Note (HBN 26) [1] provides standards for the theatre environment that supports clinical, diagnostic, and invasive procedures within the UK. Therefore, theatre design is an essential component of the perioperative pathway, allowing surgical interventions to be carried out safely and efficiently.

The operating department is a complex area containing a suite of rooms designed to facilitate surgical interventions and navigate patients safely through their perioperative journey. Healthcare provision and the services offered have developed at a rapid pace since the birth of the NHS in the UK, in 1948 [2]. Theatre facilities have evolved in response to surgical pathways such as elective, trauma, obstetrics, and dedicated day surgery units. This, in turn, has influenced their design and layout, which should be planned to increase theatre efficiency and to facilitate the smooth flow of patients as they receive care [1, 3]. Advances in technology, treatments, and techniques such as minimally invasive laparoscopic surgery and robotics require existing theatres to be redesigned and refurbished to make the best use of available space. Issues that arise from retrofitting existing spaces present challenges, such as interruption and delays to services, and the UK government's 'Health Infrastructure Plan' recognises the need to increase NHS capital spending by building new hospitals and investing in new and existing facilities [4].

Good design should enable staff to deliver high standards of patient care within a well-structured department, allowing for a positive patient experience. Designers must respond creatively, while ensuring operating theatres meet the minimum standards set out by the Department of Health and Social Care [4], and these criteria guide health providers as they grow and develop services to meet the increased demands for surgical provision. Furthermore, the NHS is navigating a complex journey towards reducing its carbon footprint and national ambition to achieve net-zero targets, and healthcare facilities will need to achieve decreases in energy consumption that impact greenhouse gas emissions [1]. In addition to the layout, which must be functional and comply with infection control principles, essentials such as power supply, lighting, equipment, and storage are part of a much larger list of perioperative-centred elements. Theatre efficiency and increased staff morale are commensurate with well-designed surroundings that adhere to workplace ergonomics, emphasising the link between a good working environment, staff performance, and patient satisfaction [5]. Throughout this chapter, elements of theatre design will be explored, highlighting how careful planning can enhance the patient experience and ensure safe care is delivered.

Location of Operating Theatres

Within modern hospitals, where ground space is a premium commodity, the location of the theatre suite requires careful planning. Operating theatres cannot function in isolation from the rest of the hospital and depend on collaboration with a range of related departments for the smooth transition of patient care, such as sterile services, imaging departments, and the pharmacy. It is beneficial for the operating theatres to be placed near to the surgical wards for convenience, safety, and improved patient satisfaction. Dedicated day surgery units serving a population of 300,000 are designed to function independently and to incorporate preoperative, intraoperative, and postoperative facilities, including a discharge lounge, patient and staff facilities, and administrative offices [6]. Day surgery is defined as a patient being admitted, operated on, and discharged home the same calendar day. Operating departments serving regional trauma centres should be near to the accident and emergency department, diagnostic imaging, and the intensive care unit. This allows patients to access critical care facilities while reducing delays in treatment. It means patients are spared the associated risks of lengthy journeys down hospital corridors during intra-hospital transfers, which can be stressful for both staff and patients. Well-located facilities improve workflow and ease logistical issues for staff, helping them to deliver quality care.

Security

While accessibility is central when planning the location of theatres, the design should prevent public access, safeguarding the security of the department, its staff, and patients while maintaining confidentiality. Access to theatres should be controlled via the theatre admissions unit; however adequate provision may be restricted in departments where building limitations present issues of space. Due to the sensitive nature of the care delivered within the operating department, security is a priority.

Departments should be located away from public areas and include restricted access to ensure patient safety is maintained. Coded doors or swipe key entry are common methods, allowing for appropriate healthcare staff to freely enter [1]. Once access is gained, a reception area should restrict further access until appropriate attire has been donned. For visitor access and external contractors, there should be a communication system based within the reception area incorporating either a closed-circuit television or an intercom in order to communicate with those wishing to enter the department [1]. This facility allows for reception staff to ensure appropriate entry, and the security of the department is maintained.

Departmental Layout

All surgical departments should be laid out with the patient journey in mind. This consists of three key areas – clean, sterile, and dirty. Clean areas are designated as such, to ensure the transition from outlay areas to sterile areas is progressive and minimises infection risks. Clean areas include patient entry points, anaesthetic rooms, and storage areas. The patient, staff, and surgical equipment should all arrive within this area at the start of the journey and progress towards the sterile area via their individual route.

The sterile area is where all three elements – patient, staff, and surgical equipment come together immediately prior to the commencement of the surgical procedure. Once surgery has been completed, the patient is transferred to the post-anaesthesia care unit (PACU) or recovery department. The sterile area is fully restricted to those directly involved in the surgical intervention and is specifically designed to meet strict infection control standards. Upon completion of the procedure, staff prepare the sterile environment for the next patient while the used surgical instruments and waste are transferred to the dirty area for collection and processing. This flow of patients, staff, and equipment allows for the separation of contaminated and used surgical equipment, reducing the risks of both cross-infection and the potential for increased anxiety associated with patients seeing waste products prior to their surgery (see Figure 6.1).

Admissions Lounge

There is a growing trend to include an admissions lounge, where patients can be admitted directly to the operating department in preparation for their surgery. This can help to alleviate the pressure experienced by surgical wards as they prepare patients for surgery. As well as reducing infection rates and bettering the patient experience [1], this could, at least

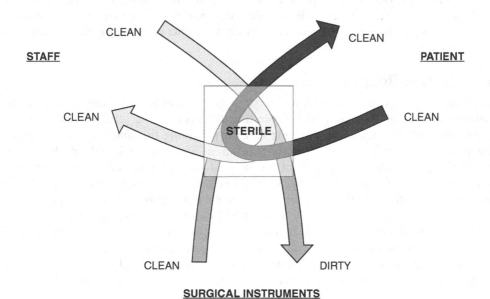

Figure 6.1 Sterile-zone flow

theoretically, improve theatre efficiency. The lounge is typically adjacent to theatres and can be utilised for preoperative preparation, such as baseline observations and tests, pre-surgery consultations with the surgical and anaesthetic team, and preoperative checklists. Seating and/or bed spaces are allocated to each patient, allowing for relatives to stay with the patient prior to their departure for the anaesthetic room.

Anaesthetic Room

Within the clean area is the anaesthetic room where patients will be administered an anaesthetic prior to surgery. Anaesthetic room usage varies worldwide and while the UK currently maintains this approach many other countries have opted to anaesthetise patients directly within the operating theatre [1]. The anaesthetic room should be adjacent to the operating theatre and have soundproof doors to ensure privacy. The room itself should be a minimum of 19 m^2 in size, creating sufficient space for the staff and the complex anaesthetic equipment used [1]. A minimalistic design approach to reduce unnecessary stimulation can contribute to the patient experience, through a calm and quiet environment [7]. Work surfaces should be flush mounted to the wall, with sufficient cupboard space to allow for equipment storage. As part of this storage, lockable drug cupboards and a fridge are required to securely store a range of medications including controlled drugs [8]. Piped medical gases supply oxygen, nitrous oxide, and medical air to Schrader valves for connection to the anaesthetic machine, alongside anaesthetic gas scavenging [9]. A clock should be clearly visible to all staff within the room, allowing for timed interventions to be administered. The emergency alarm bell should be accessible to staff within the room and the door clearly numbered, allowing for prompt identification in the event of a clinical emergency [10].

Double doors with a minimum opening width of 1,600 mm will allow access to the anaesthetic room, creating sufficient entry for all hospital beds [1]. Fitting doors with a soft close function included to facilitate quiet closing reduces disturbance for staff and patients, with each door containing a viewing window that has blinds for privacy. Clear signage identifying when the room is 'in use' is necessary to restrict entry during the induction of anaesthesia.

Preparation Room

Preparation rooms are used to prepare surgical equipment and sterile sets prior to commencement of the procedure. Separating the area allows scrub staff to 'set up' before the patient enters the operating theatre; providing this ancillary space reduces infection rates and increases theatre efficiency. The room should ideally be of a suitable size to accommodate all of the surgical sets required and current standards are between 12 m^2 and 20 m^2 [1]. Ventilation within the preparation room should match the theatre ventilation system and, where ultra-clean ventilation systems are present, the preparation room may be omitted in favour of laying up surgical trolleys under the ventilation canopy [9]. In such cases, a dedicated anaesthetic room should be included in the design. This will avoid the unnecessary movements of anaesthetic staff in theatre, which could risk contaminating instruments, and will prevent patient anxiety associated with witnessing the preparation process, thus disturbing the induction of anaesthesia.

Scrub Rooms

Some operating rooms contain dedicated scrub rooms although this is not an essential component within the design. If chosen, the room should be large enough to accommodate six people, three of whom would be scrubbing, with sufficient space in-between to prevent contamination [1]. To support the practice of scrubbing, sinks should be appropriately placed to aid in the process without compromising sterility. Sinks with internal lips should be avoided to reduce contaminated water from dripping back into the working area, creating an increased infection risk. Splash backs should be present behind the sink, minimising the risk of contaminated areas associated with dirty-water collection. The scrub taps are specific in design and are required to be operated via touchless sensors or elbow operated, with sufficient space underneath to wash hands and arms.

Operating Theatre/Operating Room

Surgical procedures are undertaken within the operating room and the space should be of sufficient size to accommodate the patient, multidisciplinary team, and range of equipment required to facilitate the intervention. While no minimum size is specified, 55 m^2 is recommended, and planning should consider future developments in surgical techniques. New facilities should be constructed to ensure progress in surgery is not hindered by limited space [1].

Lighting

Lighting within the operating room is a vital component of theatre design, requiring a combination of specialist illumination that allows staff to function effectively. The visual demands on the multidisciplinary team require lighting to be adjustable and controllable for brightness. Good illumination contributes to the accurate perception of tissue hue, enabling surgeons to see in sufficient detail to distinguish anatomical structures, and arterial and venous blood flow. Members of the anaesthetic team assess pallor and signs of cyanosis throughout anaesthesia and require adequate ambient and adjustable lighting to perform interventions such as cannulation, intubation, and nerve blocks. Poor lighting can be detrimental to the delivery of patient care, with the most notable effects being eye strain and fatigue caused by glare.

Natural light can be limited or non-existent within many operating theatres and this can have a negative impact on the well-being, morale, and productivity of staff who cannot gain access to daylight while on duty. A way to alleviate this issue, is to install daylight bulbs, which are understood to minimise these effects. All lighting units should be integrated seamlessly within the facility; this will avoid the collection of dust upon high structures associated with contamination and disruption of airflow. In surgeries where bright light may impair surgical views, such as during laparoscopic procedures, dimmable units should be incorporated. Ceiling-mounted lights and the ability to adjust their position and brightness is beneficial for awake patients in relation to their perioperative experience. Fixed and unmovable lights placed directly over treatment areas are deemed unsuitable and may result in patients staring uncomfortably into bright lights during regional or local anaesthetic procedures [1].

Operating lights must provide the surgeon with a detailed, shadowless view of the surgical site and body cavity regardless of patient position. They should be designed to reduce heat generation; this heat contributes to the evaporation of tissue fluid during surgery and causes discomfort for those working within the surgical field. Modern operating lights are constructed using LED (light-emitting diode) systems to reduce power consumption while achieving a heatless projection of shadow-free light. These are dimmable and easily moved to accommodate the required view. Being able to focus the light beam produced by the operating light is an essential component and is built into the control panel, enabling the accurate application of light within the surgical cavity. The recommended illuminance levels for operating lights are 10,000 to 100,000 lux, measured at a 1-m distance between the light and the surgical cavity. This is significantly brighter than the surrounding light, which is recommended to be measured at 1,000 lux, although this remains within expectations of clinical environments [11]. Whereas other areas such as the recovery room and preoperative area should be lit by sources delivering 500 lux [11]. The quality of light provided by these units is required to deliver true colour rendering and is essential for accurate observation of skin hue and tissue perfusion [1].

Ventilation

Ventilation is integral within building design and is necessary to replace stale air with fresh air. Ventilation provides occupants with clean air by diluting and removing potentially harmful impurities; in addition, comfort, health, and well-being are factors associated with a well-ventilated space. Broadly, ventilation can be classified as natural or mechanical, and building regulations require healthcare premises and enclosed workspaces to be ventilated by the appropriate method. These systems should be inspected annually to ensure they are compliant with the minimum standards [9]. Operating theatre ventilation has four distinct functions: to control temperature and adjust humidity when required; to reduce airborne microbial contaminants; to contribute to the dilution and removal of fumes, odours and waste anaesthetic agents; and to influence the movement of air to direct airborne contaminants from clean to less-clean areas. The theatre suite is considered unsuitable for natural ventilation methods, where opening windows and doors would compromise security and risk contamination from external pollutants. Conditions must also be controllable and consistent to allow optimal conditions for surgery; windows in theatre are double glazed and hermetically sealed and doors must be adjusted for door-gap leakage to ensure airflow is uninterrupted. Surgical site infections (SSIs), which are among the most preventable of healthcare associated infections [12], are a prime concern within the operating theatre and the focus of design and construction throughout the department. Therefore, specialist ventilation systems, which may incorporate air conditioning, are selected to provide a managed environment that is safe and comfortable for both patients and staff.

The primary legislation applicable to ventilation installations is the 1974 Health and Safety at Work Act [13] and ventilation systems contribute to the range of measures used to prevent contamination and reduce exposure to hazards while closely controlling the environment. Air quality is measurable according to characteristics such as air pollution, temperature, and relative humidity. Activities undertaken within the department impact theatre air quality, where there is a constant movement of staff, patients, and equipment. The use of electrical equipment generates heat, and clinical treatments including irrigation and processes such as wet chemical cleaning can create excess moisture. Anaesthetic and surgical procedures may cause occupants to be exposed to substances such as gases, surgical smoke, vapours, aerosols, and airborne pathogens. These elements have the potential to cause harm and the Control of Substances Hazardous to Health (COSHH) regulations [14] require employers to assess potential risks and provide measures to reduce harm to health.

A key principle in the design of theatre ventilation systems is that air should always flow from clean to less-clean areas. Conventional mechanical ventilation aims to decrease airborne pollution, by generating a positive air pressure with a mixed or turbulent flow, which directs contaminated air away from the operating site. Ventilation systems are designed by pulling air from outside the theatre suite, typically the roof, and directing it through a series of fans where particles including bacteria are removed by filters. Ultra-clean ventilation (UCV) is a specialist system used in surgeries with a moderate to increased risk of infection, such as orthopaedic surgeries and joint arthroplasty. Ultra-clean air is defined internationally as containing less than 10 colony-forming units per cubic meter (<10 cfu/m^3) and is cleaned by high-efficiency particulate air (HEPA) filters [15]. Ventilation systems replace the air and are measured in air changes per hour (AC/h); the statutory requirement is for a minimum of 22 AC/h in the operating theatre.

There is a hierarchy of room cleanliness, which dictates the pathway of airflow and the amount of ACPH [9] (see Figure 6.2).

The choice of ventilation system will consider the key principles: dilution of airborne contaminants, air movement control from less-clean to cleaner areas, temperature and humidity control, and assisting the removal and dilution of waste anaesthetic gas. The notion of 'dilution being the solution to pollution', along with the ability to control the movement and condition of air, is the concept behind the design of conventionally ventilated operating theatres. Types of airflow systems used include plenum and laminar flow.

Plenum Flow

A plenum flow system is typically found in operating theatres, because it is suitable for most applications. The plenum system requires greater air pressure within the theatre, than

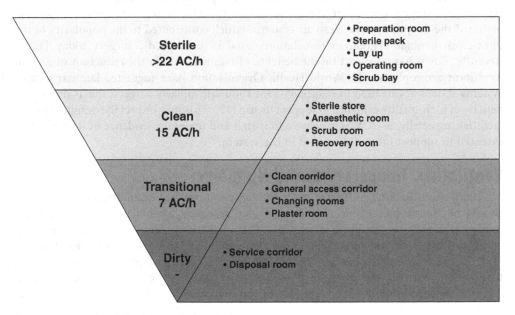

Figure 6.2 Hierarchy of cleanliness including air changes

outside. Clean air enters via ceiling or wall diffusers, flowing downward or across the surgical area and exits the room through weighted vents located above the level of the floor; the system is usually expected to produce approximately 22 AC/h. Maintaining an aseptic environment can be compromised by the movement of staff and the opening of doors, which allows air pressure to fall, decreasing the efficiency of the plenum system.

Laminar Flow

The ultra-clean laminar air flow system delivers a high volume, 450–500 ACPH of HEPA filtered air, either horizontally or, more commonly in the operating room, vertically (flowing downwards) over the operating site [15]. Filtered air continuously streams in uninterrupted parallel lines with minimal turbulence, from the outlets to the area in which the surgery is performed, significantly increasing the effect of dilution. Air is removed under positive pressure through return air grills located around the periphery of the operating room, constantly removing contaminants. Orthopaedic theatres with vertical systems are commonly fitted with ceiling canopies with a minimum size of 2.8 m × 2.8 m; the area beneath should be demarcated as the clean operating zone [14]. Air outside of this zone cannot be guaranteed to be ultra-clean; nonetheless, the level of microbiological contamination will be lower than in theatres with standard ventilation.

Factors that compromise the efficacy of UCV systems can result from air disturbance at the boundary, where the column of UCV meets the surrounding room air. Staff movement and their positioning can increase the mixing of boundary air, resulting in the surrounding particulate becoming entrained into the air within the operating zone. Therefore, limiting staff to essential personnel only, reducing movements, and keeping doors closed can help to mitigate the effect of boundary mixing.

Ultra-Clean Ventilation and SSIs

Professor Sir John Charnley is best known for his pioneering development of total hip replacement surgery during the 1960s and 1970s [16]. His strategies to reduce sepsis also included the development of clean air systems, which contributed to the popularity of the ultra-clean laminar ventilation installations used in orthopaedic surgery today [1, 4]. Recently, doubt has been cast on the benefits of laminar flow in the reduction of SSIs in total joint arthroplasty. The World Health Organization have suggested laminar airflow systems should not be used to reduce SSIs for total arthroplasty surgery; this is due to the paucity of high-quality evidence to support its use [12]. This may impact the design of future facilities, especially as UCV is expensive to install and maintain; evidence of its benefits is essential to support future investment in the system.

Ventilation, Temperature, and Humidity

Mechanical ventilation can help to moderate temperatures and humidity, and parameters should be controllable to facilitate increases or decreases when required. The ambient theatre temperature should be at least 21 °C until patient warming is established, and control of the environment is essential for patients unable to maintain thermoregulation [17]. Increased temperatures may be required during specialist procedures such as the treatment of patients with burns, and paediatric or elderly patients. Staff comfort within the working environment is also a factor and temperature and humidity can impact performance and productivity. Low humidity has a drying effect on tissues and increases static electricity. Humidity should therefore be regulated despite temperature changes, with an optimum 40–60% being desirable. This offers a suitable level of comfort without promoting the growth of microorganisms such as mould and bacteria, related to higher humidity environments [18].

Power Supply

Within an environment where multiple electrical outputs are required, an adequate supply of outlets should be provided. A minimum of 12 plug sockets of 240 V should be available and offer an uninterrupted supply of power [1]. This is achieved through the integration of two separate ring mains to provide power even in the event of supply failure. This is further supported with the use of a backup generator that creates a failsafe system that ensures patient safety is always preserved. Tertiary power supplies for use in the event of generator failure can be found in the form of battery power supplies, incorporated within both the clinical equipment and as part of the organisational structure [19]. Electrical outlets should be placed at an appropriate height to avoid fluid ingress and spacing should provide access without the need for trailing cables. This may incorporate 'booms' that are ceiling suspended, delivering power closer to the operative field. In addition to the power supply, sufficient internet points should be included within the construction, allowing for electronic data to be accessed such as patient records and imaging.

Recovery/Post-Anaesthetic Care Unit

The perioperative journey is concluded within the PACU and the design should consider its capacity, ensuring efficient patient flow in and out of the department. Flexible facilities are becoming more important as the recovery department increasingly treats patients who require critical care following surgery. Therefore, recovery bays should be large enough to accommodate hospital beds and additional equipment. Providing double the number of bed spaces per theatre will alleviate potential system blockages and costly delays in the operating list. Each bay should be self-contained, with equipment to support patients as they emerge from the effects of anaesthesia and are prepared for discharge to the ward. This self-contained design provides a dedicated space where the patient's privacy and dignity can be preserved. While self-contained bays promote individualised care, this can lead to practitioners becoming isolated from the rest of the care team and wall-mounted alarm bells are required to summon help in the case of a clinical emergency.

Within the PACU there should be disseminated areas for gender separation as well as a specific paediatric space, to ensure patient dignity is maintained and the Department of Health guidelines are upheld [1]. Children should expect to be recovered in a segregated area, which should be planned to accommodate parents and guardians. Natural light is a positive feature and should be factored into the PACU design where possible. Artificial lighting that is adjustable is recommended, to provide dark spaces that will improve comfort during the patient's immediate post-anaesthetic recovery.

Flooring

Throughout the whole department, flooring should be smooth and seamless while being constructed of non-porous material. At the junction between the floor and the wall there should be a rounded transition with the flooring material rising 4 to 6 inches, allowing for thorough cleaning, and the minimising of joints that may compromise the effectiveness of the process. No carpeted areas should be observed anywhere within the department due to the cleaning requirements and infection risks associated with surfaces that cannot be washed [1].

Walls

All building regulations relating to the operating theatre should be adhered to and the wall colour is an important yet rarely considered element. Wall surfaces should be painted in a neutral/pastel colour, using washable and non-reflective paint. While white or bright-coloured walls may appear to present a clean clinical image, poorly considered colour choice may cause problems. Reflective glare can result in staff fatigue through prolonged exposure.

Dirty Utility Room/Sluice

Many operating departments have utility areas designated for the disposal and handling of items such as urine bottles and bed pans. These rooms may be attached to an individual theatre or serve several theatres, and they typically house a disposal unit and bucket sink allowing for dirty equipment to be processed [1]. Within this area there should be adequate extraction ventilation and hand-washing facilities.

Staff Areas

Staff well-being within the operating department is fundamental to high-quality care delivery and therefore adequate changing, showering and, rest facilities must be included within the basic theatre design. Staff undertake long shifts and may not be able to leave the department, potentially resulting in increased fatigue; therefore, natural daylight is a welcome design feature in staff areas. Comfortable facilities designated for personal time should provide seating areas and amenities for refreshments during breaks.

Modular Theatres

With the ever-increasing demand for surgical interventions, there are incremental pressures on current operating theatres to perform beyond capacity [20]. To support this shift towards additional care delivery, modular operating theatres are becoming more frequently used. This innovative approach to surgical provision incorporates a 'mobile' operating theatre being stationed within the hospital site and integrated within the service delivery. These self-contained operating theatres provide the requirements needed to deliver surgical care across a range of specialities and services. External plant feeds such as medical gases can be piped in, or integrated cylinder supplies and manifolds can deliver the required elements.

Summary

Theatre design is essential to the delivery of high-quality care and every surgical department must be compliant with building regulations to ensure the safety of patients and the efficiency of the service they provide [1]. Also, for theatre staff, the importance of good design to this specialist environment cannot be underestimated. The setting in which the team works is an important factor that influences their productivity and morale, and ultimately their retention.

References

1. NHS Estates. (HBN 26) Facilities for surgical procedures in acute general hospitals. Available from: www.england.nhs.uk/publication/facilities-for-surgical-procedures-in-acute-general-hospitals-hbn-26/.

2. Nuffield Trust. Health and social care explained: an entry point into the many facets of the health and social care system in the UK. Available from: www.nuffieldtrust.org.uk/health-and-social-care-explained/nhs-reform-timeline/.

3. The Royal College of Anaesthetists. Perioperative medicine: the pathway to better surgical care. Available from: www.rcoa.ac.uk/sites/default/files/documents/2019-08/Perioperative%20Medicine%20-%20The%20Pathway%20to%20Better%20Care.pdf.

4. Department of Health and Social Care. Health infrastructure plan: a new, strategic approach to improving our hospitals and health infrastructure. Available from: https://assets.publishing.service.gov.uk/government/uploads/system/uploads/attachment_data/file/835657/health-infrastructure-plan.pdf.

5. L. Aiken, D. Sloane, J. Ball, et al. Patient satisfaction with hospital care and nurses in England: an observational study. *British Medical Journal Open* 2018; **11**; DOI 10.1136/bmjopen-2017-019189.

6. Department of Health. Surgery, health building note 10–02: day surgery facilities. Available from: https://assets.publishing.service.gov.uk/government/uploads/system/uploads/attachment_data/file/142696/HBN_10-02.pdf.

7. Department of Health. Specialist services: health technical memorandum 08–01: acoustics. Available from: https://assets.publishing.service.gov.uk/government/uploads/system/uploads/attachment_data/file/144248/HTM_08-01.pdf.

8. Royal Pharmaceutical Society. Professional guidance on the safe and secure handling or medicines. Available from: www.rpharms.com/recognition/setting-professional-standards/safe-and-secure-handling-of-medicines/professional-guidance-on-the-safe-and-secure-handling-of-medicines.

9. NHS Estates. *Heating and Ventilation Systems: Health Technical Memorandum 03–01. Specialised Ventilation for Healthcare Premises*. London: Department of Health 2007.

10. V. Patil, S. Joachim, M. Kuma, et al. Guidelines for the provision of anaesthesia services for interoperative care: the Royal College of Anaesthetists, guidelines for the provision of anaesthetic services, chapter 3. Available from: www.rcoa.ac.uk/safety-standards-quality/guidance-resources/guidelines-provision-anaesthetic-services.

11. British Standards Institute. *Light and Lighting – Lighting of Work Places. Part 1: Indoor Work Places, BS EN 12464–1*. London: British Standards Institute, 2011.

12. World Health Organization. Global guidelines for the prevention of surgical site infection. Available from: www.who.int/gpsc/global-guidelines-web.pdf.

13. Health and Safety at Work Act etc. 1974. Available from: www.legislation.gov.uk/ukpga/1974/37/contents.

14. Health and Safety Executive. Control of Substances Hazardous to Health (COSHH). Available from: www.hse.gov.uk/coshh/.

15. Department of Health. Heating and ventilation systems health technical memorandum 03–01: specialised ventilation for healthcare premises. Part B: operational management and performance verification. Available from: https://assets.publishing.service.gov.uk/government/uploads/system/uploads/attachment_data/file/144030/HTM_03-01_Part_B.pdf.

16. B. M. Wroblewski. Professor Sir John Charnley (1911–1982). *Rheumatology* 2002; **41**: 824–825.

17. National Institute for Health and Care Excellence. Hypothermia: prevention and management in adults having surgery. Available from: www.nice.org.uk/guidance/cg65/resources/hypothermia-prevention-and-management-in-adults-having-surgery-pdf-975569636293.

18. J. Green and I. Dyer. Measure of humidity. *Anaesthesia and Intensive Care Medicine* 2009; **10**: 45–47.

19. Department of Health. Electrical services supply and distribution health technical memorandum 06-01. Available from: https://assets.publishing.service.gov.uk/government/uploads/system/uploads/attachment_data/file/608037/Health_tech_memo_0601.pdf.

20. NHS Improvements. Operating theatres: opportunities to reduce waiting lists, February 2019. Available from: https://allcatsrgrey.org.uk/wp/download/surgery/Theatre_productivity_report__Final.pdf.

Fundamentals of Infection Prevention and Control in the Operating Department

Joanne Fielding and Mark Milligan

Introduction

Despite being relatively common and often harmless, infection can have potentially life-changing consequences for patients. Infections in surgical wounds are associated with longer stays in hospital, further surgical treatment, admissions to intensive care, and higher rates of mortality [1]. As a result, the prevention of infections is a paramount aspect of patient care in the perioperative environment [2]. Infections occur when pathogens overcome a patient's natural defences and colonise their tissue or systems. Pathogenic organisms are made up of five main types: viruses, bacteria, fungi, protozoa, and worms.

A patient's risk of infection is dependent on several intrinsic and extrinsic factors [3]. Intrinsic factors include age, birth weight, pre-existing conditions, and the health and nutritional status of the patient. Practitioners often have very little control over these factors, although the patient should be optimised, and care planning should consider any intrinsic factors [4]. Practitioners are more able to control the extrinsic factors that contribute towards infections. These include environmental factors, the cleanliness of the theatre, staff, and equipment. This is a key part of limiting extrinsic risk, and is known as asepsis This term describes the processes by which pathogenic microorganisms from the environment, personnel, and instruments are eliminated. Where possible this should also incorporate barriers to transmission – gloves, gowns, and surgical drapes [4].

The link between infections and extrinsic factors was first identified by Ignaz Semmelweis in 1847, who demonstrated that good hand hygiene could prevent the spread of infection. Although his theory was not well received at the time, he was later vindicated by the work of Louis Pasteur and Joseph Lister, who showed that infections were caused by pathogenic microorganisms [5]. The elimination of as many pathogens as possible from the surgical environment is achieved by several methods including cleaning, ventilation, decontamination, and sterilisation.

Chain of Infection

Health organisations and practitioners alike have a legal and ethical obligation to provide patients with safe care and treatment in an environment and with equipment that is maintained to a high standard of cleanliness [6, 7]. To ensure that these standards are maintained, all health organisations must undertake adequate auditing of their infection and prevention systems on a regular basis, with input from dedicated infection and prevention teams [6, 8]. To comply with and deliver this essential element of patient care, healthcare practitioners must understand how their daily activities and omissions can aid in the spread of microorganisms. The 'chain of infection' outlines a series of links in which the potential for microorganism growth and transmission can be understood:

(1) the infectious agent;

(2) the reservoir;

(3) the portal of exit from the reservoir;

(4) the mode of transmission;

(5) the portal of entry into the host; and

(6) the susceptible host.

Knowledge of these links allows for an understanding of how to interrupt the sequence and reduce the spread of infection to the patient, environment, and colleagues. They are summarised in Figure 7.1.

Infectious Agent

The infectious agent is any organism that has the potential to cause infection (pathogenicity) and the capability of the agent to infect a host (virulence). The likelihood of pathogenicity is increased in those patients with compromised immunity [3, 9, 10].

Reservoir

The reservoir can be defined as an area (human, animal, or environment) where microorganisms can readily reside, offering them moisture, nutrients, and an ability to thrive and multiply [3]. These areas can be further categorised into endogenous and exogenous sources [11]. Endogenous sources are those where local resident microbial flora can be found in body sites of patients such as the skin, mouth, nose, gastrointestinal tract, and vagina [11]. Exogenous sources can be defined as those areas outside of the patient, such as the environment, equipment, healthcare workers, and visitors [3, 11]. In the perioperative environment, exogenous sources can include the skin crevices and nail beds of a health practitioner's hands, or a dry environment with little to no moisture such as medical equipment, where pathogenic microorganisms are reported to survive for extended periods [9, 12, 13].

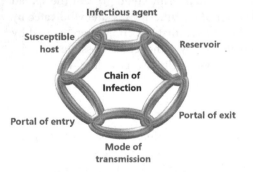

Figure 7.1 Chain of infection

The Chain of Infection

Portal of Exit from the Reservoir

The portal of exit describes the route by which a microorganism exits the reservoir [3]. For example, the release of bodily fluids as seen with a cough, releasing aerosol from the respiratory tract; other examples include urine, blood, faeces, vomit, saliva, or exudate from an open wound.

Mode of Transmission

The mode of transmission refers to the route by which the organism is spread and can be divided into direct and indirect transmission [3, 11]. Direct transmission occurs with exposure to and contact with potentially infected body fluids, secretions, and openings in the skin membrane. Indirect transmission within the healthcare environment may be primarily vehicle-borne, or airborne [11]. Vehicle-borne transmission can be via environmental sources such as contaminated equipment surfaces. Airborne transmission can be via particulates such as dust, fluid droplets which can be directly inhaled, or through touch on inanimate surfaces [3].

Portal of Entry into the Host

The portal of entry into the host includes transmission via breaks in the dermis, surgical wounds, indwelling devices, or entry via mucous membranes such as the mouth, eyes, and nostrils [3, 11].

Susceptible Host

The susceptible host includes anyone undergoing surgery from the elderly or paediatric population, any immunocompromised patient, anyone with a co-morbidity, or any other individual with increased susceptibility [3]. The introduction of pathogenic microorganisms via a break (indwelling catheter) in a susceptible host's natural protective barriers can potentially culminate in an acquired infection.

Care should also be taken with personal items being brought into clinical areas that could potentially harbour pathogens, most notably staff lanyards, bags, and other such personal belongings [14]. For practitioners, this should reinforce the need for vigilance in countering the spread of infection not just within the confines of the operating theatre but also by those items unsuspectingly bought in. Prevention and control of cross-contamination entails the provision of the correct equipment, appropriate training of staff and patients, and the utilisation of standards in preventative techniques, as well as a robust system for auditing and reporting compliance in infection control [15].

Healthcare-Associated Infection

A healthcare-associated infection (HCAI), otherwise termed a 'nosocomial' infection, is the global term used to define an infection that has been acquired by a patient during a healthcare intervention [11, 15]. Contracting an infection may be attributed to exposure with surrounding surfaces, and/or interventions of care that compromise the patient's natural protective barriers. Such infections can occur during surgery or the insertion of indwelling devices, where suboptimal care may lead to the migration of exogenous (external origin) or endogenous (internal origin) microorganisms [16]. HCAIs are defined as any infection contracted 72 hours post admission, and any infection arising within 48 hours post discharge [17]. The most prevalent HCAIs are urinary tract infections (UTIs), surgical site infection (SSIs), hospital-acquired pneumonia (HAP), ventilator-associated pneumonia (VAP), and healthcare-associated bloodstream infection (BSI) [17]. Any patient is at risk of contracting an HCAI, but there are increased risk factors for: those aged greater than 65 years; patients admitted to an intensive care unit or the emergency department; hospital inpatients with stays greater than 7 days; those having surgery; patients with indwelling devices; those with burns, trauma-induced immunosuppression, neutropenia, impaired functional, or coma status; and patients with co-morbidities [17].

Numerous UK and international campaigns have been promoted to improve public and health professionals' knowledge and practice in reducing the incidence of methicillin-resistant *Staphylococcus aureus* (MRSA) bacteraemia and other HCAIs over the course of 17 years, from 'Winning ways', published in 2003 [18] to 'Save lives: clean your hands' [19], first published in 2009. High-impact interventions implemented by the Department of Health in the UK, such as the 2005 'Saving Lives' tool kit, have been successful in reducing the numbers of HCAIs [20]. In 2019, Public Health England [21] reported a general decline in reported cases of MRSA and *Clostridium difficile* infection rates from when surveillance was initiated in 2011. HCAIs such as *Klebsiella pneumoniae* and *Pseudomonas aeruginosa* bacteraemia remain a challenge and as of 2018 have been included in the ongoing national point prevalence survey of HCAIs [21].

SSIs are the second highest reported type of HCAI in Europe and the United States [22], with 50% of SSIs being reported as only becoming evident following discharge from care [19]. The overall impact of an HCAI to the patient and their family is significant; with infection comes an increased risk of morbidity and suffering, causing undue stress, trauma, and financial burden [14, 17]. It is estimated that HCAIs can increase hospital admissions from 5 to 29.5 days [17], and the overall impact costs the National Heath Service in the UK £2.7 billion annually, with an estimated death toll of 28,500 for 2016/17 [23]. Guidance suggests that to prevent HCAIs all healthcare workers must comply with and maintain professional development on the appropriate and current ideologies in infection prevention and control, and includes compliance with local and national guidelines on the provision and use of personal protective equipment [15].

How to Prevent Surgical Site Infections

Acknowledging that we often have little control over the intrinsic infection risks, perioperative practitioners must focus on the extrinsic factors which contribute to SSIs. These can be reduced or eliminated by several different strategies within the operating department. By looking at each of these in turn, we can see that they are related to personal factors, the patient, and the theatre environment, including equipment.

Personal Factors

The most important aspect of personal hygiene related to the prevention of infections is hand washing and surgical scrubbing [24]. These two practices are separate to each other and should not be confused. Good hand washing is described as one of the standard infection control precautions that is vital to reduce the transmission of infectious agents that can cause hospital-acquired infections [25]. Hand washing should be carried out before touching a patient, before any clean or aseptic procedure, after any exposure to body fluid, after touching a patient or their surroundings; these are known as the five moments for hand hygiene [24]. They are universal and should be applied in the operating theatre in the same way they are in any other parts of the hospital.

Surgical scrubbing before participating in a sterile surgical procedure is a more thorough process, which the Association for Perioperative Practice describes as an extension of handwashing [26]. Surgical scrubbing uses antibacterial solutions containing chlorhexidine or povidone-iodine rather than simple soap and can involve the use of a brush or pick to clean the nails. The purpose of surgical scrubbing is to remove transient microorganisms and reduce the number of resident microorganisms that make up the body's natural flora. This is to minimise the risks of patients developing SSIs [27]. Surgical scrubbing should not be limited to the surgical team at the operating table; anyone undertaking a sterile procedure, for example, an anaesthetist when conducting a sterile procedure such as the insertion of an arterial line, should also be 'scrubbed up'. The WHO has produced clear guidelines on the correct ways to carry out both hand washing and surgical scrubbing [24].

The use of alcohol-based gels for washing visibly clean hands has become common in all healthcare settings, and their use is now starting to move into theatres, as part of surgical hand preparation. Surgical hand rubbing is sanctioned [24], and supported by evidence [28, 29]. Despite the importance of hand washing and scrubbing, on their own they are insufficient to protect the patient from infection. Attention should also be paid to the correct theatre dress. In the operating department, everyone should be wearing scrubs, which should be clean every shift, and should be changed when contaminated with bodily fluids or when in contact with a known infectious patient [30]. Scrubs should not be worn outside of the theatre suite, unless responding to an emergency call, and theatre shoes should not be worn outside of the department. Scrub hats should always be worn in theatres; and, where disposable masks are worn, they should be carefully removed using the tapes and disposed of immediately on leaving theatre. Non-sterile gloves should be worn for anticipated contact with blood or other body fluids, broken skin, or mucous membranes, and should be removed immediately following the end of patient care [31]; see Figure 7.2 for further information.

The Patient

Although fit and healthy patients are usually well protected from infection by their immune system, surgical patients do not always fall into this category. And, even when they do, additional precautions need to be taken to prevent them from becoming infected by their own naturally occurring skin flora, as well any pathogens present in the air or on surfaces in the theatre. Scrubbing up and the wearing of sterile gloves and gowns alone is insufficient to do this, and further precautions also need to be taken.

To ensure that the risk of infection is minimised, patients need to be properly prepared for surgery once they arrive in theatre. This preparation must be based on the best available evidence; for example, despite shaving of the surgical site being common practice for over 100 years [32] it is no longer recommended unless necessary [33]. When pre-surgical shaving is done, hair should only be removed using electric clippers with a single-use blade. This is to reduce the damage to the skin that can be caused by a razor, and the resulting increased risk of developing an SSI [33].

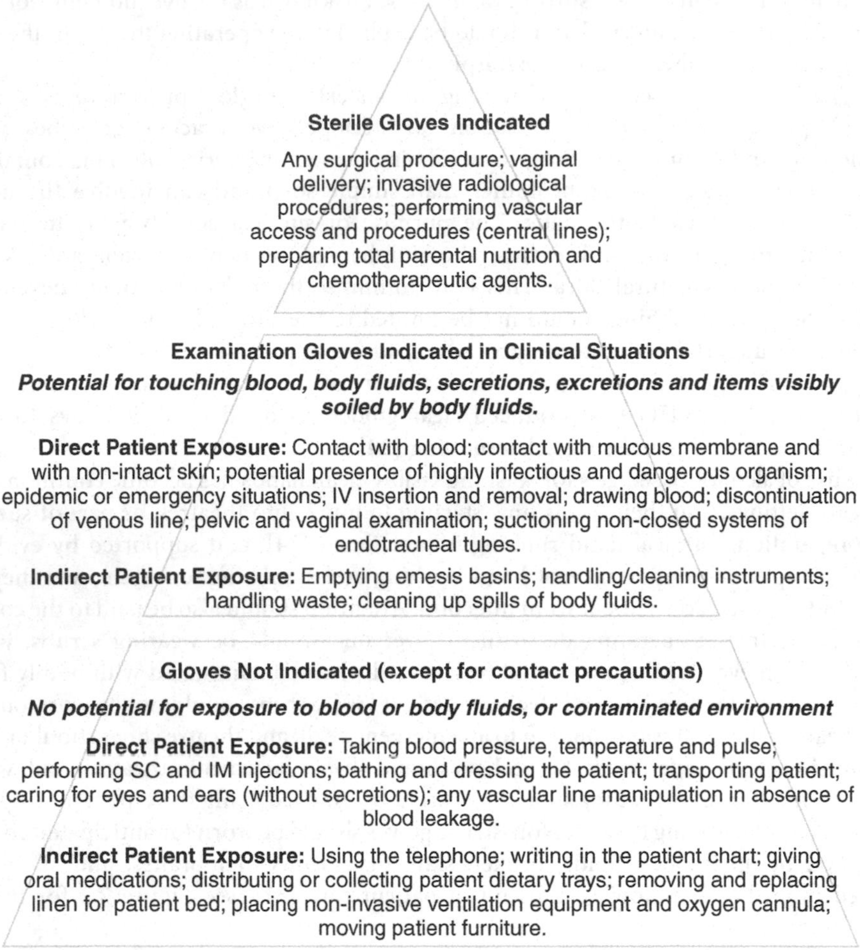

Sterile Gloves Indicated

Any surgical procedure; vaginal delivery; invasive radiological procedures; performing vascular access and procedures (central lines); preparing total parental nutrition and chemotherapeutic agents.

Examination Gloves Indicated in Clinical Situations

Potential for touching blood, body fluids, secretions, excretions and items visibly soiled by body fluids.

Direct Patient Exposure: Contact with blood; contact with mucous membrane and with non-intact skin; potential presence of highly infectious and dangerous organism; epidemic or emergency situations; IV insertion and removal; drawing blood; discontinuation of venous line; pelvic and vaginal examination; suctioning non-closed systems of endotracheal tubes.

Indirect Patient Exposure: Emptying emesis basins; handling/cleaning instruments; handling waste; cleaning up spills of body fluids.

Gloves Not Indicated (except for contact precautions)

No potential for exposure to blood or body fluids, or contaminated environment

Direct Patient Exposure: Taking blood pressure, temperature and pulse; performing SC and IM injections; bathing and dressing the patient; transporting patient; caring for eyes and ears (without secretions); any vascular line manipulation in absence of blood leakage.

Indirect Patient Exposure: Using the telephone; writing in the patient chart; giving oral medications; distributing or collecting patient dietary trays; removing and replacing linen for patient bed; placing non-invasive ventilation equipment and oxygen cannula; moving patient furniture.

Figure 7.2 Glove pyramid

Whether a patient has been shaved or not, the usual first step in any surgery is the preparation of the surgical site with an antiseptic solution. These solutions are either chlorhexidine or povidone-iodine based. Povidone-iodine solutions can be either alcohol or aqueous based. As alcohol, itself an antiseptic, is considered preferable except for preterm infants or when there is contact with mucus membranes, where the alcohol can cause damage [34]. It is usual for an antiseptic solution to be applied using a disposable applicator or a swab, gauze, or a sponge moving away from the centre of the site of the incision.

Only once the skin preparation is dry can the drapes be placed on the patient. Surgical drapes are sterile sheets of material, used to cover the patient and the operating table completely except for the area of the surgery, which has been prepped with antiseptic solution [35]. Drapes in the past were made from cotton and had to be clipped to each other to hold them in place. But now they are mostly self-adhesive and made from paper, making them disposable. Modern drapes are treated, making them impervious to fluids

[36], and procedure packs are often assembled and sterilised in advance, containing the correct number and sizes of drapes for a particular surgical procedure. If it becomes necessary to move or replace drapes, they should only be moved away from the surgical field, never towards; if a drape becomes contaminated or has a hole, a second clean drape should be placed over it [26].

One of the final key patient-related activities that can be undertaken to reduce infections is the use of antibiotic prophylaxis. This is the administration of antibiotics that are specifically recommended against infections at the site of the surgery. Not all surgeries require antibiotics but the insertion of implants and surgery where there is a risk of contamination from the gastrointestinal tract routinely do. The choice of antibiotic, and the dose, timing, and duration, are governed by local antibiotic formularies which combine the latest evidence and the best clinical judgement of pharmacists [37]. This forms part of the UK Department of Health's antimicrobial stewardship program, which aims to reduce antimicrobial resistance by providing a framework to guide prescribers [2].

Theatre Environment

The last extrinsic factor that needs to be considered in relation to reducing SSIs is the theatre environment itself. Key to this is the cleanliness of the theatre, the discipline of the theatre team in maintaining the hygiene, and the security of the environment and its ventilation [38].

A theatre suite can be divided into two distinct spaces, and access to both should be limited to patients and staff members wearing scrubs and theatre shoes. First, the area around the theatre, the corridors, storage facilities for consumables and instruments, and patient reception areas. Second, within the theatres themselves, where there is a higher level of cleanliness, head coverings must be worn and face masks may be required, particularly when trays of instruments are uncovered [39].

Within the theatre environment, cleaning should take place at the start of the day and following the departure of every patient. The level of cleaning required following procedures is dictated by local policy but will include the use of antibacterial or sporicidal wipes as well more technological tools such as ultraviolet light or hydrogen peroxide vaporisation. A rolling program of deep cleaning using equipment of this type should also be in place [40].

The movement of staff, patients, and equipment in and out of the theatre, as well as the number of staff present, can increase the risk of a patient acquiring a SSI. Research shows that there is a link between door opening and surgical site infections [41, 42]. For this reason, the traffic in and out of the theatre during surgery should be strictly controlled. Related to this is the movement of patients, instruments, and waste from the surgical environment. The design of operating theatres should incorporate a system of entry and exit routes that separates soiled or contaminated items from clean or sterile ones, preventing cross-contamination of patients and equipment from case to case [43].

The ventilation in theatres is the final environmental factor in reducing SSIs. Ventilation can be broadly divided into two distinct types: plenum and laminar flow. Both reduce the contamination of wounds and surgical instruments by airborne particles, such as skin cells, dust, and fibres from clothing, and the moisture from exhaled breath, which can normally be found circulating in the air [38]. Plenum ventilation works along a pressure gradient with the highest-pressure air flowing into one part of the operating suite, usually the lay-up room, and from there into the operating theatre, and out through the anaesthetic room and sluice. The airflow is controlled by a series of weighted pressure-stabilising vents connecting the rooms, which close automatically if the pressure in one room drops, for example when a door is opened [44].

Laminar ventilation or air flow channels highly filtered air down directly from the centre of the operating theatre, at a pressure greater than the air in the rest of the room, preventing airborne contaminants from entering the surgical field [45]. As laminar flow has a greater number of air exchanges in an hour it is generally considered to be superior to plenum ventilation. Maintaining a clean as possible surgical environment is decisive in the fight against SSIs. Regular cleaning, good surgical-team discipline, and modern ventilation will contribute towards minimising the SSI risk to patients. A multifaceted approach that also includes patient optimisation, preparation, cleaning, and draping, and in some cases the use of antibiotic prophylaxis, is also necessary. Combining this with effective surgical scrubbing and careful gloving and gowning is crucial for the prevention of infection.

Antibiotic Resistance

Medicines such as antibiotics can be used to destroy or inhibit the growth of a range of bacterial microorganisms. Resistance to these antimicrobials occurs as microorganisms evolve and adapt, through processes of genetic mutation and natural selection. This inevitable resistance has been accelerated and attributed to the inappropriate use of antimicrobials, and the broad-spectrum antimicrobial use in human, animal, and environmental industries [46, 47]. At present, 700,000 deaths per year are reported to occur globally due to antimicrobial resistance (AMR) [47, 48]. Various organisations have raised [47–49] concerns that, if professionals do not take AMR seriously, treatment for diseases will become limited, and inevitably result in prolonged illness, together with an increase in the psychological and socioeconomic impact on patients and their families, as well as leading to an increase in the costs of providing healthcare. As AMR increases, routine operations will potentially become far more hazardous options for patients [46, 49]. A major factor contributing to this problem is the fact that there have been no new classes of antibiotics discovered since the 1980s. As a result, those readily available today could soon be rendered ineffective in the fight against infection [46, 47, 49]. Prevalent multidrug resistant organisms (MDROs) encountered in healthcare organisations today are:

- MRSA;
- vancomycin-resistant *Enterococci* species;
- extended-spectrum beta-lactamase gram-negative organisms;
- carbapenems-resistant Enterobacteriaceae; and
- multi-resistant *Acinetobacter baumannii* [46, 21].

In response to the threat presented by MDROs, the UK government [48] has released a national framework outlining initiatives to enhance AMR awareness, including the promotion of responsible prescribing, and the utilisation of effective infection and prevention measures such as those described in this chapter to curtail spread of microorganisms. To further support this, a robust monitoring and reporting system has been put in place to develop a greater understanding of the indications for antibiotic use, dosages, and adherence to guidelines [50]. The aim of this project is to reduce as much as possible the need for antibiotic use.

On a global as well as a national scale, funding has been ring-fenced for further research into new pharmaceuticals, diagnostic tools, and vaccines to combat infection [47, 50]. Until these are readily available, healthcare professionals can aid in tackling the AMR burden by ensuring that their practice is guided by effective infection and prevention measures and antimicrobial stewardship [47].

Summary

Although practitioners cannot necessarily control the intrinsic patient factors associated with infection, they can influence the management of infection through appropriate supervision of the surgical environment and patient intervention. With continued application of infection and control practice in their daily activities, practitioners can contribute towards the drive to lower the incidence of HCAI today.

References

1. European Centre for Disease Prevention and Control. Healthcare-associated infections: surgical site infections, annual epidemiological report for 2017. Available from: www.ecdc.europa.eu/en/publications-data/healthcare-associated-infections-surgical-site-infections-annual-1#no-link.

2. Public Health England. Start smart – then focus: antimicrobial stewardship toolkit for English hospitals. Available from: https://assets.publishing.service.gov.uk/government/uploads/system/uploads/attachment_data/file/417032/Start_Smart_Then_Focus_FINAL.PDF.

3. D. Weston. *Fundamentals of Infection Prevention and Control: Theory and Practice*, 2nd ed. Chichester: John Wiley & Sons Ltd, 2013.

4. C. Thomas. Intrinsic and extrinsic sources and prevention of infection (in surgery). *Surgery* 2019; 37: 26–32.

5. J. Cavaillon and F. Chrétien. From septicaemia to sepsis 3.0: from Ignaz Semmelweis to Louis Pasteur. *Genes and Immunity* 2019; 20: 371–382.

6. The Care and Quality Commission. Health and Social Care Act 2008 (Regulated Activities) Regulations 2014: Regulation 12. Available from: www.cqc.org.uk/guidance-providers/regulations-enforcement/regulation-12-safe-care-treatment.

7. Health and Care Professions Council. Standards of proficiency: operating department practitioners. Available from: www.hcpc-uk.org/standards/standards-of-proficiency/operating-department-practitioners/.

8. The Health and Social Care Act 2008: code of practice on the prevention and control of infections. Available from: www.gov.uk/government/publications/the-health-and-social-care-act-2008-code-of-practice-on-the-prevention-and-control-of-infections-and-related-guidance.

9. D. Chowdhury, S. Tahir, M. Legge, et al. Transfer of dry surface biofilm in the healthcare environment: the role of healthcare workers' hands as vehicles. *Journal of Hospital Infection* 2018; 100: 85–90.

10. World Health Organization. Evidence of hand hygiene to reduce transmission and infections by multi-drug resistant organisms in health-care settings. Available from: www.who.int/gpsc/5may/MDRO_literature-review.pdf.

11. C. G. Mayhall. *Hospital Epidemiology and Infection Control*. Philadelphia, PA: Wolters Kluwer Health, 2011.

12. K. Ledwoch, S. J. Dancer, J. A. Otter, et al. Beware biofilm! Dry biofilms containing bacterial pathogens on multiple healthcare surfaces; a multicentre study. *Journal of Hospital Infection* 2018; 100: 47–56.

13. F. Parvin, H. Hu, G. S. Whiteley, et al. Difficulty in removing biofilm from dry surfaces. *Journal of Hospital Infection* 2018; 100: 85–90.

14. K. French. Ten unusual sites in healthcare facilities harbouring pathogens that have been reported in the *Journal of Hospital Infection*. *Journal of Infection Control* 2018; **100**: 361–362.

15. National Institute for Health and Care Excellence. Healthcare-associated infections: prevention and control in primary and community care. Available from: www.nice.org.uk/guidance/cg139/resources/healthcareassociated-infections-prevention-and-control-in-primary-and-community-care-35109518767045.

16. National institute for Health and Care Excellence. Infection prevention and control, quality standard [QS61] . Available from: www.nice.org.uk/guidance/qs61.

17. World Health Organization. Report on the burden of endemic health-care-associated infection worldwide, January 2011. Available from: www.who.int/publications/i/item/report-on-the-burden-of-endemic-health-care-associated-infection-worldwide.

18. Department of Health. Winning ways: working together to reduce healthcare associated infection in England. Available from: https://webarchive.nationalarchives.gov.uk/20120510091859/http://www.dh.gov.uk/prod_consum_dh/groups/dh_digitalassets/@dh/@en/documents/digitalasset/dh_4064689.pdf.

19. World Health Organization. Save lives: clean your hands. Available from: www.who.int/gpsc/5may_advocacy-toolkit.pdf?ua=1.

20. Department of Health. Saving lives: a delivery program to reduce healthcare associated infections including MRSA. Available from: https://webarchive.nationalarchives.gov.uk/ukgwa/+/www.dh.gov.uk/en/Publicationsandstatistics/Publications/PublicationsPolicyAndGuidance/DH_4113889.

21. Public Health England. Annual epidemiological commentary: gram-negative bacteraemia, MRSA bacteraemia, MSSA bacteraemia and *C. difficile* infections, up to and including financial year April 2018 to March 2019. Available from: www.gov.uk/government/statistics/mrsa-mssa-and-e-coli-bacteraemia-and-c-difficile-infection-annual-epidemiological-commentary.

22. B. Allegranzi, P. Bischoff, S. de Jonge, et al. Surgical site infections 1. New WHO recommendations on preoperative measures for surgical site infection prevention: an evidence-based global perspective. *Lancet Infectious Diseases* 2016; **16**: e276–287.

23. J. Guest, T. Keating, D. Gould, and N. Wigglesworth. Modelling the annual NHS costs and outcomes attributable to healthcare-associated infections in England. *British Medical Journal* 2020; **10**: e033367.

24. World Health Organization. WHO guidelines on hand hygiene in health care, 2009. Available from: https://apps.who.int/iris/bitstream/handle/10665/44102/9789241597906_eng.pdf;jsessionid=C1D950BB42FE9CA543C751149797DA77?sequence=1.

25. National Health Service, Standard infection control precautions: national hand hygiene and personal protective equipment policy, 2019. Available from: www.england.nhs.uk/publication/standard-infection-control-precautions-national-hand-hygiene-and-personal-protective-equipment-policy/.

26. Association for Perioperative Practice. *Standards and Recommendations for Safe Perioperative Practice*, 4th ed. Harrogate: Association for Perioperative Practice, 2016

27. J. Tanner. Surgical hand antisepsis: the evidence. *Journal of Perioperative Practice* 2008; **18**: 330–339.

28. G. G. Gaspar, M. G. Menegueti, A. E. R Lopes, et al. Alcohol-based surgical hand preparation: translating scientific evidence into clinical practice. *Antimicrobial Resistance and Infection Control* 2018; **7**: 80.

29. Y. H. Ho, Y. C. Wang, E. W. Loh, and K. W. Tam. Antiseptic efficacies of waterless hand rub, chlorhexidine scrub and povidone-iodine scrub in surgical settings: a meta-analysis of randomized

controlled trials. *Journal of Hospital Infection* 2019; **101**: 370–379.

30. Department of Health. Uniforms and workwear: guidance for NHS employers, 2020. Available from; www.england.nhs.uk/wp-content/uploads/2020/04/Uniforms-and-Workwear-Guidance-2-April-2020.pdf.

31. World Health Organization. Glove use information leaflet, 2009. Available from: www.who.int/gpsc/5may/Glove_Use_Information_Leaflet.pdf.

32. O. H. Wangensteen and S. D. Wangensteen. *The Rise of Surgery from Empiric Craft to Scientific Discipline.* Minneapolis, MN: University of Minnesota Press, 1978.

33. National Institute for Health and Care Excellence. Surgical site infections: prevention and treatment. Available from: www.nice.org.uk/guidance/ng125.

34. One Together. Surgical skin preparation: quality improvement resource. Available from: www.onetogether.org.uk/downloads/Surgical%20Skin%20Preparation%20Quality%20Improvement%20Guide_AW.pdf.

35. World Health Organization. Global guidelines for the prevention of surgical site infection. Available from: www.who.int/gpsc/global-guidelines-web.pdf.

36. T. H. A. Arumlampalam. Principles and techniques of operative surgery including neurosurgery. In C. R. G. Quick, S. Biers, and T. H. A. Arumlampalam (eds.), *Essential Surgery*, 6th ed. London: Elsevier, 2020, pp. 124–151.

37. National Institute for Health and Care Excellence. Surgical site infection, quality standard [QS49], 2013. Available from: www.nice.org.uk/guidance/qs49/resources/surgical-site-infection-pdf-2098675107781.

38. One Together. Surgical environment: quality improvement resource. Available from: www.onetogether.org.uk/downloads/OneTogether%20Surgical%20Environment%20QIR_2019.pdf.

39. M. C. Roy. The operating theatre. In G. M. L. Bearman, M. Stevens, M. B. Edmond, and R. P. Wenzel (eds.), *A Guide to Infection Control in the Hospital*, 5th ed. Boston, MA: The International

Society for Infectious Diseases (ISID), 2014, pp. 137–145.

40. Association of Anaesthetists. *Guidelines, Infection Prevention and Control 2020.* London: Association of Anaesthetists, 2020.

41. P. Perez, J. Holloway, L. Ehrenfeld, et al. Door openings in the operating room are associated with increased environmental contamination. *American Journal of Infection Control* 2018; **46**: 954–956.

42. C. Wang, S. Holmberg, and S. Sadrizadeh. Impact of door opening on the risk of surgical site infections in an operating room with mixing ventilation. *Indoor and Built Environment* 2021; **30**: 166–179.

43. C. Spry. Infection prevention and control. In J. C. Rothrock (ed.), *Alexander's Care of the Patient in the Surgical Environment*, 15th ed. St Louis, MO: Elsevier, 2015.

44. Department of Health (United Kingdom). Heating and ventilation systems health technical memorandum 03–01: specialised ventilation for healthcare premises. Part B: operational management and performance verification. Available from: https://assets.publishing.service.gov.uk/government/uploads/system/uploads/attachment_data/file/144030/HTM_03-01_Part_B.pdf.

45. M. Kiernan. Infection prevention. In K. Woodhead and L. Fudge (eds.), *Manual of Perioperative Care, An Essential Guide.* Oxford: Wiley Blackwell, 2012, pp. 43–55.

46. House of Commons Health and Social Care Committee. Antimicrobial resistance: eleventh report of session 2017–19. Available from: https://publications.parliament.uk/pa/cm201719/cmselect/cmhealth/962/962.pdf.

47. National Institute for Health and Care Excellence. NICE impact antimicrobial resistance. Available from: www.nice.org.uk/media/default/about/what-we-do/into-practice/measuring-uptake/nice impact-antimicrobial-resistance.pdf.

48. HM Government. Tackling antimicrobial resistance 2019–2024: the UK's five-year

national action plan HM Government. Available from: www.gov.uk/govern ment/publications/uk-5-year-action-plan-for-antimicrobial-resistance-2019-to-2024.

49. World Health Organization. Global action plan on antimicrobial resistance. Available from: www.who.int/publications/i/item/9789241509763.

50. Public Health England. English Surveillance Programme for Antimicrobial Utilisation and Resistance (ESPAUR): report 2020–2021. Available from: https://assets .publishing.service.gov.uk/government/uploads/system/uploads/attachment_data/file/843129/English_Surveillance_Programme_for_Antimicrobial_Utilisation_and_Resistance_2019.pdf.

Chapter

8 Fundamentals of Cardiovascular Physiology

Dominic Nielsen and James Ip

Anatomy of the Cardiovascular System

The cardiovascular system consists of the heart, arteries, veins, and capillaries. The heart is a muscular organ with four chambers. The atria are the two smaller chambers, and the two larger chambers are the ventricles.

The cardiovascular system can be sub-divided into the systemic and pulmonary circulations, supplied by the left and right ventricles, respectively. Blood flows from the right atrium to the right ventricle through the tricuspid valve; so called because it consists of three leaflets or cusps. The right ventricle pumps blood to the lungs through the pulmonary valve, which prevents the flow of blood back into the right ventricle. After releasing carbon dioxide and taking up oxygen in the lungs, blood is returned to the left atrium. It then flows through the mitral valve into the left ventricle. The mitral valve is the only heart valve that has two leaflets rather than three, although the aortic valve can also be bicuspid in 1–2% of humans. All the valves act to allow blood to flow in one direction only. The left ventricle then pumps oxygenated blood out into the aorta. The aorta and left ventricle are separated by the aortic valve. The aorta supplies all the tissues of the body via several increasingly small branches. The smallest of these, arterioles, then connect with capillaries, where oxygen is delivered to the tissues. Oxygen is unloaded passively into the tissues from red blood cells and carbon dioxide is taken up. The capillaries then drain into venules, which in turn drain into veins. These veins combine to form the inferior vena cava (containing blood from the lower limbs and abdomen) and the superior (carrying blood from the upper limbs, head, and neck) which drain into the right atrium [1, 2]. Figure 8.1 illustrates the arrangement of the heart, systemic, and pulmonary circulations.

The Pulmonary Circulation

The pulmonary circulation consists of the right atrium, right ventricle, pulmonary arteries, pulmonary capillaries, and pulmonary veins. It is a much lower pressure system than the systemic circulation, with pulmonary artery pressures typically 25/10 mmHg compared to 120/80 mmHg in the systemic circulation. This lower pressure is a consequence of the lower resistance of the pulmonary vascular bed. The walls of these vessels have around a third as much muscle in them as the aorta and its branches. Therefore, the right ventricle is smaller, thinner walled, and less muscular than the left ventricle, as less work is required of it. The total volume of blood within the pulmonary circulation at any time is normally around 1 litre, compared to 4 litres for the systemic circulation.

Blood entering the right atrium has a lower oxygen content (is deoxygenated) and has a higher carbon dioxide content than blood leaving the left side of the heart, with typical

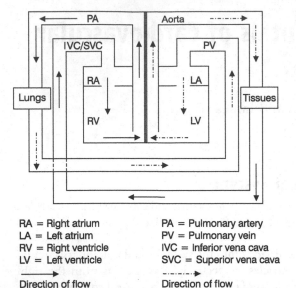

Figure 8.1 The heart and circulation

RA = Right atrium
LA = Left atrium
RV = Right ventricle
LV = Left ventricle

PA = Pulmonary artery
PV = Pulmonary vein
IVC = Inferior vena cava
SVC = Superior vena cava

Direction of flow
(Deoxygenated blood)

Direction of flow
(Oxygenated blood)

oxygen saturations in the right atrium at 75%, compared to nearly 100% in the left atrium. Thus, approximately 25% of the total oxygen content leaving the left heart is utilised by the tissues, leaving 75% returning unused to the heart.

The Systemic Circulation

The systemic circulation consists of the left atrium, left ventricle, the aorta and its branches, arterioles, capillaries, and all the veins draining the body. It supplies oxygenated blood to the body. The left ventricle is a much thicker and more muscular structure than the right ventricle, due to the requirement to supply blood to the whole body, including the heart itself, rather than just the lungs. It is also working against a much greater resistance than the right ventricle.

Arterial oxygen saturations are typically 96–98% in health. Blood flow to the various organs is regulated by local variations in arterial tone under the control of the autonomic nervous system and circulating catecholamines. Some organs (notably the brain, spinal cord, heart, and kidney) can regulate their own flow by autoregulation, so in a healthy individual, the cerebral blood flow is constant between mean arterial pressures of 60 and 160 mmHg. However, in chronic hypertension (high blood pressure), these limits increase. Therefore, patients with long-standing hypertension may require a greater mean arterial pressure to ensure adequate perfusion of their vital organs. This is demonstrated graphically in Figure 8.2 [1].

The Cardiac Cycle

The cardiac cycle consists of two phases: diastole and systole. These phases occur simultaneously for both sides of the heart; the left and right sides relax and contract together.

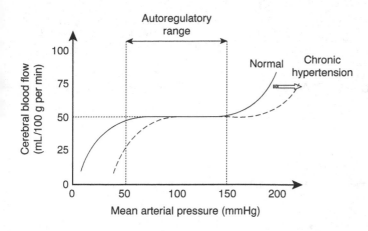

Figure 8.2 Autoregulation of cerebral blood flow

Diastole is the period when the chambers are relaxed and filling, while systole is when they contract and eject blood. Diastole is also the period when most of the flow down the coronary arteries to the heart occurs. During diastole, blood flows from the atria into the ventricles, mostly passively, with the final 10–15% being ejected by contraction of the atria [1]. Flow from the right atrium to the right ventricle is through the tricuspid valve and flow from the left atrium to the left ventricle (LV) is through the mitral valve.

In systole, the ventricles contract to eject blood into the pulmonary artery and the aorta, for the right and left ventricles, respectively (see Figure 8.3). The increase in pressure from ventricular contraction causes the mitral and tricuspid valves to close, preventing flow back into the atria. This occurs at point A in Figure 8.3. When listening with a stethoscope, these closures are heard as the first heart sound, S_1. Shortly afterwards, the pressure in the ventricles further increases until it is greater than the pressure in the pulmonary artery and the aorta, opening the pulmonary and aortic valves and allowing blood to leave the ventricles (point B in Figure 8.3). Once ventricular contraction has finished, the ventricles relax (ventricular diastole) and the pressure in the ventricles falls (point C in Figure 8.3). The pressure gradient between the ventricles and the great arteries is then reversed, closing the pulmonary and aortic valves and giving rise to the second heart sound, S_2 (point D in Figure 8.3). During ventricular systole, the atria are filling with blood returning from the body and lungs. After systole, the ventricular pressure falls to below the pressure in the atria, and the tricuspid and mitral valves open; ventricular filling commences again and the cardiac cycle repeats.

The Cardiac Conduction System

The conduction system of the heart facilitates the transmission of impulses from the atria to the ventricles, allowing coordinated contraction of the chambers to occur. Impulses originate in the sinoatrial (SA) node, which is located at the junction of the superior vena cava and the right atrium. The impulse then propagates across the atria, stimulating them to contract. It then travels to the atrioventricular (AV) node. The AV node acts to regulate the transmission of atrial impulses to the ventricles, allowing atrial and ventricular contractions

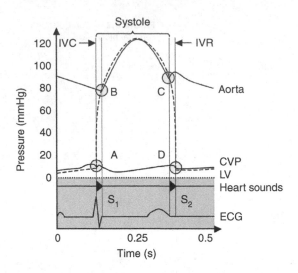

Figure 8.3 Cardiac-cycle diagram; CVP, central venous pressure; IVC, inferior vena cava; IVR, idioventricular rhythm; LV, left ventrical

to be well coordinated. The AV node or surrounding tissue can also generate impulses, giving rise to a junctional rhythm. After passing through the AV node, the impulse travels down the bundle of His (pronounced *Hiss*), located within the interventricular septum. Part way down the interventricular septum, the bundle of His divides into the left and right bundle branches which supply the left and right ventricles, respectively. The bundle branches terminate in Purkinje fibres, which are specialised conducting cells distributing the electrical impulse to the contractile cells of the heart.

The Electrocardiogram

A three-lead electrocardiogram (ECG) is part of the standard, mandatory continuous monitoring requirements under anaesthesia [3]. Use of the ECG allows the measurement of heart rate as well as detection of rhythm disturbances and signs of myocardial ischaemia. The three leads are colour-coded red, yellow, and green and are usually positioned with the red lead on the right shoulder, yellow lead on the left shoulder and the green lead positioned on the patient's left lower chest.

The ECG only records the electrical activity of the heart, with no information on cardiac contraction. The normal ECG trace consists of a P wave and, after a short interval, this is followed by a QRS complex. After a further short interval is the T wave. The sequence of P, QRS, and T then repeats. P waves are an upwards (positive) deflection that represents the contraction of the atria (atrial systole). The QRS complex can comprise several different waves. Q waves are any negative deflections following the P wave. R waves are positive deflections after the P wave, and S waves are negative deflections after the R wave.

The time interval between the start of the P wave and the start of the QRS complex is known as the PR interval. The normal duration of the PR interval is 120–200 milliseconds. The QRS complex is usually an upwards deflection and represents ventricular systole. The normal duration of the QRS is 80–120 milliseconds. Following the QRS complex is the T wave, which is another upwards deflection, of lower height and broader than the QRS complex. The T wave represents the repolarisation of the ventricles in preparation for their next contraction. Repolarisation of the atria occurs at approximately the same time as the contraction of the ventricles. Due to the much greater size of the ventricles relative to the atria, this atrial repolarisation is not normally seen on the ECG as it is masked by the QRS complex.

The standard settings used intraoperatively for ECG display are the same as those used for recording ECGs on paper. This is a sweep speed of 25 mm/s and an amplification of 1 cm per mV. By convention, it is displayed as a green waveform on monitors.

Cardiac Muscle

There are three main types of muscle in the human body. Smooth muscle maintains tone in areas such as the vasculature and lung. It functions constantly but is not especially powerful. Skeletal muscle is powerful but suffers from fatigue under constant use. Cardiac muscle fibres are constantly working but must not fatigue. Cardiac muscle is powerful like skeletal muscle but is structured differently. The junctions between the individual cells (myocytes) are known as gap junctions. This allows the electrical impulse to spread between the myocytes so that they function as a single unit (syncytium). In contrast, the junctions between individual cells elsewhere in the body are tight junctions, where there is almost no separation between the cells, and which only allow some ions to pass across them.

Determinants of Cardiac Output

Cardiac output is defined as the volume of blood ejected by the heart per unit time. It is measured in litres per minute and can be calculated from the following equation:

cardiac output = heart rate × stroke volume.

The heart rate is the number of contractions of the ventricles per unit time and the stroke volume (SV) is the volume of blood ejected with each beat. In a healthy adult with a resting heart rate of 70 beats per minute and a stroke volume of 70 mL, this will be approximately 5 L per minute. The SV will be determined by preload (i.e., fluid status) myocardial contractility and arterial resistance. Cardiac output can be compared between patients of different sizes by dividing it by the patient's body surface area. This value is known as the cardiac index. In adults this is normally 2.7–4.0 L/min per m^2.

Maintenance of an adequate cardiac output during anaesthesia is important because the cardiac output is an essential determinant of total oxygen delivery to the body's tissues (the others being haemoglobin concentration and arterial oxygen saturation). The heart rate is controlled by the balance of autonomic innervation to the heart and the level of circulating adrenaline in the blood (secreted by the adrenal glands). Sympathetic stimulation (acting via noradrenaline) leads to an increase in the heart rate. The heart rate and stroke volume will both increase, leading to an increase in cardiac output. The opposite occurs when the pacemaker receives parasympathetic stimulation; the discharge of the pacemaker is slower and the heart rate falls (see Figure 8.4). Changes in heart rate are termed positive (increase in rate) and negative (decrease in rate) chronotropic actions (changes to time and rhythm).

Along with the changes in heart rate due to sympathetic stimulation, the stroke volume also increases. Sympathetic stimulation will lead to a greater force of contraction for the same fibre length, with parasympathetic stimulation having the opposite effect. This is

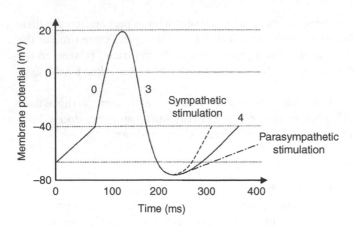

Figure 8.4 Pacemaker action potential

termed positive and negative inotropy, respectively. The heart's force of contraction is also influenced by its preload and afterload. The preload is the cross-sectional wall tension in the ventricle at end diastole (or how 'filled' the ventricle is), while the afterload is the cross-sectional wall tension at end systole. The preload can be inferred from the central venous pressure (CVP) for the right ventricle and the pulmonary capillary wedge pressure (PCWP) for the left ventricle. The afterload encompasses not just resistance from the arterial tree, but also resistance from aortic valve disease, for example, aortic stenosis. The relationship between the preload and stroke volume is described by Frank–Starling's law of the heart. This states that the stroke volume will increase in response to an increase in the preload if all other factors remain static, until the point of overstretch of the myocytes, at which stage the relationship will fail and the stroke volume will decrease, leading to heart failure. This can be shown via a Frank–Starling curve, as shown in Figure 8.5.

In very simple terms, the cardiovascular system can be compared to an electrical circuit with Ohm's law applied to it. Ohm's law can be stated mathematically as

$$V = I \times R,$$

where V = voltage (potential difference), I = current flow, and R = resistance. In relation to systemic circulation, the voltage becomes the difference between mean arterial pressure (MAP) and the CVP, the current flow is cardiac output (CO), and the resistance is the systemic vascular resistance (SVR). The equation for calculation of CO is:

$$CO = (MAP - CVP) \times 80/SVR.$$

where SVR is measured in dynes seconds (dyn s) per cm^5; 80 is a correction factor to convert the value calculated into dyn s/cm^5.

Blood pressure is hence controlled through the alteration of vascular tone and cardiac output. Blood pressure is sensed by baroreceptors in the aortic arch, carotid sinus, and atria, which feed into several control mechanisms [1]. A sudden fall in blood pressure will be detected by baroreceptors, resulting in sympathetic stimulation, causing an increase in

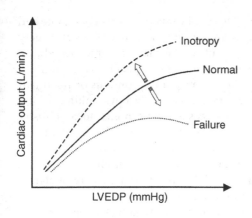

Figure 8.5 Frank–Starling law; LVDEP, left-ventricular end-diastolic pressure

vascular tone to increase the preload and SVR as well as positive chronotropic and inotropic effects on the heart, increasing cardiac output. Longer-term regulation of blood pressure includes fluid and electrolyte homeostasis mediating renal output to control intravascular and extracellular fluid volumes via such mediators as renin, angiotensin, atrial natriuretic peptide, and aldosterone.

Problems Occurring during Anaesthesia

The most common changes in the cardiovascular system under anaesthesia are a reduction in heart rate and blood pressure. However, due to autoregulation, flow to vital organs such as the brain and kidneys is usually maintained at an adequate level to prevent insufficient perfusion, reduced oxygen delivery, and end-organ damage. However, sometimes the reductions in cardiac output and subsequent oxygen delivery can be such that organ damage will occur if this is not treated.

The reduction in cardiac output can be attributed to several causes. These can be categorised: 'pump', 'vessel', and 'volume' problems. Pump problems are those due to the heart's function either from a low heart rate, force of contraction (contractility), or abnormal rhythm (dysrhythmias). Vessel problems are due to low vascular tone, which can be due to multiple causes. Volume problems are those related to insufficient intravascular volume, commonly due to preoperative starvation or bleeding.

Most intravenous induction agents and volatile anaesthetics cause a reduction in heart rate, contractility, and vascular tone. Combined, these lead to a fall in cardiac output and blood pressure. Bradycardia can be treated using agents that increase the heart rate (e.g., glycopyrronium and atropine). Vasodilation can be treated by alpha-adrenergic agents such as phenylephrine and metaraminol. Increased contractility can be achieved with agents that activate beta-adrenergic receptors (e.g., ephedrine, which also exhibits alpha-adrenergic effects).

During central venous cannulation (where the target vessel is punctured with a needle, a guidewire is inserted, a tract dilated, and the catheter then advanced over the guidewire), the sinoatrial node is at risk of stimulation by the wire as it is advanced. This can manifest as extra (ectopic) beats or other dysrhythmias including ventricular fibrillation. Withdrawal of the guidewire slightly will usually resolve the problem.

Certain surgical sites, when stimulated, can lead to significant decreases in heart rate and therefore blood pressure/cardiac output. This is commonly seen in gynaecological surgery when the cervix is stimulated, or carbon dioxide is insufflated for laparoscopic procedures. The ensuing bradycardia can be severe, even causing asystole and requiring cardiopulmonary resuscitation. This can usually be treated by the removal of the stimulus or treatment with an anticholinergic agent to increase the heart rate, such as glycopyrronium, or, if a more rapid response is required, atropine. For this reason, some prefer to administer prophylactic glycopyrronium to these patients prior to surgery starting. The other surgical site associated with bradycardia is the posterior fossa of the brain, particularly the medulla, due to this being the origin of the vagus nerve. When stimulated surgically, it leads to a decrease in the heart rate. Neurosurgeons are aware of this and thus are aware of alarms from anaesthetic monitors during posterior fossa procedures.

Reductions in systemic vascular resistance may be particularly notable in patients on certain antihypertensive agents such as angiotensin-converting enzyme (ACE) inhibitors (e.g., ramipril) and angiotensin-2 receptor blockers (e.g., losartan). This hypotension can be treated with alpha-adrenergic agonists to directly counteract the fall in systemic vascular resistance. The previously mentioned drugs ephedrine and metaraminol will act upon these receptors to increase the blood pressure. The agent most used in obstetric anaesthetic practice, phenylephrine, is a pure alpha-adrenergic agonist; therefore, the patient's heart rate may fall in response to its administration, an effect known as reflex bradycardia.

Preoperative fasting for patients to prevent regurgitation and aspiration of gastric contents leads to intravascular volume depletion in nearly all patients. This can be compensated through the administration of intravenous fluids given to patients during anaesthesia. During prolonged operations with exposed body cavities such as open intra-abdominal procedures, there can be considerable loss of water by evaporation, which can be of particular concern in children. This can be replaced with intravenous fluid, but rates of 10 mL/kg per hour are sometimes required to keep up with evaporative losses. In procedures with significant haemorrhage, such as cardiac, vascular, and obstetric procedures, hypotension is frequently due to intravascular volume depletion. After initial volume resuscitation with intravenous crystalloid solutions, blood (as packed red cells) and/or blood products are administered to restore the intravascular volume. Additionally, blood suctioned from the surgical site can be collected and reinfused to the patient through the process known as cell salvage. This has the benefit of reducing exposure to other patients' blood and the possibility of the transmission of blood-borne infections such as HIV and hepatitis C [4, 5].

References

1. K. E. Barrett, S. M. Barman, J. Yuan, and H. L. Brooks. *Ganong's Review of Medical Physiology*. New York: McGraw-Hill Education, 2019.

2. N. Herring, D. J. Paterson, and J. R. Levick. *Levick's Introduction to Cardiovascular Physiology*, 6th ed. Boca Raton, FL: CRC Press, 2018.

3. A. A. Klein, T. Meek, E. Allcock, et al. Recommendations for standards of monitoring during anaesthesia and recovery 2021. *Anaesthesia* 2021; DOI https://doi.org/10.1111/anae.15501.

4. P. S. Myles, S. Andrews, J. Nicholson, et al. Contemporary approaches to perioperative IV fluid therapy. *World Journal of Surgery* 2017; **41**: 2457–2463.

5. A. A. Klein, C. R. Bailey, A. J. Charlton, et al. Association of Anaesthetists guidelines: cell salvage for peri-operative blood conservation 2018. *Anaesthesia* 2018; **73**: 1141–1150.

Chapter 9	# Recognition and Interpretation of the Electrocardiogram

Kully Sandhu

Introduction

The electrocardiogram (ECG) is a non-invasive representation of the activity of the cardiac electrical conducting system. ECGs are widely available in all hospitals and therefore interpretation is of great importance. They allow assessment of cardiac rate, recognition of conduction blocks, myocardial ischaemia, life-threatening arrhythmias, and the effects of drugs. Therefore, ECGs provide a wealth of information allowing safe and appropriate treatment strategies for patients. This chapter summarises the most salient features of common arrhythmias seen in clinical practice.

ECGs are widely available and provide a vast quantity of information. Rapid ECG recognition and interpretation is crucial in the diagnosis and treatment of patients in the perioperative environment. Therefore, a systematic approach to ECG interpretation is vital. Always seek advice if in doubt about ECG interpretation.

ECG Monitoring

All unwell patients or patients undergoing any surgical procedure require cardiac monitoring. ECG monitoring must be used before and during the administration of general anaesthesia [1]. There are three main methods of ECG monitoring: 12 leads, defibrillator pads, and modified limb leads (also known as three-lead monitoring). Their advantages and potential disadvantages are summarised in Table 9.1.

The electrode positionings for 12 leads, defibrillator pads, and modified limb leads are placed at specific anatomical landmarks, as detailed in Table 9.2. Table 9.3 shows the positionings for three-lead ECGs. ECG electrodes and defibrillator pads are available in a range of sizes to accommodate neonates to adults, and it is is important to use the correct size for an optimum output.

Defibrillator pads will usually be labelled with an image, and the correct placement identified (see Figure 9.1). They should be placed beneath the right clavicle and the other on the mid-left-axillary line. Extra care must be taken with placements of defibrillator pads in patients with pacemakers or implantable cardioverter-defibrillator (ICDs). It is recommended that the defibrillator pads are positioned 8 cm from any pacemaker or ICD unit to minimise the risk of burns or other harm [2].

The Cardiac Conducting System

The coordinated contraction of the atria followed by the ventricles is made possible due to the cardiac conducting system. This conducting system is composed of specialised cells that allow the passage of electrical signals in the form of cell-membrane depolarisation from the

Table 9.1 The advantages and potential disadvantages of three different types of cardiac monitoring

Type of monitoring	Advantages	Disadvantages
12 leads	Provides information on different territories of the heart and additional details that enhance rhythm interpretation.	Cumbersome, time consuming to attach all 12 leads to patients. Unable to keep on continuously.
Defibrillator pads	Easily applied and therefore easily used in emergencies. They are also capable of shock delivery for electrical cardioversions.	Only provides rhythm information.
Three leads (modified limb leads)	Quick to attach to patients, provide ample space on chest to allow chest compressions. Therefore ideal in emergencies. Unlike 12-lead ECG, three-lead rhythm strips may have continuous monitoring and provide real-time monitoring.	Does not provide as much detail as 12-lead ECGs.

Table 9.2 Twelve-lead ECG electrode placement

Electrode label	Electrode position
V_1	In the fourth intercostal space just to the right of the sternum
V_2	In the fourth intercostal space just to the left of the sternum
V_3	Between leads V_2 and V_4
V_4	In the fifth intercostal space in the mid-clavicular line
V_5	Horizontally even with V_4, in the left anterior axillary line
V_6	Horizontally even with V_4 and V_5 in the mid-axillary line
Right arm	On the right arm – avoiding thick muscle
Left arm	On left arm – avoiding thick muscle
Right leg	On the right leg – lateral calf muscle
Left leg	On the left leg – lateral calf muscle

Table 9.3 Three-lead ECG electrode placement

Electrode label	Electrode position
Red	Right-shoulder prominence
Green	In the fourth intercostal space just to the left of the sternum
Yellow	Left-shoulder prominence

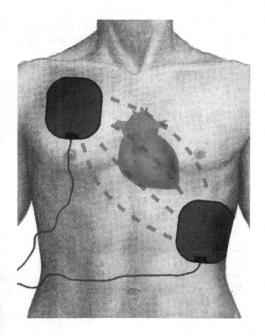

Figure 9.1 Position of electrodes during defibrillation/cardioversion, position of heart, flow of intrathrocical energy during shock (by PhilippN, licensed under CC BY-SA 3.0)

atria to the ventricles. The depolarisation originates in the sinoatrial (SA) node located on the wall of the right atrium, near the entrance of the superior vena cava. The SA node comprises a group of cells that generate a regular depolarisation, initiating the heartbeat. This depolarisation then travels through the atria causing contraction, pushing blood into the ventricles. This is seen as P waves on an ECG. The electrical impulses then reach the atrioventricular (AV) node, which is a specialised group of cells between the atria and ventricles within the atrial septum, forming the electrical connection between the atria and ventricles. The AV node can initiate its own signals if none arrive from the atria, giving rise to 'nodal' or 'junctional' rhythm, usually at a slow rate of 40–60 beats per minute (bpm).

The electrical impulses are then conducted via Purkinje fibres to both ventricles via specialised conducting tissue called the bundle of Hiss and, finally, left and right bundle branches. The right bundle branch carries electrical impulses that allow depolarisation of the right ventricle, causing contraction and ejection of blood into the pulmonary arteries. The left bundle branch carries electrical impulses that allow depolarisation of the left ventricle, and hence contraction. The left ventricle has a large muscle mass that splits into two, the anterior and posterior fascicles, to allow faster and more coordinated left-ventricular contraction into the aorta, hence supplying the body. The conducting system is summarised in Figure 9.2.

The conducting system is represented on the ECG and gives rise to important intervals and durations. ECG paper is calibrated and standardised. In the UK, standard paper speed is 25 mm per second. This corresponds to each small square representing 0.1 mV in height and 40 milliseconds (ms) duration with each large square representing 0.5 mV in height and 200 ms in width. Therefore five large or 25 small squares correspond to 1 second.

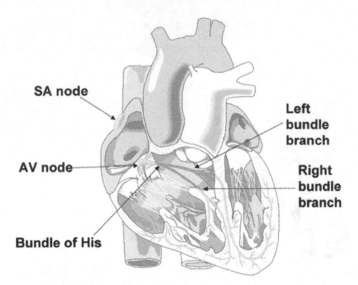

Figure 9.2 Conducting system of the heart (reproduced with kind permission of the Resuscitation Council (UK))

SA node

Left bundle branch

AV node

Right bundle branch

Bundle of His

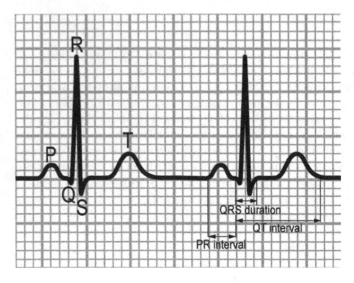

Figure 9.3 Three main deflections on an ECG recording ((reproduced with kind permission of the Resuscitation Council (UK))

There are three main deflections on ECG recordings (see Figure 9.3). The first deflection is the P wave and corresponds to atria contraction. The second deflection corresponds to ventricular contraction and is called the QRS complex. Finally, the T wave corresponds to ventricular repolarisation or relaxation.

Table 9.4 ECG interval and duration times

Feature	Description	Normal duration
RR interval	Interval between an R wave and next R wave. Used to calculate the cardiac rate (see below).	0.6–1.2 s
P wave	Corresponds to electrical impulse from the SA node towards the AV node with atrial depolarisation and contraction (atrial systole).	80 ms
PR interval	Measured from the beginning of the P wave to the beginning of the QRS complex. The interval corresponds to the time taken for the electrical impulse to travel from the SA node through the AV node to the ventricles. The PR interval is a useful indicator for describing the various types of cardiac heart block (see below).	120–200 ms Less than five small squares
QRS complex	Usually, the largest complex seen on the ECG tracing and represents the depolarisation of the ventricles (ventricular systole).	80–120 ms Less than three small squares
ST segment	Represents the period when the ventricles are depolarised. This segment is of pivotal importance when considering myocardial ischaemia.	80–120 ms
T wave	Represents the repolarisation of the ventricles. The absolute refractory period corresponds to beginning of the QRS complex to the apex of the T wave. The relative refractory period corresponds to the apex of the T wave to the iso-electrical line.	160 ms

The most important intervals and duration of ECGs are summarised in Table 9.4. Analysing these assists in recognising many abnormalities and rhythm disturbances.

Cardiac Rate

The normal cardiac rate for an adult is between 60 and 100 bpm. Bradycardia is defined as a cardiac rate less than 60 bpm and tachycardia greater than 100 bpm. Figure 9.4 shows an example of sinus rhythm with each P wave preceding every QRS complex.

There are several different methods to calculate cardiac rate. The most common method is to divide 300 by the number of large squares between two QRS complexes. In the ECG strip in Figure 9.4, the number of squares between the R waves = 4; therefore 300/4 = 75 bpm.

Using an alternative method, in the standard ECG paper speed, 30 large squares equates to 6 seconds. Therefore, if the number of R waves are counted within 30 large squares and then multiplied by 10, this gives the number of R waves in 1 minute and therefore the heart rate.

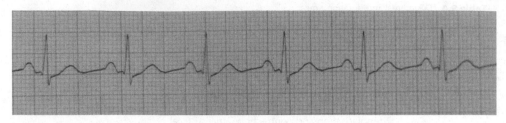

Figure 9.4 Sinus rhythm (reproduced with kind permission from Laerdal Medical)

The above are reliable methods if the cardiac rate is constant; however, it is not so accurate if an irregular rate such as atrial fibrillation is present. In such cases, two main methods used are to:

- calculate the 'average heart rate' as in the above method by choosing the QRS interval that appears to be an average length; or
- identify the shortest RR interval and longest RR intervals. Then divide 300 by each and give the heart rate as a range.

The longest RR interval is approximately three large squares, and the shortest RR interval is approximately two large squares. Therefore, the cardiac rate is in the range of 300/3 to 300/2 = 100–150 bpm.

Cardiac Arrhythmias

Bradycardias and tachycardias are referred to sinus rhythm, with rates of less than 60 bpm and greater than 100 bpm, respectively. In contrast to these are cardiac arrhythmias that occur due to abnormal cardiac conduction. These arrhythmias can be identified by QRS complex duration, regularity, and any relationship with P waves if P waves are present. They can broadly be divided into tachycardias or bradyarrhythmias.

Tachyarrhythmias

There are two main categories of tachyarrhythmia: narrow and broad complex, depending on the QRS duration.

Narrow Complex Tachyarrhythmia

These are identifiable by having normal QRS duration (less than three small squares on standard ECG paper). There are three common narrow complex tachyarrhythmias: atrial fibrillation, atrial flutter, and supraventricular tachyarrhythmias.

Atrial Fibrillation

Atrial fibrillation is the most common arrhythmia seen in clinical practice, with an overall population prevalence in England of 2.5–3.5% [3, 4]. Figure 9.5 shows an example of atrial fibrillation.

The two pathognomonic features are:

- the absence of P waves; and
- irregularly irregular QRS complexes.

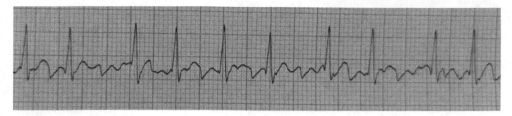

Figure 9.5 Atrial fibrillation (reproduced with kind permission from Laerdal Medical)

Atrial fibrillation may be acute (sudden), chronic (constant), or paroxysmal (occasional), and patients may experience no symptoms. It can cause problems, however, as fibrillating atria do not contract properly, allowing blood to become immobile and therefore causing blood clots (mural thrombus) to accumulate. Such clots can pass through the heart and be ejected into the body as an embolus, stopping blood supply to the affected organ such as the brain, where a cerebrovascular accident (a stroke) will occur. Furthermore, as the fibrillating atrium is no longer contributing to ventricular filling, cardiac failure can be provoked. This can be worsened by the tendency for atrial fibrillation to cause a tachycardia, which in elderly patients may not permit enough time for the ventricles to fill properly, further reducing cardiac output and making cardiac failure more likely. It is frequently found on a preoperative ECG and may require management prior to elective surgery, especially if cardiac failure is suspected. Management strategies include attempting to stabilise the rhythm by antiarrhythmics such as amiodarone, rate control using drugs such as digoxin to treat tachycardia, and the use of anticoagulants such as warfarin to reduce embolism and stroke risk. Acute atrial fibrillation may be due to simple electrolyte disturbance such as hypokalaemia (low potassium) or fluid depletion but may benefit from direct current (DC) cardioversion, which has been shown to be a safe and effective treatment for atrial fibrillation and to restore sinus rhythm, especially if treated soon after onset [5].

Atrial Flutter

Atrial flutter is also an arrhythmia that originate in the atria. However, unlike atrial fibrillation, atrial flutter has a regular positive 'P' deflection, which will be best seen in lead II, III, and aVF (inferior leads). These regular positive deflections are often referred to as 'saw-tooth' waves due to their regular pattern. These give rise to a regular relationship between P waves and QRS complexes that may be 1:1, 2:1, 3:1, or greater. The atria contract very quickly in atrial flutter and the ventricles will struggle to keep up and may only respond on every second atrial depolarisation (2:1 heart block), every third atrial depolarisation (3:1 heart block), or even less frequently. Ventricular filling is severely impacted either by tachycardia (preventing the ventricles from having enough time to fill properly) or by the lack of coordination between atrial and ventricular pumping. This can cause the heart to fail. Figure 9.6 shows a typical atrial flutter ECG pattern.

Broad Complex Tachyarrhythmias

The QRS complex represents ventricular depolarisation and contraction and, as stated above, the normal duration is 80–120 ms. A narrow complex tachyarrhythmia (three squares or less across) arises from the atria and suggests normal but rapid ventricular activity. A broad complex tachycardia (more than three squares wide) suggests a ventricular

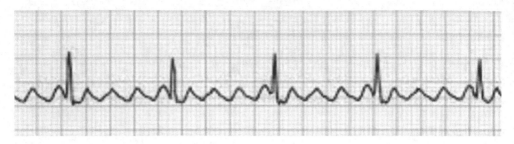

Figure 9.6 Atrial flutter (reproduced with kind permission from Laerdal Medical)

problem and can indicate a significant medical emergency. The two most important life-threatening arrhythmias arising from the ventricle are ventricular tachycardia and fibrillation. Both are life-threatening broad complex tachyarrhythmias (>120 ms or three squares wide, hence 'broad') and require urgent medical attention.

Ventricular Tachycardia

Ventricular tachycardia is a regular broad complex tachyarrhythmia. The most common causes are: myocardial scarring, acting as a substrate for arrhythmia; myocardial infarction; and drug toxicity and electrolyte abnormalities. Treatment depends on the haemodynamic status of the patient. If patients have any of the following – chest pains, syncope, clinical cardiac failure, or hypotension – then emergency synchronised electrical cardioversion are required. If, however, none of the above are present then medical therapy such as beta blockers or amiodarone may suffice. A patient with ventricular tachycardia must be constantly monitored and observed in case electrical cardioversion becomes necessary, either because one of the above indications develops or because the rhythm progresses to ventricular fibrillation.

Features supporting the diagnosis of ventricular tachycardia:

- regular pattern; and
- broad QRS.

Figure 9.7 shows a typical ECG for ventricular tachycardia.

Ventricular Fibrillation

Ventricular fibrillation consists of chaotic electrical activity that is incompatible with cardiac output and therefore life threatening, requiring immediate electrical cardioversion. Please refer to the Resuscitation Council (UK) guidelines for current advice. Causes of ventricular fibrillation include myocardial ischaemia, electrolyte abnormalities, drug toxicity, and congenital syndromes. A typical ECG for ventricular fibrillation is shown in Figure 9.8.

Bradycardias and Heart Blocks

Sinus bradycardia is demonstrated by every P wave being followed by a QRS of normal duration and, like other bradyarrhythmias, can be caused by numerous intrinsic and extrinsic factors. A mild bradycardia such as a resting heart rate of 40–50 bpm may be a

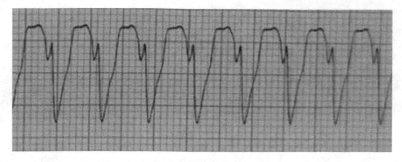

Figure 9.7 Monomorphic ventricular tachycardia (reproduced with kind permission from Laerdal Medical)

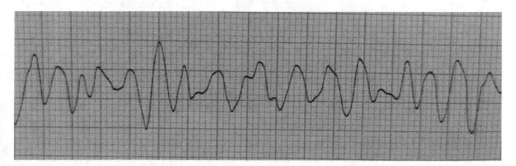

Figure 9.8 Ventricular fibrillation. Reproduced with kind permission from Laerdal Medical

normal occurrence in healthy subjects, especially athletes, but in less healthy patients it will reduce cardiac output and can cause hypotension and heart failure.

Bradycardia due to vagal stimulation slowing the SA node may commonly be provoked around the time of surgery by intra-abdominal stimulation, in which case it may respond to anticholinergic drugs such as atropine. In severe cases, it may even progress to complete stopping of the heart (asystole), requiring cardiopulmonary resuscitation.

Bradycardia may also result from the slowing down of the cardiac rate due to heart block, which is due to a failure of the electrical communication from the atria to the ventricles. There are three main types of heart block, increasing in severity from first to second and third degree blocks. Patients with symptomatic heart block will usually require fitment of a pacemaker to stimulate a suitable heart rhythm.

First-Degree Heart Block

First-degree heart blocks have fixed a PR interval that is greater than 200 ms (five small squares; see Figure 9.9). In this example, the PR interval is greater than five small squares. This condition is often entirely asymptomatic.

Second-Degree Heart Block

In second-degree heart block, not all P waves are followed by a QRS complex. It is categorised into two types by the Mobitz classification.

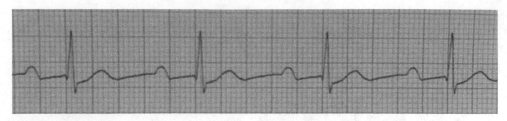

Figure 9.9 First-degree heart block (reproduced with kind permission from Laerdal Medical)

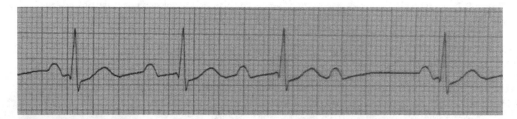

Figure 9.10 Mobitz type 1 (reproduced with kind permission from Laerdal Medical)

In **Mobitz type 1** second-degree heart block, there is progressive prolongation of the PR interval on consecutive beats until there is a P wave with a 'dropped' QRS complex. After the dropped QRS complex, the PR interval resets and the cycle repeats, with this cycle being known as the 'Wenckebach period'. It is described in terms of the ratio of atrial to ventricular beats, such as 'Mobitz type 1 with 3:2 block' meaning that, for every three atrial beats, the atrium only beats twice (see Figure 9.10). In this example, note the gradual prolongation of the PR interval until the fourth P wave not being followed by a QRS complex. Then the cycle is repeated. This would be called a 4:3 block. It can be very difficult to discern the increasing prolongation of PR intervals if there are frequent dropped beats such as a 2:1 block.

Mobitz type 1 block may occur in healthy young patients, especially in sleep, but becomes more common in older age. It rarely progresses to a more severe block, in which case an artificial pacemaker may be required.

Mobitz type 2 heart block is characterised by a 'dropped' QRS complex. Unlike Mobitz type 1, there is no lengthening of the PR interval; rather, the PR interval remains constant, then there is a dropped QRS complex. This is almost always a disease of the distal conduction system (His–Purkinje system). The significance of this type of AV node block is that it may progress rapidly to complete heart block. The definitive treatment may include an artificial pacemaker.

Figure 9.11 shows a typical ECG pattern for a Mobitz type 2 heart block. Note the fixed PR interval, then the fourth P wave with a dropped QRS complex.

Third-Degree or Complete Heart Block

A third-degree AV node block is also known as complete heart block. There is no electrical connection between the atria or ventricles. The typical features are bradyarrhythmia with broad and regular QRS complexes, which have no relationship with the P waves (see Figure 9.12). This can cause severe bradycardia and heart failure as the bradycardia may not provide an adequate cardiac output. These patients are very likely to require an artificial pacemaker.

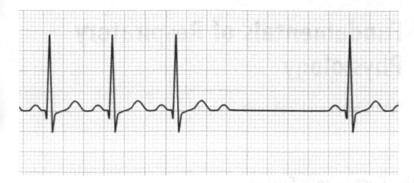

Figure 9.11 Mobitz type 2 (reproduced with kind permission from Laerdal Medical)

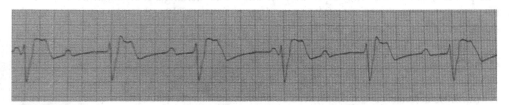

Figure 9.12 Third-degree or complete heart block (reproduced with kind permission from Laerdal Medical)

References

1. A. A. Klein, T. Meek, E. Allcock, et al. Recommendations for standards of monitoring during anaesthesia and recovery 2021. *Anaesthesia* 2021; DOI https://doi.org/10.1111/anae.15501.

2. Resuscitation Council UK. *Advanced Life Support*, 8th ed. London: Resuscitation Council UK, 2021.

3. N. J. Adderley, R. Ryan, K. Nirantharakumar, et al. Prevalence and treatment of atrial fibrillation in UK general practice from 2000 to 2016. *Heart* 2019; **105**: 27–33.

4. National Institute for Health and Care Excellence. Atrial fibrillation: how common is it? Available from: https://cks.nice.org.uk/topics/atrial-fibrillation/background-information/prevalence/#:~:text=Complications%20and%20prognosis-,How%20common%20is%20it%3F,to%20be%20undiagnosed%20and%20untreated.

5. J. P. Piccini and L. Fauchier. Rhythm control in atrial fibrillation. *Lancet* 2016; **388**: 829–840.

Chapter 10

Fundamentals of Respiratory Physiology

Sarah John and Tahzeeb Bhagat

Function of the Respiratory System

The primary function of the respiratory system is gas exchange. It transports oxygen from the atmosphere to the blood and carbon dioxide from the blood to the atmosphere. The transport of these gases into the lungs is known as ventilation.

Secondary functions of the lungs include:

- acid–base balance;
- metabolic factors; and
- immune defence.

Anatomy of the Respiratory System

The primary components of the respiratory system are the airways and the lungs. These can be separated into areas that do not participate in gas exchange, the conducting airways; and areas that do participate in gas exchange, the respiratory airways [1].

Conducting Airways

The conducting airways comprise the following:

- Upper airways – including the nose, mouth and pharynx. They are responsible for conduction of air to the larynx, and they warm, filter, and humidify incoming air.
- Larynx – responsible for phonation and conducts air to the trachea. It is located at the junction of the trachea and the oesophagus. Closure of the vocal cords in the larynx protects the lower airway from aspiration of foreign material.
- Tracheobronchial tree – a series of branching small tubes starting from the single trachea, branching into the right and left main bronchi at the carina. These tubes each continue to branch into smaller tubes. They function to conduct air to the respiratory airways.

Intubation

Endotracheal intubation involves inserting a tube through the nose or mouth, through the larynx and into the trachea. The tip of the endotracheal tube (ETT) should sit below the larynx but above the carina. Insertion too far risks the ETT entering the left or, more commonly, the right main bronchus, resulting in only one lung being ventilated. This can be seen by falling oxygen saturations a few minutes after intubation and is why the position of the ETT at the teeth is always noted at intubation.

Respiratory Airways

The final branches of the tracheobronchial tree are the respiratory bronchioles. These terminate in small air-filled sacs known as alveoli. Each alveolus is thin walled and surrounded by capillaries, allowing oxygen to diffuse in, and carbon dioxide out, of the blood.

The lungs are surrounded by two membranes, the pleura. One layer, the pulmonary, or visceral, pleura, covers the surface of the lung. The second, the parietal pleura, is attached to the inside of the chest wall. Usually, these two membranes are in close proximity, separated only by a small amount of fluid to reduce friction. Fluid or air can enter this space during illness or injury. Air entry into this space, known as a pneumothorax, can cause collapse of that lung. Excess fluid in the pleura space is known as a pleural effusion [1].

Control of Respiration

Respiration occurs spontaneously and rhythmically due to the integration of three basic components [2]:

(1) Sensors – gather information to send to the controller:

- Receptors in the blood vessels and the brain respond to the amount of oxygen and carbon dioxide in the blood. The most important receptors are the central chemoreceptors in the brain, which respond to the amount of carbon dioxide in the blood.
- Receptors in the lungs respond to the degree of stretch of the lung tissue and to any irritation from inhaled irritants.

(2) Controller – responsible for the spontaneous automaticity of respiration, integration of the incoming signals, and sending impulses to the effectors.

- The main respiratory control centre is located in the medulla in the brainstem.
- It receives signals from other parts of the brain, allowing some voluntary control over respiration.

(3) Effectors – the respiratory muscles.

The main muscle of inspiration is the diaphragm, a large, dome-shaped muscle that separates the thorax from the abdomen. During inspiration, it contracts, moving downwards. At the same time, the intercostal muscles between the ribs contract, pulling the chest wall up and out. The combined action of these muscles increases the volume of the thorax, drawing air into the lungs. During quiet expiration, the passive relaxation of the diaphragm pushes the air back out again [3].

When the work of breathing increases, extra muscles are recruited to increase the force of inspiration and expiration. These muscles are known as the accessory muscles. They include muscles to pull the rib cage up during inspiration, sternocleidomastoid and scalene muscles, and muscles to push the diaphragm up during expiration, including the abdominal wall muscles.

Nerves send signals between each of these three components to coordinate respiration. The most important nerve of respiration is the phrenic nerve, which supplies the diaphragm. It originates from nerves exiting the spinal cord at the cervical vertebrae C5, C6, and C7. Spinal cord injuries at or above this level can result in the inability to breathe.

Lung Volumes

The lungs can be divided up into volumes which can be measured with a spirometer. The sum of more than one volume is known as a capacity. The following are the most important in the anaesthetic context [2]:

- Tidal volume (TV) – the volume of air that enters the lungs during quiet respiration. At rest in an adult, it is about 500 mL.
- Total lung capacity (TLC) – the volume of air occupying the lungs at maximal inspiration (about 6 L).
- Vital capacity (VC) – the volume of air that enters the lungs from maximum expiration to maximum inspiration (about 4.5 L).
- Expiratory reserve volume (ERV) – the maximum volume that can be voluntarily exhaled after a normal expiration (about 1.5 L).
- Inspiratory reserve volume (IRV) – the maximum extra volume that can be inhaled at the end of a normal inspiration (about 2.5 L).
- Residual volume (RV) – the volume of air that is left in the lungs at the end of maximal expiration (about 1.5 L).
- Functional residual capacity (FRC) – the volume of air that is left in the lungs at the end of normal expiration (about 3 L).

Functional Residual Capacity

If someone stops breathing, for example, after induction of anaesthesia, the volume of air that remains in the lungs is the FRC. Under normal circumstances the FRC is roughly composed of normal inspired air (i.e., 21% oxygen). When someone stops breathing (apnoea), the oxygen in the FRC can continue to diffuse into the capillaries acting as an

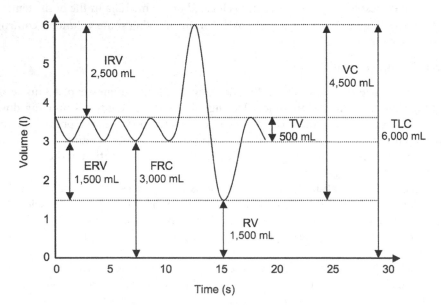

Figure 10.1 Lung volumes

oxygen reservoir to maintain oxygenation during periods with no ventilation. This can be improved by two mechanisms:

(1) Increase the amount of oxygen in the FRC by pre-oxygenation. Allowing a patient to breath high-concentration oxygen before induction of anaesthesia increases the amount of oxygen in the FRC.

(2) Increase the size of the FRC. The FRC is decreased by lying a patient flat, obesity, pregnancy, and anaesthesia. Therefore, sitting a patient up while pre-oxygenating them further increases the oxygen reservoir.

Optimisation of these two factors increases the amount of time that oxygenation can be maintained without ventilation [2].

Ventilation

Minute ventilation is the volume of air that is inhaled per minute. Described in terms of the lung volumes above, it is the tidal volume multiplied by the number of breaths per minute (respiratory rate). Not all inspired air reaches alveoli to take part in gas exchange. Some remains in the conducting airways, and some will enter alveoli that are not perfused. This volume of air that is inhaled but does not take part in gas exchange is known as the dead-space volume. The air that reaches the alveoli is known as the alveolar volume:

tidal volume = dead-space volume + alveolar tidal volume.

Dead space is particularly problematic in anaesthesia as the patient's natural 'anatomical' dead space (around 140 mL) is added to by the 'mechanical' dead space of the breathing apparatus. In this instance, no useful alveolar ventilation would take place at a tidal volume of less than the sum of the anatomical and mechanical dead space. If the tidal volume is less than the total dead space then there is effectively no gas exchange. Therefore, ventilation must ensure that the tidal volume is sufficient to provide a good alveolar tidal volume after the dead space has been ventilated. As only alveolar volume participates in gas exchange, a reduction in alveolar ventilation will result in a fall in gas exchange, shown by a fall in oxygen saturations and a rise in carbon dioxide levels.

In a mixture of gases, the sum of all their individual partial pressures is the total pressure. This is expressed as Dalton's law [4]. For example, in a sample of room air at the standard atmospheric pressure of 101 kPa, 78 kPa is due to the nitrogen and 21 kPa is due to oxygen, with the remaining partial pressure being due to other gases such as argon and carbon dioxide. The partial pressure of oxygen in the blood is related to oxygen saturation by a sigmoid (S-shaped curve) relationship, shown by the oxygen dissociation curve (see Figure 10.2). As can be seen, the haemoglobin saturation is relatively flat ('saturated') until the partial pressure of oxygen has fallen significantly. This means that during periods of reduced alveolar ventilation the oxygen saturations will not initially fall. However, when they start to decline, they will fall rapidly. Thus, a fall in oxygen saturation from 100% to 95% represents very little change in actual oxygen carriage by the blood but a fall from 90% to 85% represents a very significant reduction in oxygenation and requires immediate intervention.

On the other hand, carbon dioxide levels in the blood are related to alveolar ventilation by a linear inverse relationship. For a fixed production rate of carbon dioxide, halving the alveolar minute volume would theoretically result in a doubling of alveolar carbon dioxide. Carbon dioxide almost immediately equilibrates between the capillaries and the alveoli,

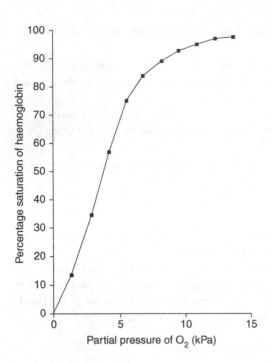

Figure 10.2 Haemoglobin disassociation curve

therefore the partial pressure of carbon dioxide in the blood is approximately equal to the expired carbon dioxide. The expired carbon dioxide can easily be measured with capnography and can therefore be used as an indirect measure of the adequacy of alveolar ventilation. This can be seen during anaesthesia: too high a minute ventilation (hyperventilation) results in falling expired carbon dioxide levels, while too low a minute ventilation (hypoventilation) results in rising expired carbon dioxide levels [2].

The ventilation of the lung is not uniform throughout, with the bases receiving more ventilation than the apices. This is primarily to do with two related factors [1]:

(1) Gravity – the weight of the lung presses down on itself, compressing the bases of the lungs compared to the apices. Like a spring suspended from above, the coils at the base are relatively compressed compared to the top. When stretched, this spring will increase in size to a greater extent at the base.

(2) Compliance – the change in volume per unit pressure. Higher compliance means a greater change in volume for the same change in pressure (i.e., more stretchy). Compliance changes with lung volume. Think of a balloon, it is much easier to inflate once there is some air in it, it is hardest to inflate at the extremes of volume, either empty or full. The same is true of the lungs: compliance is greatest with a small amount of air remaining in the lungs. At the end of normal expiration, the apical alveoli remain almost full of air, while the basal alveoli only have a small amount of air remaining. Thus, during normal inspiration, the compliance of the basal alveoli is much greater than the apical alveoli.

Perfusion

The pulmonary circulation originates at the pulmonary artery, which exits from the right side of the heart. This artery branches multiple times, terminating in the capillaries that surround the alveoli to take part in gas exchange. These capillaries are numerous and very thin walled to maximise the surface area available for gas exchange [1].

Not all blood that leaves the right side of the heart will reach ventilated alveoli for gas exchange. Some blood will supply the airways themselves, and some will supply alveoli that are currently not being ventilated. This blood that returns to the left side of the heart having not taken place in gas exchange is known as shunt. Similar to ventilation, the perfusion of the lung is not uniform throughout, with perfusion being greater at the base than at the apex due to gravity. The lung bases are below the heart, while the apices are above, resulting in gravity aiding perfusion of the bases.

The natural consequence of the weight of the lung's tissue and of the surface tension of the wet surface of the alveoli is a tendency for alveoli to collapse under their own weight, especially at the bases. The resulting atelectasis would give rise to hypoxia as the alveoli contain liquid but no oxygen, so any blood passing through their capillaries returns to the heart without becoming oxygenated. Fortunately, in the healthy and conscious patient, such activities as deep breathing, talking, coughing, and postural changes prevent atelectasis becoming a serious problem. However, in the unconscious and anaesthetised patient, these protections are absent, and atelectasis can lead to hypoxia, especially in patients who are obese, pregnant, or who suffer from lung disease.

This problem can be reduced by appropriate ventilation strategies such as the mainten- ance of constant positive airway pressure (CPAP) or positive end airway pressure (PEEP). If these should fail then a 'recruitment procedure' may be successful in reinflating the lost alveoli. This involves the application of a higher ventilation pressure for several seconds, either manually using bag ventilation or mechanically via the ventilator. Great care should be exercised when performing this procedure as the haemodynamic effects of increasing the intra-thoracic pressure can be considerable, especially in the unstable of fluid-depleted patient. There is also a risk of 'barotrauma', which is lung damage from hyperdistension of the alveoli due to the application of excessive pressure.

Ventilation–Perfusion Relationship

For ideal gas exchange, the ventilation (V) and perfusion (Q) of each individual alveolus should be matched. That is to say, the V/Q ratio is 1. Both an increased V/Q ratio (more ventilation than perfusion) and decreased V/Q ratio (more perfusion than ventilation) can result in hypoxia.

As described above, during normal respiration, both ventilation and perfusion are increased in the bases of the lungs compared with the apices. The result of this is to direct ventilation to the best perfused areas of the lung, improving V/Q matching, thus improving gas exchange.

Anaesthesia impairs the body's normal mechanisms for maintaining V/Q matching, impairing gas exchange. During anaesthesia, the bases of the lungs tend to collapse, known as atelectasis. The result of this is an increase in shunt. There will be a larger amount of blood that enters the lungs which does not meet ventilated alveoli (i.e., a low V/Q ratio). This blood will then return to the left side of the heart without being oxygenated. The resulting hypoxia will not improve with the administration of oxygen, as that portion of blood will never come into contact with ventilated alveoli.

Spontaneous vs Mechanical Ventilation

During spontaneous ventilation, air is drawn into the lungs by a negative pressure produced by the increase in volume, as described above. The reverse is true during mechanical ventilation, also known as positive-pressure ventilation. Positive-pressure ventilation has several consequences [4]:

- There is an increase in airway and alveolar pressures.
- It preferentially ventilates non-dependent, less-well-perfused regions of the lung, impairing V/Q matching and gas exchange.
- The increase in alveolar pressure can occlude pulmonary capillaries, restricting blood flow to these well-ventilated lung regions.
- The increased intra-thoracic pressure can reduce blood flow returning to the heart from the rest of the body, lowering cardiac output and therefore blood pressure.

Positioning during Mechanical Ventilation

The following positions may be used during mechanical ventilation:

- Lateral – mechanical ventilation in the lateral position preferentially ventilates the upper (non-dependent) lung, while the lower lung (dependent) is better perfused. This increases the amount of ventilation–perfusion mismatch, impairing gas exchange.
- Trendelenburg – this position forces the abdominal contents up onto the diaphragm, restricting diaphragmatic movement and compressing the lung bases. This impairs ventilation, particularly of the lung bases, resulting in increased ventilation–perfusion mismatch, reduced compliance and reduced functional residual capacity.
- Prone – mechanical ventilation in the prone position may improve ventilation–perfusion matching compared to in the supine position, especially in patients with severe lung disease such as acute respiratory distress syndrome (ARDS). This is due to the more uniform distribution of both ventilation and perfusion throughout the lung fields; this position also permits the reinflation and recruitment of previously unventilated alveoli. This has been found to be of particular benefit in acute lung injuries and in the obese, and has become a mainstay of intensive care ventilation strategy, although the improvement in oxygenation is usually temporary and may require the patient to be returned to the supine position after a while. Prone ventilation poses many technical problems of its own, such as the pressure area care, and the difficulty of safely turning a critically ill patient and of cardiopulmonary resuscitation in a prone patient.

References

1. J. B. West and A. M. Luks. *West's Respiratory Physiology. The Essentials*, 10th ed. Philadelphia, PA: Lippencott Williams and Wilkins, 2015.

2. D. Chambers, C. Huang, and G. Matthews. *Basic Physiology for Anaesthetists*, 2nd ed. Cambridge: Cambridge University press, 2019.

3. G. H. Mills. Respiratory physiology and anaesthesia. *British Journal of Anaesthesia* 2001; 1: 35–39.

4. T. Smith, C. Pinnock, and T. Lin. *Fundamentals of Anaesthesia*, 4th ed. Cambridge: Cambridge University Press, 2017.

Introduction to General Anaesthesia

James Ip and Jo Han Gan

Introduction

The term anaesthesia was first used by Oliver Wendell Holmes in 1846 from the Greek 'anaisthesis' [αισθησις], meaning 'without sensation' [1]. The aim of anaesthesia is to allow diagnostic or interventional procedures to be done with minimal to no patient discomfort and no recall of intraoperative events. Anaesthesia can broadly be divided into general, regional, and local anaesthesia.

General anaesthesia is a reversible state of unconsciousness induced by pharmacological agents. Regional anaesthesia involves administering a local anaesthetic to a group of nerves or the spinal cord to render a region of the body insensate without impairing consciousness. Local anaesthesia is the infiltration of local anaesthesia to the tissue at the site of surgery to produce a localised area of numbness.

General Anaesthesia

Sedation and general anaesthesia can be viewed as a spectrum of unconsciousness. At one end of this spectrum, a patient may be lightly sedated to undergo a painless imaging procedure. Conversely, a patient may need to be deeply anaesthetised for major intra-cavity surgery. The transition between sedation and general anaesthesia can be vague but a useful demarcation is the loss of verbal contact and the absence of awareness or explicit recall.

Increasing the depth of anaesthesia results in a progressive depression of protective and autonomic reflexes. These reflexes are essential to help maintain physiological homeostasis and avoid harm. For example, a person touching a hot dinner plate would automatically withdraw their hand very quickly. This is the withdrawal reflex, which originates from the spinal cord and serves to protect the body from injuries. Reflexes more pertinent to anaesthesia include airway reflexes (e.g., closure of the vocal cords to avoid aspiration), corneal reflexes (e.g., blinking in response to corneal stimulation), respiratory reflexes, and cardiovascular reflexes. Loss of airway reflexes is particularly significant as failure to protect the airway under anaesthesia may result in aspiration of gastric contents, leading to severe pneumonitis.

It is important to distinguish the presence of intact reflexes from consciousness (or awareness) during anaesthesia as an individual may be unconscious but still maintain some degree of protective reflex. Different protective reflexes are lost at different depths of anaesthesia. For example, airway reflexes are usually diminished at a greater depth of anaesthesia compared to corneal reflexes. This also explains how a patient may exhibit a withdrawal reflex under anaesthesia during initial incision but have no recollection of the event.

History of Anaesthesia

Prior to the discovery of anaesthesia, surgery was often limited to amputations, removal of bladder stones, and superficial surface surgery. Due to the lack of anaesthesia and the extreme pain involved, surgery was often seen as the last option for the moribund or in patients in severe distress.

The first attempts to alleviate pain from disease or to facilitate surgery were often crude, with variable levels of effectiveness. Most involved ingestion of ethanol and/or herbal mixtures. Nitrous oxide was discovered in 1772 by Joseph Priestley and was first used by Horace Wells in 1844 to facilitate a tooth extraction. Diethyl ether (known simply as ether; first used 1846) and chloroform (first used 1847) subsequently replaced nitrous oxide as they were considered more potent, safer, and were readily produced in bulk. More anaesthetic agents were introduced after the 1930s (cyclopropane in 1930, trichlorethylene in 1941, and halothane in 1956) after it was found that ether and chloroform had significant disadvantages, such as prolonged recovery, nausea, and vomiting as well as flammability (ether) and cardiac arrhythmias (chloroform).

Propofol, the currently most widely used intravenous anaesthetic drug, was originally developed in the UK by Imperial Chemical Industries following research into the sedative effect of phenol derivatives in animal models. It was first licensed for clinical use in 1986 and very quickly became the induction agent of choice due to patients' rapid recovery of cognitive and psychomotor function and its favourable side-effect profile.

Modern inhalational agents are derivatives of ether that have been halogenated and are therefore less toxic and non-flammable. Halogenation means that a chemical reaction has occurred where a compound or material has gained one or more halogens. Halothane was the first halogenated anaesthetic agent to be introduced in 1956. It was non-irritant to the airway and pleasant smelling, which was especially useful for inhalational induction in children. Isoflurane and desflurane were introduced as alternatives to halothane due to concerns over hepatitis and arrhythmias, but they have the disadvantage of being unpleasant smelling and irritant, rendering them unsuitable for inhalational induction. The advent of sevoflurane (benign side-effect profile, non-irritant, with rapid onset of anaesthesia) rendered halothane obsolete.

Looking to the future, xenon gas displays many properties of being an ideal anaesthetic agent. These properties include rapid induction and emergence, cardiovascular stability, cerebral protection, not a greenhouse gas, and not triggering malignant hyperpyrexia. It is currently only used for research purposes due to its high cost. There will need to be major advances in scavenging and 'recycling' of xenon before it can be used widely.

Mechanism of Action

In 1984, Franks and Lieb showed that most general anaesthetics inhibit the lipid-free enzyme, firefly luciferase, indicating that they act directly at a protein receptor in a hydrophobic site [2]. Thus, it is now thought anaesthetic agents exert their effects via specific neuronal receptors, in particular inhibitory gamma-aminobutyric acid A (GABA$_A$) receptors within the central nervous system. GABA$_A$ receptors are ligand-gated ion channels consisting of five subunits arranged around a central pore. These GABA$_A$ complexes form chloride anion channels and are molecular targets for benzodiazepines, barbiturates, and volatile inhalational agents. Activation of the GABA$_A$ receptor leads to post-synaptic hyperpolarisation of the cell membrane, inhibitory post-synaptic currents, and inhibition of neuronal activity.

Modulation of $GABA_A$ receptors alone incompletely accounts for the mechanism of action of all anaesthetics. Ketamine, N_2O, and xenon have a minimal effect on $GABA_A$ receptors and deliver their effects through inhibition of N-methyl-D-aspartate (NMDA) receptors on excitatory glutaminergic neurons. Other potential targets of anaesthetic agents include two-pore potassium channels and extra-synaptic $GABA_A$ receptors.

The Concept of Balanced Anaesthesia

'Balanced anaesthesia' is the concept of using a combination of techniques and drugs to provide the optimal conditions to facilitate surgery. It was first described by Lundy in 1926, who suggested that a balance of agents and techniques can be used to produce the three main components of anaesthesia: hypnosis, analgesia, and muscle relaxation, which are also known as the 'triad of anaesthesia' [3].

Today, induction of anaesthesia is commonly achieved using intravenous anaesthetic agents such as propofol or thiopentone. The inclusion of opioids significantly reduces the dose of anaesthetic agent required to achieve loss of consciousness. In addition, opioids decrease somatic and autonomic responses to airway manipulations, improve haemodynamic stability, and provide immediate postoperative analgesia.

Inhalational anaesthetic agents can then be used to maintain loss of consciousness. Despite anaesthesia, skeletal muscle tone is relatively unaffected, which is a problem with intra-abdominal and intra-thoracic surgery. Neuromuscular blocking agents (muscle relaxants) prevent reflex muscle contraction, thereby allowing a much lower dose of anaesthetic agent to be used, sufficient to induce only the loss of consciousness. Additionally, regional and local anaesthetic techniques can also be used in combination with general anaesthesia. Such techniques may further reduce the need for opioids intraoperatively and can provide very effective analgesia postoperatively.

Phases of Anaesthesia

General anaesthesia may be divided into three phases: induction, maintenance, and emergence. In the UK, induction of anaesthesia is commonly performed in the anaesthetic room before transferring the anaesthetised patient into theatre. Emergence from general anaesthesia begins in theatres and patients are transferred to the post-anaesthetic care unit (PACU). In the PACU, the patient's airway is supported as necessary. Once consciousness has fully returned, further analgesia and antiemetics are given if necessary to ensure patient comfort, before being transferred back to the ward.

Induction

Induction of anaesthesia is the transition from an awake to an anaesthetised state. The endpoint is difficult to define; however, in 1937, Arthur Ernest Guedel proposed a widely cited system for describing the depth of anaesthesia, based on clinical signs [4].

Depth of Anaesthesia

The Guedel classification was described in the context of ether used as a sole agent in patients premedicated with morphine and atropine. This classification was divided into four

Table 11.1 Guedel classification of depth of anaesthesia

Stage	Description
1 Stage of analgesia or disorientation	Begins at the induction of anaesthesia until the point of loss of consciousness.
2 Stage of excitation/ delirium	From loss of consciousness to automatic breathing. Eyelash reflexes are lost but airway reflexes remain. Patient may struggle, vomit, or exhibit breath holding.
3 Stage of anaesthesia	From automatic breathing to respiratory paralysis. Laryngeal reflexes are lost. Intercostal muscle paralysis occurs in the early part, followed by diaphragmatic paralysis at the end of Stage 3. The desired depth of anaesthesia when muscle relaxants are not used is where regular diaphragmatic respiration still occurs with absent laryngeal and pupillary light reflexes.
4 Overdose	From respiratory paralysis to death. Death occurs due to medullary paralysis, resulting in respiratory arrest and cardiovascular collapse.

stages, based on respiratory pattern, ocular and pharyngeal reflexes, pupillary response, and muscle tone. The four stages are described in Table 11.1.

This classification is of limited application with modern drugs as intravenous anaesthetics have a very quick onset of action within one arm–brain circulation; this describes the time it takes for a drug to travel from the injection site to the brain. Patients traverse from a state of full consciousness to Stage 3 anaesthesia within seconds, bypassing stages 1 and 2 rapidly. They are then maintained at Stage 3 for the duration of the procedure.

Nonetheless, knowledge of Guedel classification is still essential when conducting gas induction and during emergence. Any airway intervention, such as the insertion of an airway adjunct or tracheal extubation should be avoided in Stage 2, when patients are at most risk of laryngospasm, breath holding, or vomiting.

Process of Induction

Anaesthesia can be induced using either an intravenous or inhalational agent. The choice is made by the anaesthetist depending on clinical circumstances. The anaesthetist is assisted by an anaesthetic assistant (usually an operating department practitioner or anaesthetic nurse). It is the responsibility of the anaesthetist and the anaesthetic assistant to ensure that all drugs and equipment are prepared and checked, and the anaesthetic plan discussed in advance.

Induction begins with the application of non-invasive monitoring. The Association of Anaesthetists has provided minimum monitoring standards for all patients undergoing general anaesthesia or sedation [5]. Minimum monitoring data (heart rate, blood pressure, pulse oximetry, end-tidal carbon dioxide, and anaesthetic gas concentration) must be recorded at least every 5 minutes, and more frequently if the patient is clinically unstable. The Association of Anaesthetists also recommend that patient temperature should be documented every 30 minutes.

Induction of anaesthesia using intravenous agents is generally quicker and smoother than an inhalational induction. An opioid may be used as a co-induction agent to reduce the dose of hypnotic required. A muscle relaxant may also be used if intubation is required. An alternative method of inducing anaesthesia is with a volatile agent. The anaesthetic gas is delivered via a face mask until the patient becomes unconscious. Inhalational induction is most frequently used when anaesthetising children because of the challenges of cooperation and gaining intravenous access. Nitrous oxide is commonly used as an adjunct to the volatile agent as it speeds up the induction process. Unlike an intravenous induction, patients who are subject to inhalational induction may enter the excitatory stage (Stage 2 of Guedel's planes), which, although the patient will not recall the experience, may be upsetting for parents or guardians who may be present during the induction process. Pre-warning chaperones in advance will help to alleviate any distress or alarm they may experience.

Rapid Sequence Induction

Rapid sequence induction (RSI) is a specifically adapted induction technique used when rapid intubation of the trachea with a cuffed tube is required to minimise risk of regurgitation and pulmonary aspiration of stomach contents. Aspiration remains the largest cause of anaesthesia-related death in the UK – the risk of aspiration is as high as 1 in 600–800 for emergency surgery [6, 7]. RSI is commonly used when there is a likelihood of a full stomach and other factors associated with a high risk of aspiration. These factors include but are not limited to unfasted patients, raised intra-abdominal pressure, intestinal obstruction, pregnancy, hiatus hernia, and gastro-oesophageal reflux disease. A 'classical' RSI involves delivering a pre-calculated dose of thiopentone and suxamethonium after adequate pre-oxygenation. Cricoid pressure is applied to the larynx as consciousness is lost to control passive regurgitation of gastric contents by occluding the upper end of the oesophagus, and this is maintained until the anaesthetist has verified a cuffed tracheal tube is *in situ*.

Cricoid pressure is achieved by compressing the cricoid cartilage against the bodies of the cervical vertebrae. Brian Sellick described the use of cricoid pressure in 1961 and this led to its widespread adoption and is why it is sometimes called 'Sellick's manoeuvre' [8]. The place of the classical RSI has become more contentious over the past few years due to the development of new drugs, especially propofol and rocuronium (with a large dose of sugammadex available to reverse rocuronium) in case of a failed intubation, as well as the lack of evidence over the efficacy of Sellick's manoeuvre [9]. There is significant variation in the application of RSI, and preferences on patient positioning, the use of a nasogastric tube (which if left in place must be suctioned), the choice of induction agent and neuromuscular blocking drug, and the application of cricoid pressure can differ widely [10, 11]. The use of RSI remains the standard practice to reduce the risk of aspiration but there is a paucity of good-quality evidence to support its use.

Airway Maintenance

Under general anaesthesia, the soft tissues of the airway relax, and airway patency may be lost. Protective airway reflexes are also suppressed. Manual manoeuvres and simple adjuncts such as a chin tilt, jaw thrust, and Guedel airway are used to achieve airway patency. Airway patency is then maintained for the duration of the procedure with supraglottic airway devices such as laryngeal mask airway (LMA) or an endotracheal tube. Endotracheal intubation is the most secure option where a cuffed endotracheal tube is passed through the vocal cords into the trachea and the cuff inflated within the trachea to ensure an airtight seal. This allows full ventilatory control and prevents any aspiration of gastric contents. An LMA is a supraglottic device, which sits above the vocal cords and keeps the airway open but offers no protection against aspiration. Both endotracheal tubes and LMAs come in a variety of shapes and sizes to suit individual patient needs.

Muscle Relaxation

Muscle relaxation (or muscle paralysis) may occasionally be required during anaesthesia particularly for intra-abdominal or intra-thoracic procedures. The earliest documented use of muscle-relaxant drugs was by indigenous tribes of the Amazon Basin in South America who used poison-tipped arrows that produced death by skeletal muscle paralysis in the sixteenth century. This plant-based poison, known today as curare, has tubocurarine as its active ingredient and competitively blocks acetylcholine (ACh) at the neuromuscular junction. Tubocurare-derived drugs were first used in clinical practice in 1942, transforming the delivery of anaesthesia.

This discovery led to the development of multiple agents that can be broadly divided into two groups: depolarising muscle relaxants and non-depolarising muscle relaxants. Normally, an action potential reaching the nerve terminal of the neuromuscular junction causes ACh to be released. Acetylcholine crosses the cleft and binds to post-synaptic nicotinic ACh receptors, causing opening of ion channels and depolarisation of the motor end plate, with subsequent muscle contraction.

A depolarising agent (e.g., suxamethonium) binds to the post-synaptic ACh receptors, resulting in transient receptor activation and widespread muscle contraction (fasciculation) followed by a refractory period of muscle relaxation. On the other hand, non-depolarising agents are competitive antagonists of ACh at the post-synaptic nicotinic receptor. Blocking the ion channels prevents end-plate depolarisation and muscle activation.

Neuromuscular junction function can be monitored using a peripheral nerve stimulator. Supramaximal stimulation stimulates all the nerve fibres to produce a consistent muscular response. The number and relative strength of the resultant muscle twitches provides information, to ensure good intraoperative muscle relaxation as well as confirming the restoration of neuromuscular function at the end of the procedure.

A 'reversal agent' may be used to reverse the effect of non-depolarising muscle relaxants at the end of an operation. The most widely used is neostigmine, which increases the concentration of acetylcholine at the neuromuscular junction, allowing normal function to return. A more recent addition is sugammadex, which can be used to quickly reverse neuromuscular blockade induced by rocuronium and vecuronium.

Maintenance of General Anaesthesia

Maintenance of general anaesthesia refers to keeping the patients anaesthetised for the duration of the procedure. This can be achieved using inhaled volatile agents or intravenous agents (either by continuous infusion or intermittent boluses).

Volatile agents remain the most commonly used method to maintain anaesthesia. They are delivered via vaporisers located on the back bar of the anaesthetic machine which feeds into the breathing system. The expired end-tidal concentration of volatile agent is measured and is assumed to approximate the alveolar concentration, which in turn approximates the concentration at the site of action in the central nervous system. This can then be used as a surrogate marker for the depth of anaesthesia.

The minimum alveolar concentration (MAC) is the alveolar concentration of a volatile agent which, when given alone, prevents movement in 50% of healthy volunteers to a standard surgical stimulus. It is therefore an indicator of the relative potency of the various volatile agents (a lower MAC indicating higher potency). MAC values can therefore be used to compare the potencies of different volatile agents. An agent with a high MAC value will require a greater concentration to achieve a given depth of anaesthesia than one with a low MAC value. The MAC values for the most used volatile agents are as follows:

- isoflurane 1.15%;
- sevoflurane 2.00%; and
- desflurane 6.35%.

Isoflurane is thus the most potent and desflurane the least. The MAC value for a given agent is affected by other pharmacological and physiological factors, such as age, temperature, presence of other drugs (e.g., opioids).

The maintenance of total intravenous anaesthesia can be achieved by infusion of propofol delivered via a syringe pump programmed with one or more pharmacokinetic models (termed a 'target-controlled infusion' pump). These models require basic patient demographics to calculate the clearance and volume of distribution. It will then deliver the drug as a bolus and infusion to achieve and maintain the target plasma or effector site concentration (hence, the term 'target-controlled' infusion). Further information on the various models, benefits, and limitations are explored in Chapter 15.

Depth of Anaesthesia Monitoring

The depth of anaesthesia monitoring is a potentially useful tool to prevent awareness during the maintenance of general anaesthesia. Anaesthetic awareness is a serious complication and can be classified into explicit awareness or implicit awareness. Explicit awareness is defined as the conscious recollection of events and experiences during the intraoperative period. It may occur with or without the sensation of pain. On the other hand, implicit awareness is the perception of 'something', without spontaneous recall of events. It is much harder to define but may have equally distressing psychological repercussions. In 2014, results of a national audit project showed that the incidence of accidental awareness under general anaesthesia is 1:19,000 but ranges from ~1:8,000 when neuromuscular blockers are used to 1:136,000 when they are not used [12]. Cardiac surgery (1:8,600) and Caesarean sections (1:670) are associated with a higher risk of accidental awareness.

There are multiple techniques to monitor the depth of anaesthesia. Subjectively, monitoring for clinical signs of tachycardia, hypertension, tachypnoea, sweating, and lacrimation may be used. However, these can be masked by some drugs (e.g., beta blockers). Objectively, the isolated forearm technique has previously been used to monitor the depth of anaesthesia. A tourniquet on the patient's upper arm is inflated above systolic blood pressure prior to giving muscle relaxant. This arm theoretically receives no muscle relaxant and can move if the patient is awake. The patient is then asked to move their arm during anaesthesia and if a positive response is detected, this will constitute awareness. However, this is often a late and unreliable sign of awareness.

Electroencephalogram (EEG) monitoring is another method that can be used to monitor the depth of anaesthesia. However, it is time consuming, impractical, and complex to interpret. The bispectral index (BIS) is a similar concept to EEG but using only frontal-temporal electrodes to obtain an EEG trace. The trace is transformed using a proprietary formula into a dimensionless number on a scale of 0–100; 100 represents normal brain activity, 0 represents complete absence of cerebral function. A BIS value of between 40 and 60 corresponds to a low risk of awareness. The evidence that BIS monitoring reduces the risk of intraoperative awareness remains unclear [13].

Perioperative Care

Anaesthetists are also responsible for ensuring that the body's homeostatic mechanisms are maintained during anaesthesia. Patients are susceptible to hypothermia under anaesthesia because of vasodilation causing redistribution of heat from core to periphery, via convection, radiation, conduction, and evaporation. Hypothermia may result in coagulopathy, arrhythmias, and increased risk of postoperative infections. It is of particular concern in neonatal and paediatric patients due to their high body surface area to weight ratio. Exposure should be minimised, and the temperature monitored throughout the perioperative period. Forced air warmers and warmed fluids can be used to offset heat loss and maintain an optimal body temperature.

Preoperative fasting may render a patient hypovolaemic before induction of anaesthesia. The effect of hypovolaemia is compounded by the vasodilatory effects of induction agents resulting in significant hypotension with haemodynamic compromise. The anaesthetist can manipulate the volume status of a patient using intravenous fluids and/or vasoconstrictors where appropriate. Multiple tools can be used to estimate cardiac output such as pulse contour analysis (e.g., a PiCCO (Pulse index Continuous Cardiac Output) device), Doppler flow (e.g., a CardioQ monitor), and thermodilution techniques (e.g., a Swann–Ganz catheter) may aid the assessment of fluid status. Each of these devices requires training to interpret results, respond appropriately, and to be aware of its limitations. Ultimately, the goal is to ensure good tissue perfusion and oxygen delivery.

Patients are vulnerable to nerve and pressure-point injury under anaesthesia and protection of these areas is the responsibility of the anaesthetist. Patients should ideally be in a neutral position with padding used to support at-risk areas. Eye protection is also crucial during anaesthesia (particularly important when the patient is in the prone position) as the protective blink reflex is lost during general anaesthesia, leading to a risk of accidental injury such as corneal abrasion or anterior ischaemic optic neuropathy.

Emergence and Recovery

During emergence, the patient regains consciousness in a controlled manner. This is achieved by lowering the concentration of anaesthetic agent and switching it off completely at the end of the procedure. Adequate analgesia and antiemesis should be ensured, and the return of neuromuscular function ensured if a muscle relaxant has been used.

Emergence can be a time of physiological disturbance. Patients waking from anaesthesia may be agitated or exhibit breath holding and/or laryngospasm, particularly if there is a noxious stimulus to the airway. It is therefore crucial to ensure that the airway is clear of secretions and debris, and to time tracheal extubation appropriately. Extubation can be performed either awake, when airway reflexes have returned and the patient is obeying commands, or while they are still deeply anaesthetised. Deep extubation may reduce the risk of coughing while airway reflexes are returning and may improve the stability of systemic blood and intracranial pressure but carries the risk of aspiration, airway obstruction, and hypoventilation.

The patient is then transferred to the post-anaesthetic care unit (PACU) or a critical care unit, depending on their clinical needs. The PACU is an intermediate place of safety between the operating theatre and the ward where early surgical or anaesthetic complications can be detected and managed. Vital signs, pain scores, and other potential problems such as postoperative nausea and vomiting are monitored closely and dealt with immediately. Patients are discharged to the ward when they are fully awake, normothermic, maintaining their own airway, obeying commands, have pain and nausea well controlled, and are haemodynamically and cardiovascularly stable.

References

1. R. P. Haridas. The etymology and use of the word 'anaesthesia': Oliver Wendell Holmes' letter to W. T. G. Morton. *Anaesthesia and Intensive Care* 2016; **44**: 38–44.

2. N. Franks and W. Lieb. Do general anaesthetics act by competitive binding to specific receptors? *Nature* 1984; **310**: 599–601.

3. J. S. Lundy. Balanced anesthesia. *Minnesota Medical Journal* 1926; **9**: 399–404.

4. A. E. Guedel. Stages of anesthesia and a re-classification of the signs of anesthesia. *Anesthesia and Analgesia* 1927; **6**: 157–162.

5. A. A. Klein, T. Meek, E. Allcock, et al. Recommendations for standards of monitoring during anaesthesia and recovery 2021. *Anaesthesia* 2021; DOI https://doi .org/10.1111/anae.15501.

6. C. Wallace and B. McGuire. Rapid sequence induction: its place in modern anaesthesia. *Continuing Education in Anaesthesia Critical Care and Pain* 2014; **14**: 130–135.

7. C. P. H. Kalinowski and J. R. Kirsch. Strategies for prophylaxis and treatment for aspiration. *Best Practice and Research: Clinical Anaesthesiology* 2004; **18**: 719–737.

8. A. S. Moied and J. Pal. Cricoid pressure: a misnomer in pediatric anaesthesia. *Journal of Emergencies, Trauma and Shock* 2010; **3**: 96–97.

9. C. M. Algie, R. K. Mahar, H. B. Tan, et al. Effectiveness and risks of cricoid pressure during rapid sequence induction for endotracheal intubation. *Cochrane Database of Systematic Reviews* 2015; **11**: CD011656.

10. M. Zdravkovic, J. Berger-Estilita, M. Sorbello, et al. An international survey about rapid sequence intubation of 10,003 anaesthetists and 16 airway experts. *Anaesthesia* 2020; **75**: 313–322.

11. J. Klucka, M. Kosinova, K. Zacharowski, et al. Rapid sequence induction. *European Journal of Anaesthesiology* 2020; **37**: 435–442.

12. J. J. Pandit, J. Andrade, D. G. Bogod, et al. On behalf of the Royal College of Anaesthetists and the Association of Anaesthetists of Great Britain and Ireland, 5th National Audit Project (NAP5) on accidental awareness during general anaesthesia: summary of main findings and risk factors. *British Journal of Anaesthesia* 2014; **113**: 549–559.

13. S. R Lewis, M. W. Pritchard, L. J. Fawcett, and Y. Punjasawadwong. Bispectral index for improving intraoperative awareness and early postoperative recovery in adults. *Cochrane Database of Systematic Reviews* 2019; **9**: CD003843.

Fundamentals of Airway Management

Rebecca Sherwood

Introduction

Perioperative practitioners should be able to recognise the need for and be able to perform potentially life-saving airway management. This is necessary because of the increased risk of airway compromise in those undergoing anaesthesia or surgery. Practitioners should be familiar with the techniques and equipment used within the clinical area and undertake regular training to maintain the currency of their clinical skills.

Airway Anatomy

The airway can be divided into what is termed the upper airway and lower airway. The upper airway consists of the airway passages that lie above the level of the vocal cords, and the lower airway consists of the airway passages that lie below the vocal cords. The upper airway is described as consisting of the nasal cavity and pharynx (see Figure 12.1).

The nasal cavity is separated into right and left portions by a midline nasal septum and is supported by bone and cartilage. It is lined by the highly vascular nasal mucosa, which warms and humidifies air as it passes through. The pharynx is divided into the nasopharynx, oropharynx, and laryngopharynx, which lie posterior to the nasal cavity, oral cavity, and larynx, respectively.

The larynx enables phonation due to the presence of the vocal cords and consists of nine cartilages. The most significant structures in terms of airway management are the epiglottis, composed of elastic cartilage; and the thyroid, cricoid, and arytenoid cartilages, composed of hyaline cartilage. The epiglottis protects the airway from the accidental inhalation of food and fluids by closing over the laryngeal inlet during swallowing. The thyroid cartilage can be manipulated by the anaesthetist or anaesthetic assistant to obtain a more favourable view of the vocal cords. This manoeuvre is referred to as backwards upwards retrograde pressure (BURP) and can help visualise the vocal cords during laryngoscopy. The cricoid cartilage – being the only complete ring of cartilage in the trachea – can be manipulated to occlude the oesophagus to prevent passive regurgitation of gastric contents entering the pharynx and subsequently into the lungs, during a rapid sequence induction. The cricoid and thyroid cartilages are connected by a cricothyroid membrane, which can be cannulated for front-of-neck access in an emergency.

The trachea is a cartilaginous tube supported by C-shaped rings that are continuous with the larynx (at the level of C6). The trachea eventually bifurcates at the carina (level of T4), which branches into the right and left main stem bronchi. The primary bronchi continue to divide into secondary bronchi, tertiary bronchi, and then bronchioles of continually decreasing diameter. These eventually lead to the alveoli ducts and alveoli, where gas exchange takes place.

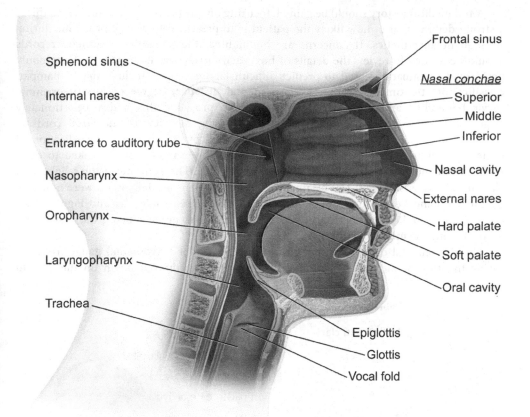

The Upper Respiratory System

Figure 12.1 Upper respiratory system (Blausen.com staff (2014). Medical gallery of Blausen Medical 2014. *WikiJournal of Medicine* 1 (2). DOI 10.15347/wjm/2014.010. ISSN 2002-4436)

The passageways of the respiratory tree serve to supply the three lobes of the right lung and two lobes of the left lung with air. As these passageways become smaller, they consist of less cartilage, which becomes replaced with smooth muscle tissue until the terminal respiratory bronchioles are reached, when the walls are entirely composed of epithelial tissue. Unintentional intubation of the right main bronchus is not uncommon due to the main bronchi having a slightly wider diameter, more vertical in orientation, and shorter in length [1].

Preoperative Airway Assessment

When a patient is administered a sedative or anaesthetic drug, their level of consciousness, muscle tone, and respirations will gradually reduce as the dose of drug administered increases. When a patient experiences a reduced level of consciousness (from any cause), the airway is at risk until it has been secured with a suitable airway device. The time between anaesthetic induction and the establishment of a definitive airway should be as short as possible to minimise this risk.

A full medical history should be gained, focusing on any previous anaesthetics, as this is a strong determinant of how likely the patient is to present with airway problems during subsequent anaesthetics. If concerns are highlighted, the patient's anaesthetic records should be located to review the details of how their airway was managed [2]. Commonly performed examinations used to predict difficult laryngoscopies include the Mallampati classification, thyromental distance, sternomental distance, degree of mouth opening, cervical mobility, and jaw protrusion. Mallampati proposed that a disproportionately large tongue base could be responsible for obscuring the view of the vocal cords at laryngoscopy, and this poor view could be predicted by the degree of visualisation of structures within the oral cavity. The patient faces the examiner and is asked to open their mouth and protrude their tongue as far as possible. The examiner using a light then classifies the view obtained. The original three classifications of Mallampati were modified by Samsoon and Young to give four Mallampati classes (see Table 12.1 and Figure 12.2), corresponding indirectly to the four grades of intubation, grade 1 being the easiest and grade 4 being the most difficult [3, 4].

The thyromental distance is measured using a ruler or thyromental gauge from the inside mentum of the lower mandible, to the top of the thyroid notch on the thyroid

Table 12.1 Mallampati classification

Mallampati class	Structures visualised
1	Soft palate, fauces, uvula, pillars
2	Soft palate, fauces, uvula
3	Soft palate, base of uvula
4	Soft palate not visible

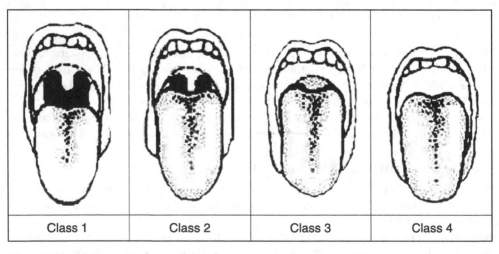

| Class 1 | Class 2 | Class 3 | Class 4 |

Figure 12.2 Mallampati classification (taken from M. A. Sewell, Managing difficult intubations. In B. Smith, P. Rawling, P. Wicker, and C. Jones. *Core Topics in Operating Department Practice: Anaesthesia and Critical Care* (2007). Cambridge: Cambridge University Press, p. 112)

Table 12.2 Factors associated with difficult intubation and ventilation

Co-morbidities/conditions increasing the risk of difficult intubation	Characteristics associated with difficult mask ventilation
High BMI	High BMI
Rheumatoid arthritis	Presence of a beard
Ankylosing spondylitis	Facial deformities
Obstructive sleep apnoea	Obstructive sleep apnoea
Pregnancy	Mallampati classes 3 or 4
Tumors/trauma affecting the airway or cervical spine	Edentulous (lack of teeth)
Temporomandibular joint disorders	Male sex
Diabetes (stiff joint syndrome)	Age > 55 years
Congenital syndromes, e.g., Down's syndrome, Pierre-Robin syndrome, Treacher-Collins syndrome Micrognathia	

Adapted from [8] and [9].

cartilage when the neck is fully extended. In an adult, this distance is normally ~7 cm. A distance less than 6.5 cm is sometimes used as a predictor for difficult intubation, although less than 6 cm is more strongly associated with difficult intubation, especially when combined with other risk indicators. Accurate measurement is important, therefore the seemingly convenient rough estimate of using three finger breadths as a minimum acceptable indicator is not recommended due to the variability in finger size of anaesthetists [5]. The sternomental distance is measured from the mentum to the top of the manubrium with the neck extended. Lower than predicted values (less than ~12.5 cm) may predict a difficult laryngoscopy [6]. Other reassuring signs include a good degree of mouth opening (or inter-incisor gap), which should be at least 4 cm, and adequate jaw protrusion assessed by ensuring the patient can easily bite their top lip; whereas the presence of protruding or 'buck teeth', a body mass index (BMI) of 25 or above, and limited neck mobility suggests that the patient will be more difficult to intubate [7]. In addition, the anaesthetic team should be aware of a range of other patient conditions and characteristics associated with difficult airway management (see Table 12.2).

Basic Airway Management

In the unconscious supine patient, the primary cause of airway obstruction is the tongue falling backwards onto the posterior pharyngeal wall. This obstruction can be relieved by optimal patient positioning. The patient is placed in what is termed the 'sniffing the morning air' position. A small pillow is placed under the patient's head to slightly flex the neck. The head is then extended backwards with one hand and the chin lifted with the other. This manoeuvre, also called 'head tilt and chin lift', may be enough to pull the tongue of the posterior pharyngeal wall and relieve the obstruction. The anaesthetist can then place a suitably sized anaesthetic face mask (sizes 3–5 will fit most adult patients) over the face, ensuring a good fit before assessing airway patency. The practitioner should observe bilateral chest rise and fall, misting of the mask, and adequate movement of the reservoir bag on the anaesthetic circuit during spontaneous ventilation. The 'sniffing the morning air' position brings the oral, pharyngeal, and laryngeal axis into alignment and is therefore used as the standard position for direct laryngoscopy. If head tilt and chin lift does not result in a patent airway, additional 'jaw thrust' can be applied. Jaw thrust is achieved by placing the index fingers behind the angle of the mandible and displacing it forwards to move the base of the tongue anteriorly.

Oropharyngeal Airway

Airway obstruction caused by the tongue can also be relieved by using an oropharyngeal airway and avoids the need for prolonged jaw thrust. The most used version in clinical practice is the disposable plastic Guedel airway. A correctly sized Guedel airway should reach from the maxillary incisors to the angle of the mandible [10]. In adults, the Guedel airway is inserted into the mouth in an inverted position, until the soft palate is reached, at which point it is rotated 180° before completing insertion. The airway should only be inserted in patients with sufficient depth of anaesthesia/reduced consciousness, otherwise there is a risk of stimulating airway reflexes, causing laryngospasm, vomiting, and raised intracranial pressure [11].

Nasopharyngeal Airway

The nasopharyngeal airway is better tolerated than the oropharyngeal airway in conscious and semi-conscious patients with an intact gag reflex. This airway may also be indicated in patients with clenched jaws, wiring of the jaw, or oral trauma. Nasopharyngeal airways are made of soft plastic and usually have a large flange or are supplied with a safety pin to prevent the real risk of migration of the device into the patient's airway [12]. Although an estimate of the size to be used can be taken from measuring the airway from the nares to the tip of the tragus, it has been shown that there is a good correlation between patient height and the size of nasopharyngeal airway required, with average-height females requiring a size 6 and average-height males requiring a size 7 [13]. As the nasal mucosa is highly vascular, the nose can be prepared with a vasoconstrictor. Then, the well-lubricated airway is passed (usually into the right nostril) along the floor of the nasal cavity until the flange reaches the nostril. If obstruction is felt, the practitioner can use gentle rotation or try the left nostril, but the airway should never be forced. Nasopharyngeal airways are contraindicated in patients taking anticoagulants, who have known coagulopathies (e.g., haemophilia), or have sustained head trauma, facial fractures, or suspected basal skull fractures [14, 15].

Laryngeal Mask Airway

In 1981, the anaesthetist Dr Archibald Brain, while working at the Royal London Hospital, invented a new airway device called the laryngeal mask airway (LMA), and a prototype was first used in 1981 at the William Harvey Hospital. The LMA (Figure 12.3) allowed easier control of a patient's airway than bag–mask ventilation but was not as invasive as endotracheal intubation [16]. Since its invention, a plethora of supraglottic airway designs have entered the market, with various advantages and disadvantages. The LMA is a wide-bore

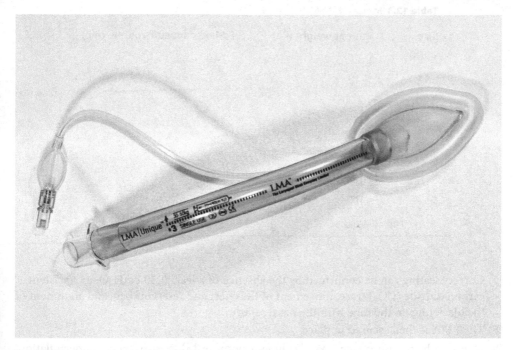

Figure 12.3 Laryngeal mask airway (author's photograph)

tube with a 15-mm connector allowing it to be connected to standard anaesthetic circuits. The tube ends in an elliptical cuff (inflated via a pilot balloon and line) that sits over the entrance to the larynx. The distal aperture contains bars to prevent the epiglottis entering the tube. Originally created as an autoclavable reusable device, disposable versions are now popular (see Table 12.3 for sizing [17]).

Use of the LMA is less fatiguing for the user than face-mask ventilation and it can be used to establish an airway quickly, without the skill required for intubation. The minimal resistance to airflow makes it suitable for patients breathing spontaneously. However, although the LMA will provide some isolation of the respiratory and alimentary tracts, it does not provide the reliable seal achieved with an endotracheal tube. This is because there is likely to be an air leak at pressures > 20 cm H_2O, and so should be avoided in patients at risk of aspiration [18]. The following describes a 'classic insertion technique' [19]:

(1) Lubricate the posterior surface of a completely deflated cuff.

(2) Position the patient in the 'sniffing the morning air position'.

(3) Hold the LMA like a pen close to the junction of the cuff and tube, introduce the LMA into the mouth with the aperture facing forward.

(4) Advance the LMA by pressing it to the surface of the hard palate until it reaches the posterior pharyngeal wall.

(5) Push the proximal end of the LMA until resistance is felt as it reaches the base of the hypopharynx.

(6) The cuff is then inflated; the tube can be seen to rise, and the larynx is pushed forward.

Table 12.3 Standard LMA Classic™ sizes

Size	Patient weight (kg)	Maximum cuff volume (mL)
1	Up to 5	4
1.5	5–10	7
2	10–20	10
2.5	20–30	14
3	30–50	20
4	50–70	30
5	70–100	40
6	>100	50

Adapted from Teleflex Inc. [17].

(7) Correct seating can be confirmed by the absence of a leak at 20 cmH$_2$O, a consistent carbon dioxide (CO_2) trace, movement of the chest and reservoir bag, and alignment of the black line on the tube with the nasal septum.

(8) The LMA is then secured in place.

Problems with the use of the LMA include a poor seal due to over- or underinflation, obstruction due to rotation of the LMA or downfolding of the tip of the LMA or epiglottis, and trauma to laryngeal and pharyngeal structures [20]. It is important to promptly identify inadequate placement, remove the device and reposition, use an alternative size, or use an alternative method.

Second-Generation Supraglottic Airway Devices

The LMA is now considered a first-generation supraglottic airway device (SAD). Newer designs incorporating enhanced safety features and functions are termed second-generation SADs. Features typical of second-generation devices include the presence of gastric channels to facilitate clearance of gastric secretions and decompress the stomach, preformed shapes, and more rigid designs to prevent rotation and allow easier insertion, integrated bite blocks, improved pharyngeal seal, and, in some cases, the ability to act as a conduit for endotracheal intubation [21].

The i-gel® supraglottic airway is made from an almost transparent thermoplastic elastomer. It has been modelled to align closely with laryngeal and perilaryngeal structures to provide an accurate anatomical fit. A gastric channel allows the detection of possible regurgitation and can be used to drain and suction gastric contents. An artificial epiglottic ridge prevents obstruction of the aperture by the epiglottis and the proximal end houses an integral bite block (a horizontal marker indicates the optimal position of the incisors once the device has been inserted). The i-gel® can be used as an emergency airway rescue device, and an endotracheal tube can be passed through its lumen to intubate the trachea [22]. The recommended adult sizes based on weight are size 3 (30–60 kg), size 4 (50–90 kg), and size 5 (>90 kg) [23].

The LMA ProSeal™ is based on the standard LMA but incorporates a second tube lateral to the main airway tube called the drain tube. The drain tube passes along the floor of the mask to open at the tip of the LMA, which (when *in situ*) will lie over the upper oesophageal sphincter. This creates a pathway for regurgitated stomach contents and gastric suctioning, an improved seal pressure (assisted by the presence of a dorsal extension of the cuff), all of which theoretically reduces the risk of gastric inflation [24]. The LMA Supreme™ is the disposable version of the LMA ProSeal™ and is made from polyvinyl chloride (PVC). Additionally, the shaft of the tube is elliptical in shape which facilitates insertion [25].

The intubating LMA Fastrach™, unlike the classic LMA®, has been designed to allow blind tracheal intubation. It is available either as a single-use device or reusable version (autoclavable up to 40 times, which must be accurately recorded). The airway tube is rigid, and a curved handle allows insertion without needing to move the head and neck. The distal aperture has an elevating bar that replaces the two bars in the standard version; this bar (not being fixed at one end) means an endotracheal tube will pass through. The LMA Fastrach™ is available in three sizes (3, 4, and 5) which correspond to the equivalent classic LMA®. All sizes comfortably allow the passage of a lubricated endotracheal tube up to 8.0 mm in diameter. The handle can be used to adjust the position of the LMA to achieve optimal ventilation before inserting a specially designed reinforced tube into the trachea. If desired, the 15-mm proximal connector can then be removed and a stabilising rod inserted into the top of the endotracheal tube to remove the LMA, while leaving the endotracheal tube in situ [26]. The device is used in cases of anticipated or unanticipated difficult intubation or in situations where head and neck movement is not desirable (e.g., a patient with a suspected or confirmed cervical spinal injury) [27]. There is also the LMA CTrach™ which is modelled on the LMA Fastrach™ but with built-in fibre optics and a detachable video screen [28].

Advanced Airway Management

Endotracheal Intubation

Endotracheal intubation involves the introduction of an endotracheal tube via the oral or nasal cavity, through the vocal cords, and into the trachea. It remains the most practiced advanced airway skill to ensure a safe and secure airway. In most cases, the inflation of a cuff within the trachea is considered the 'gold standard' approach to preventing aspiration of gastric contents and is the preferred airway management technique when positive-pressure ventilation is applied.

Endotracheal Tubes

Tracheal tubes were originally manufactured from red rubber but have subsequently been replaced in clinical practice with plastic tubes made from PVC. Some PVC tubes are siliconised, which aids the passage of suction catheters. The tubes can be seen on a chest X-ray due to the presence of a radio-opaque line running along their length. At the proximal end, the tube houses a 15-mm connector for attachment to the anaesthetic circuit or ventilating device. The body of the tube is marked at 1-cm intervals, and the internal diameter (ID) of the tube is indicated in millimetres. The distal end of the tube has a left-angled bevel that enables easier visualisation of the vocal cords during intubation, and some designs have a 'Murphy eye' (a hole cut out of the tube on the opposite side of the bevel) to allow ventilation if the distal tip becomes obstructed.

When selecting the size of endotracheal tube, several factors need to be taken into consideration; while smaller tubes are easier to insert, cause less laryngeal trauma, and reduce the occurrence of postoperative sore throats, they also increase airway resistance and make suctioning more difficult [29]. Therefore, if the patient is undergoing intermittent positive-pressure ventilation, a 6.0–6.5-mm ID for women, or a 6.5–7.0-mm ID for men, should be sufficient. However, for spontaneously breathing patients, larger diameters (7.0–7.5-mm ID for women and 8.0–8.5-mm ID for men) are recommended [30]. In all cases, a range of tube sizes should be available. The tip of the endotracheal tube should ideally be located 4–5 cm above the carina. To achieve this, in most adults the tube will be secured between 21 cm and 23 cm at the lips.

Tracheal tubes can be either cuffed or uncuffed. Cuffed tubes are more commonly used in adults than in children (especially infants and young children) due to differences in the shape of the airway. Broadly speaking, cuffs are said to be either high pressure/low volume, which are good at preventing aspiration but risk causing tracheal mucosal necrosis because of the high pressure against the mucosal wall; or low pressure/high volume, which means they can be safely inflated for longer periods of time, but wrinkles may form in the cuff so they are potentially less suited to preventing aspiration. Gel lubrication on the cuff may reduce this leakage [31]. The recommended cuff pressure lies between 20 cmH$_2$O and 30 cmH$_2$O [32]. During anaesthesia, cuff pressure can increase as nitrous oxide diffuses into the cuff and such pressure changes could cause postoperative complications. Aneroid pressure gauges are recommended to monitor the cuff pressure and keep it within safe limits [33].

Laryngoscopes for Direct Laryngoscopy

Standard rigid laryngoscopes (Figure 12.4) provide a direct line of sight for the operator in order to intubate the trachea. They consist of a handle, which houses the batteries for a light source (which in most designs is transmitted to the blade via fibre optics), and a blade, which elevates the lower jaw and tongue to enable a clear view of the laryngeal inlet. The light source switches on when the laryngoscope is 'opened'. It is important that the practitioner checks that this light is of sufficient strength prior to any intubation attempt and that a backup is available in case of failure.

The most-used laryngoscope blade in adults is the curved Macintosh blade (sizes 3 and 4). The tip of this blade is inserted into the vallecula. When the laryngoscope is lifted upwards and forwards it elevates the epiglottis, allowing the vocal cords to be seen. Alternatively, a straight blade can be used, where the blade is inserted posterior to the epiglottis for it to 'flatten' the epiglottis to view the larynx. This technique is more frequently used in small children where the epiglottis is 'floppy' [34]. Examples of straight blades include the Miller, Magill, Soper, and Wisconsin blades. A modification of the Macintosh blade is the McCoy blade, which has a hinged tip that is operated via a lever on the handle. This provides extra elevation of the epiglottis and is a useful blade for difficult intubations. Where patients have prominent chests (e.g., obesity or pregnancy) a Polio blade can be used; this sits at ~120° to the handle (as opposed to the 90° of a Macintosh blade). In these situations, a short 'stubby' handle can also allow unimpeded intubation [35].

Intubation Aids

Magill forceps (Figure 12.5) are angled for use within the oral and pharyngeal cavity and can be used to help direct tubes (particularly nasal) through the vocal cords, retrieve foreign

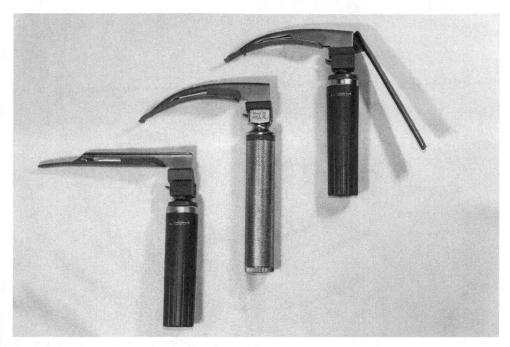

Figure 12.4 Direct laryngoscopes (from left to right with Miller blade, Macintosh blade, McCoy blade (author's photograph))

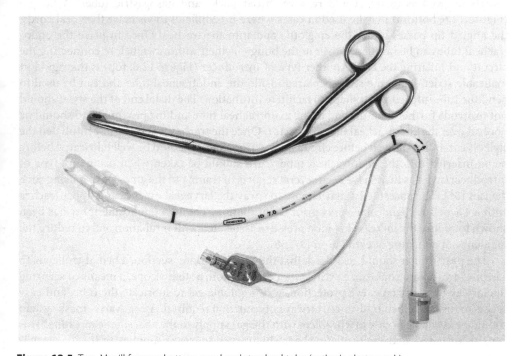

Figure 12.5 Top, Magill forceps; bottom, nasal endotracheal tube (author's photograph)

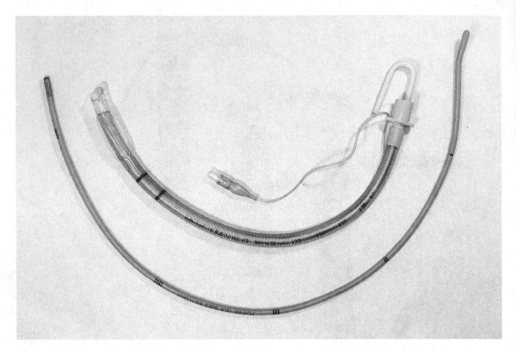

Figure 12.6 Top, reinforced tube with stylet inserted; bottom, bougie (author's photograph)

objects, as well as to insert and remove throat packs and nasogastric tubes. A bougie (Figure 12.6, bottom) may be used in cases where it is difficult to visualise the vocal cords; the angled tip passes under the epiglottis and into the trachea. Once in place the endotracheal tube can be railroaded over it; the bougie is then withdrawn before connecting the circuit and inflating the cuff. Another type of introducer (Figure 12.6, top) is the rigid but malleable stylet. Here, the stylet is placed inside the endotracheal tube and can be used to bend the tube into a desired shape to facilitate intubation. The distal end of the stylet should not protrude further than the end of the endotracheal tube and the proximal end should be hooked over the endotracheal tube connector. Once the trachea is successfully intubated the stylet is carefully removed before circuit connection. Stylets should be well lubricated before being inserted into the endotracheal tube. Care should be taken when using any type of introducer/stylet as there have been several reports of trauma to the airway when using such devices [36]. The anaesthetist may choose to spray the laryngeal mucosa and upper trachea with a 4% or 10% lignocaine spray prior to intubation. The 10% lignocaine spray has been shown to reduce the increase in blood pressure associated with intubation and to reduce the incidence of coughing at extubation [37, 38].

The practitioner should also check that they have working suction, a bed or trolley with a head-down tilt mechanism, a syringe for cuff inflation, a stethoscope, a means of securing the airway by tie or tape, eye protection, water-soluble gel to lubricate the tube, and easy access to further difficult/advanced airway equipment if required. A bag–valve–mask system should be available in case of a problem with the gas supply to the anaesthetic machine. This consists of a mask and a self-inflating bag, which when squeezed supplies air (or if oxygen is attached an air/oxygen mixture) to the patient's lungs through a one-way valve.

A typical intubation sequence is as follows [39]:

(1) The patient is pre-oxygenated and placed supine in the 'sniffing the morning air position'. A suitably sized endotracheal tube is prepared and lubricated with water-soluble gel.

(2) Holding the laryngoscope with the left hand, the blade is inserted into the right side of the mouth, ensuring that the lip does not become caught between the blade and the lower teeth.

(3) The blade is gradually brought into the midline as it is advanced, displacing the tongue to the left.

(4) The tip of the blade is placed into the vallecula, and the laryngoscope is lifted forwards and upwards until an optimal view of the laryngeal inlet is obtained.

(5) An assistant may enhance the view by gently retracting the angle of the mouth laterally.

(6) The tube is inserted into the right side of the mouth and through the vocal cords, ensuring that the cuff comes to lie 2–3 cm beyond the cords.

(7) The laryngoscope is removed and the circuit is attached to the tube. The cuff is inflated until the sealing pressure is reached (i.e., until the audible leak on ventilation ceases).

(8) Confirmation of correct tube placement is made, and the tube is secured in place.

Correct endotracheal tube placement must be confirmed to prevent potentially life-threatening complications such as oesophageal intubation, or hypoxaemia from shunting of blood, lung collapse, and barotrauma caused by bronchial intubation. The following methods are used to confirm correct tube position: directly observing that the tube passes through the vocal cords during intubation; observing bilateral chest movement and auscultating breath sounds in both axillae; checking that there are no sounds of air entry in the epigastric area; and ensuring that there is a good consistent capnography trace for at least six breaths [40]. Apart from incorrect tube placement, further complications can result from intubation attempts including laryngospasm; bronchospasm; aspiration; trauma to the lips, teeth, and tongue; jaw and arytenoid dislocation; trauma to the larynx and trachea, causing swelling and necrosis; obstruction of the tube; hypertension pressure; and arrhythmias [41].

Specialist Tubes and Techniques

Preformed tubes such as RAE (Ring, Adair, and Elwyn) and polar tubes are designed to allow greater access to the surgical field in maxillofacial and ear, nose, and throat procedures. Preformed tubes may be either north facing or south facing, cuffed or uncuffed. South-facing RAE tubes move the circuit connections to below the chin and therefore allow upper facial surgeries including nasal surgery and some oral surgery (e.g., tonsillectomy), although north-facing nasal tubes (Figure 12.5), where the tube passes over the forehead, provide far better access for oral surgeries. Disadvantages of preformed tubes are that as the bend in the tube is fixed, it does not allow for anatomical variations, increasing the risk of endobronchial intubation, and suctioning via catheters is made more difficult [42, 43]. Nasal intubations can be performed using a 'blind technique' where the nasal tube is skillfully manipulated into the trachea without the use of laryngoscopy or is performed under direct vision, similar to oral intubation. For the latter procedure, a well lubricated nasal tube of slightly smaller diameter than the oral equivalent (~1 mm) is inserted preferentially into the right nostril [44]. The tube is passed without the use of excessive force along the floor of the nose. When the tube reaches the pharynx, laryngoscopy is performed, and the tube is inserted (often with the help of Magill forceps) through the vocal cords.

In procedures where it is anticipated that blood will collect in the oral cavity, a throat pack is inserted around the tube to help prevent soiling of the trachea and lungs with blood. However, incidences have occurred where throat packs have been accidently retained post extubation, leading to airway obstruction. Therefore, practitioners should use at least one visual reminder that a throat pack is *in situ*, for example, a throat-pack sticker on the patient's forehead or airway, and one documentary check that the throat pack has been removed and included as part of the swab count record [45, 46]. All throat packs should contain a radio-opaque strip. Nasal intubation is contraindicated in certain patients, such as those with suspected base of skull fractures and coagulopathy [47].

Microlaryngeal tubes are of narrow diameter with a long length and adult-sized cuffs. They improve surgical access when operating on the larynx. Microlaryngeal tubes are made of soft plastic and are available in sizes 4.0, 5.0, and 6.0 ID [48]. Reinforced endotracheal tubes (Figure 12.6) are also used in head and neck surgery, where their increased flexibility with ability to resist kinking is seen as an advantage. Reinforced tubes incorporate a wire spiral within their walls. Due to their flexibility, an introducer may be required for insertion, and (as the tube cannot be cut) there is an increased risk of endobronchial intubation [49].

When laser surgery is performed on the airway, PVC endotracheal tubes should not be used as they ignite very easily when struck by a laser beam. Instead, laser tubes (Figure 12.7) capable of resisting the effects of CO_2 and KTP (potassium titanyl phosphate) lasers should be employed. Laser tubes greatly reduce but do not completely prevent airway fires; they come in two main designs: those that are wrapped in a metallic foil such as aluminium or

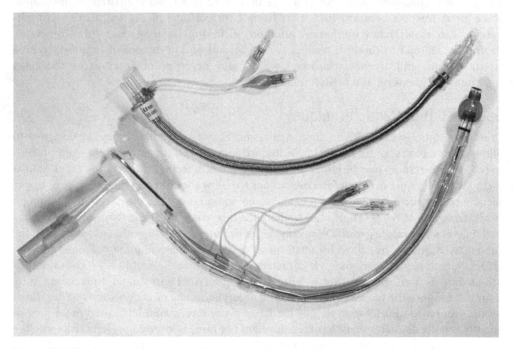

Figure 12.7 Top, laser tube; bottom, double-lumen endobronchial tube (author's photograph)

copper, or those that have a flexible stainless-steel body such as the Laser-Flex® endotracheal tube. Laser beams are deflected from the metal and defocused. The cuffed version of the Laser-Flex® tube has two cuffs which should be filled with saline rather than air, to help prevent ignition. The double-cuff system means that if one cuff bursts the patient can still be ventilated. Additionally, if methylene blue is added to the cuff, the rupture can be quickly detected [50, 51]. A disadvantage of metal tubes is that they have a smaller internal circumference for a given external diameter and may be more traumatic [52].

Double-lumen endobronchial tubes (DLTs) allow one-lung ventilation and are indicated for a range of thoracic procedures, including operations on a lung, or the deflation of a lung in order to allow visualisation and access to other intra-thoracic structures (e.g., thoracic spinal surgery, vascular surgery, or oesophageal surgery). DLTs (Figure 12.7) can be thought of as two tubes bonded together with one shorter tube ending in the trachea and the other longer tube ending in either the left or right main bronchi. Both tubes have their own cuffs and pilot balloons allowing selective ventilation of one lung with simultaneous deflation of the other. The original Robertshaw tubes were made of red rubber; now, disposable PVC tubes are preferred. The tubes are specifically designed as being left or right sided. This is necessary as the left main-stem bronchus is longer, whereas the right upper-lobe bronchus comes off the right main-stem bronchus very proximally. Placement of a left-sided tube is easier and is therefore preferred where feasible. DLTs are available in the following French gauge sizes 26, 28, 32, 35, 37, 39, and 41 [53]. DLTs can be inserted with or without the aid of a fibre-optic laryngoscope, but confirmation of correct portioning should always be made with a fibrescope, and again upon any significant change in position (such as transfer into the lateral position) [54]. DLTs are bulky and correct positioning can be difficult. This increases the risk of complications such as laryngeal trauma, cuff herniation, displacement, and bronchial rupture [55]. An alternative to the use of a DLT for one-lung anaesthesia is the endobronchial blocker. This consists of a narrow tube with a cuff, passed through or beside an endotracheal tube using fibre-optic guidance into the bronchus of the lung to be deflated [56].

Fibre-Optic Bronchoscopy

Intubation using an endotracheal tube loaded onto a flexible bronchoscope can be performed by either the oral or nasal route. Indications include anticipated or unanticipated difficult airway management, cervical spine instability, awake techniques in those with a high risk of aspiration, for confirming the positions of endotracheal, tracheostomy, and double-lumen tubes. Fibre-optic intubation can be carried out using a wide variety of techniques in both the awake patient, as well as anaesthetised patients who are either spontaneously breathing or paralysed [57]. A standard adult intubating bronchoscope consists of a body, an insertion cord, and a light cord. The body has a control lever which moves the tip of the bronchoscope. There is an eyepiece, a working channel port with a suction connector, and a valve covered by a cap. The port can be used for suction, instilling drugs or oxygen, or inserting guidewires. The insertion cord is flexible and can be loaded with an endotracheal tube to allow intubation. The insertion cord contains the light transmission bundle with ~10,000 glass fibres, the working channel, angulation wires, and distal bending section. The light cord transmits light from an external light source to the light transmission bundle in the insertion cord [58]. A camera can be attached to the bronchoscope, and the image

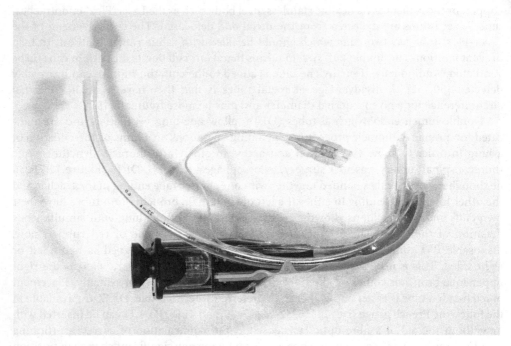

Figure 12.8 Airtraq® Avant, mounted with an endotracheal tube (author's photograph)

viewed through a monitor. Alternatively, in systems such as the single-use Ambu® aScope™, a small video camera is sited at the distal end of a flexible and steerable cord and the image is passed electronically to a video screen, avoiding the necessity for the fragile and expensive fibre optics.

Videolaryngoscopes

As in the technology used in flexible fibre-optic bronchoscopy, another form of indirect laryngoscopy in which the clinician does not directly view the larynx can be achieved using rigid videolaryngoscopes. Images obtained from video laryngoscopy can be magnified and displayed on a monitor. Videolaryngoscopes can be classified into three main categories [59]:

- those based on the Macintosh-style blade (e.g., the C-MAC® and McGRATH™);
- those with hyper-angulated blades (e.g., the GlideScope® and C-MAC® D BLADE); and
- channelled devices (e.g., the Pentax AWS® and Airtraq®); the Airtraq® Avant, which uses reusable optics and disposable blades, can be seen in Figure 12.8.

References

1. E. N. Marieb and K. Hoehn. *Human Anatomy and Physiology*, 11th ed. Harlow: Pearson, 2017.

2. C. Zhou, F. Chung, and D. T. Wong. Clinical assessment for the identification of the potentially difficult airway. *Perioperative Care and Operating Room Management* 2017; **9**: 16–19.

3. S. R. Mallampati, S. P. Gatt, L. D. Gugino, et al. A clinical sign to predict difficult tracheal intubation: a prospective study. *Canadian*

Anaesthetists' Society Journal 1985; **32**: 429–434.

4. G. L. T Samsoon and J. R. B. Young. Difficult tracheal intubation: a retrospective study. *Anaesthesia* 1987; **42**: 487–490.

5. P. A. Baker, A. Depuydt, and J. M. P. Thompson. Thyromental distance measurement: fingers don't rule. *Anaesthesia* 2009; **64**: 878–882.

6. B. Patel, R. Khandekar, R. Diwan, and A. Shah. Validation of modified Mallampati test with addition of thyromental distance and sternomental distance to predict difficult endotracheal intubation in adults. *Indian Journal of Anaesthesia* 2014; **58**: 171–175.

7. S-H. Seo, J-G. Lee, S-B. Yu, et al. Predictors of difficult intubation defined by the intubation difficulty scale (IDS): predictive value of 7 airway assessment factors. *Korean Journal of Anesthesiology* 2012; **63**: 491–497.

8. U. U. Williams and C. A. Hagberg. Preoperative airway assessment and strategies. *Trends in Anaesthesia and Critical Care* 2018; **19**: 21–24.

9. L. C. Berkow and P. Ariyo. Preoperative assessment of the airway. *Trends in Anaesthesia and Critical Care* 2015; **5**: 28–35.

10. H-J. Kim, S-H. Kim, N-H. Min, and W-K, Park. Determination of the appropriate sizes of oropharyngeal airways in adults – correlation with external facial measurements: a randomised crossover study. *European Journal of Anaesthesiology* 2016; **33**: 936–942.

11. S. Bush and D. Ray. Basic airway management. In A. Burtenshaw, J. Benger, and J. Nolan (eds.), *Emergency Anaesthesia*, 2nd ed. Cambridge: Cambridge University Press, 2015, pp. 20–29.

12. P. G. Grube, D. Fan, V. R. Pothula, et al. Prevention of aspiration of nasopharyngeal airway. *Indian Journal of Anaesthesia* 2010; **54**: 74.

13. K. Roberts, H. Whalley, and A. Bleetman. The nasopharyngeal airway: dispelling myths and establishing the facts. *Emergency Medicine Journal* 2005; **22**: 394–396.

14. D. Bullard, K. Brothers, C. Davis, E. Kingsley, and J. Waters. Contraindications to nasopharyngeal airway insertion. *Nursing* 2012; **42**: 66–67.

15. J. E. Martin, R. Mehta, B. Aarabi, et al. Intracranial insertion of a nasopharyngeal airway in a patient with craniofacial trauma. *Military Medicine* 2004; **169**: 496–497.

16. J. R. Jones. Laryngeal Mask Airway: an alternative for a difficult airway. *Journal of the American Association of Nurse Anesthetists* 1995; **63**: 444–449.

17. Teleflex Inc. LMA Classic™: the classic laryngeal mask. Available from: www .lmaco.com/sites/default/files/31817-LMA -Classic-A4Data-0214-LORES-fnl.pdf.

18. J. Räsänen. The laryngeal mask airway: first class on difficult airways. *FINNANEST* 2000; **33**: 302–305.

19. C. V. Pollack. The laryngeal mask airway: a comprehensive review for the emergency physician. *The Journal of Emergency Medicine* 2001; **20**: 53–66.

20. T. M. Cook. Maintenance of the airway during anaesthesia: supraglottic devices. In I. Calder and A. Pearce (eds.), *Core Topics in Airway Management*. Cambridge: Cambridge University Press, 2005, pp. 43–56.

21. M. B. Rosenburg, J. C. Phero, and D. E. Becker. Essentials of airway management, oxygenation, and ventilation. Part 2. Advanced airway devices: supraglottic airways. *Anesthesia Progress* 2014; **61**: 113–118.

22. N. Choudhary, A. Kumar, A. Kohli, S. Wadhawan, and P. Bhadoria. i-gel as an intubation conduit: comparison of three different types of endotracheal tubes. *Indian Journal of Anaesthesia* 2019; **63**: 218–224.

23. Intersurgical. i-gel: the supraglottic airway with the non-inflatable cuff. Available from: www.intersurgical.com/info/igel.

24. A. I. J. Brain, C. Verghese, and P. J. Strube. The LMA 'ProSeal': a laryngeal mask with an oesophageal vent. *British Journal of Anaesthesia* 2000; **84**: 650–654.

25. C. Verghese and B. Ramaswamy. LMA Supreme™ – a new single-use LMA™ with gastric access: a report on its clinical efficacy. *British Journal of Anaesthesia* 2008; **101**: 405–410.

26. M. S. Bogetz. Using the laryngeal mask airway to manage the difficult airway. *Anesthesiology Clinics of North America* 2002; **20**: 863–870.

27. N. S. Gerstein, D. A. Braude, O. Hung, J. C. Sanders, and M. F. Murphy. The Fastrach™ Intubating Laryngeal Mask Airway®: an overview and update. *Canadian Journal of Anesthesia* 2020; **57**: 588–601.

28. E. H. Liu, R. Wender and A. J. Goldman. The LMA CTrach™ in patients with difficult airways. *Anesthesiology* 2009; **110**: 941–943.

29. V. Michell and A. Patel. Tracheal tubes. In I. Calder and A. Pearce (eds.), *Core Topics in Airway Management*. Cambridge: Cambridge University Press, 2005, pp. 57–68.

30. T. Cook. Airway management. In J. Thompson, I. Moppett, and M. Wiles (eds.), *Smith and Aitkenhead's Textbook of Anaesthesia*, 7th ed. Edinburgh: Elsevier, 2019, pp. 456–506.

31. M. C. Blunt, P. J. Young, A. Patil, et al. Gel lubrication of the tracheal tube cuff reduces pulmonary aspiration. *Anesthesiology* 2001; **95**: 377–381.

32. P. Sengupta, D. I. Sessler, P. Maglinger, et al. Endotracheal tube cuff pressure in three hospitals, and the volume required to produce an appropriate cuff pressure. *BMC Anesthesiology* 2004; **4**. Available from https://bmcanesthesiol .biomedcentral.com/track/pdf/10.1186/ 1471-2253-4-8.

33. P. Sultan, B. Carvalho, B. O. Rose, and R. Cregg. Endotracheal tube cuff pressure monitoring: a review of the evidence. *Journal of Perioperative Practice* 2011; **21**: 379–386.

34. R. M. Bingham and L. T. Proctor. Airway management. *Pediatric Clinics of North America* 2008; **55**: 873–886.

35. L. Maronge and D. Bogod. Complications in obstetric anaesthesia. *Anaesthesia* 2018; **73**: 61–66.

36. S. Grape and P. Schoettker. The role of tracheal tube introducers and stylets in current airway management. *Journal of Clinical Monitoring and Computing* 2017; **31**: 531–537.

37. D. H. Lee and S-J. Park. Effects of 10% lidocaine spray on arterial pressure increase due to suspension laryngoscopy and cough during extubation. *Korean Journal of Anesthesiology* 2011; **60**: 422–427.

38. A. Mahajan, A. K. Gupta, S. Gulati, and S. Gupta. Efficacy of intravenous lignocaine 2% versus oropharyngeal topical 10% Xylocaine spray before induction of anaesthesia in attenuating the pressor response to direct laryngoscopy and endotracheal intubation. *JK Science* 2019; **21**. Available from: www.jkscience.org/arc hives/volume211/2-Original%20Article .pdf.

39. J. Henderson. Tracheal intubation of the adult patient. In I. Calder and A. Pearce (eds.), *Core Topics in Airway Management*. Cambridge: Cambridge University Press, 2005, 69–79.

40. O. Sanehi. Confirmation of tracheal intubation. In I. Calder and A. Pearce (eds.), *Core Topics in Airway Management*. Cambridge: Cambridge University Press, 2005, 81–85.

41. J. V. Divatia and K. Bhowmick. Complications of endotracheal intubation and other airway management procedures. *Indian Journal of Anaesthesia* 2005; **49**; 308–318.

42. S. K. Mishra, N. C. Ashraf, H. Balchander, and A.S Badhe. Location of the upper Murphy's eye in the uncuffed Ring, Adair, and Elwyn tube. *Journal of Anaesthesiology Clinical Pharmacology* 2012; **28**: 528.

43. W. K. Chee. Orotracheal intubation with a nasal Ring–Adair–Elwyn tube provides

an unobstructed view in otolaryngologic procedures. *Anesthesiology* 1995; **83**: 1369.

44. A. Boku, H. Hanamoto, Y. Hirose, et al. Which nostril should be used for nasotracheal intubation: the right or left? A randomized clinical trial. *Journal of Clinical Anesthesia* 2014; **26**: 390–394.

45. National Patient Safety Agency. Reducing the risk of retained throat packs after surgery, 28 April 2009: supporting information. Available from: www.medis-medical.com/content-files/NPSA-Report-Reducing-Risk-Retained-Throat-Packs-Surgery.pdf.

46. A. Gupta, R. Sharma, and N. Gupta. Throat pack: 'friend or foe' for anesthesiologist. *Journal of Anaesthesiology and Critical Care* 2018; **1**. Available from: www.imedpub.com/articles/throat-pack-friend-or-foe-pdf.pdf.

47. V. Chauhan and G. Acharya. Nasal intubation: a comprehensive review. *Indian Journal of Critical Care Medicine* 2016; **20**: 662–667.

48. A. K. Ross and D. R. Ball. Equipment for airway management. *Anaesthesia and Intensive Care Medicine* 2009; **10**: 471–475.

49. K. Jackson and T. Cook. Equipment for airway management. *Anaesthesia and Intensive Care Medicine* 2006; **7**: 356–359.

50. C. F. Haas, R. M. Eakin, M. A. Konkle, and R. Blank. Endotracheal tubes: old and new. *Respiratory Care* 2014; **59**: 933–955.

51. P. Dhar and A. Malik. Anesthesia for laser surgery in ENT and the various ventilatory techniques. *Trends in Anaesthesia and Critical Care* 2011; **1**: 60–66.

52. C. Best. Anesthesia for laser surgery of the airway in children. *Pediatric Anesthesia* 2009; **19**: 155–165.

53. M. Licker, M. Le Guen, J. Diaper, F. Triponez, and W. Karenovics. Isolation of the lung: double-lumen tubes and endobronchial blockers. *Trends in Anaesthesia and Critical Care* 2014; **4**: 47–54.

54. J. N. Wilkinson, S. H. Pennefather, and R. A. McCahon. *Thoracic Anaesthesia*. Oxford: Oxford University Press, 2011.

55. G. Jackson, N. Soni, and C. Whiten. *Practical Procedures in Anaesthesia and Critical Care*. Oxford: Oxford University Press, 2011.

56. E. Mirzabeigi, C. Johnson, and A. Ternian. One-lung anesthesia update. *Seminars in Cardiothoracic and Vascular Anesthesia* 2005; **9**: 213–226.

57. J. Wong, J. S. E. Lee, T. G. L. Wong, R. Iqbal, and P. Wong. Fibreoptic intubation in airway management: a review article. *Singapore Medical Journal* 2019; **60**: 110–118.

58. B. Al-Shaikh and S. Stacey. *Essentials of Anaesthetic Equipment*, 4th ed. Edinburgh: Churchill Livingstone, 2013.

59. J-B. Paolini, F. Donati, and P. Drolet. Review article: video-laryngoscopy – another tool for difficult intubation or a new paradigm in airway management? *Canadian Journal of Anesthesia* 2013; **60**: 184–191.

Chapter 13

Artificial Ventilation

Vicky Lester

Introduction

Artificial ventilation is the process of simulating normal breathing in a patient who is anaesthetised or unable to breathe for themselves. Anaesthetists care for anaesthetised or unconscious patients by managing their airway and providing artificial ventilation. In modern anaesthetic practice, artificial ventilation is usually provided either with use of a mask and bag or by intermittent positive-pressure ventilation (IPPV) via a ventilator.

Brief History of Artificial Ventilation

Modern ventilators and the concept of intensive care units are a product of the twentieth century. There are multiple descriptions of doctors and scientists describing artificial ventilation, dating back hundreds of years. The Greek physician Galen described artificial ventilation into the larynx of animals with a hollow cane, around the second century CE [1]. In the 1700s, William Tossach, a Scottish surgeon, described his use of mouth-to-mouth ventilation to resuscitate a suffocated coal-pit miner [2]. The Silvester method, introduced in 1858 by Dr Henry Robert Silvester, describes early artificial ventilation when moving the arms of supine patients above their head to aid inspiration by creating negative pressure, and back down, to aid expiration. This method was repeated 30 times per minute with variable results [3].

The first 'modern' ventilators were negative-pressure ventilators. These either surrounded the chest of the patient or the whole body from the neck down or consisted of a room to which negative pressure was applied. The first widely used negative-pressure ventilator was the Drinker respirator, the 'iron lung' used in 1928 to treat a child with polio. During the polio epidemic of 1952 in Denmark, positive-pressure ventilators were used for the first time in Blegdams Hospital, Copenhagen [4].

Ventilation and Ventilators

Ventilators are mechanical units that artificially move air in and out of patient airways and lungs.

Ventilators are used in a variety of settings that include the operating theatre, intensive care, emergency department, and during transfers of ventilated patients. Ventilators may be relatively simple, with limited controls, or may utilise state-of-the-art technology to drive a piston ventilator; these are more common in the intensive care setting (see Figures 13.1 and 13.2).

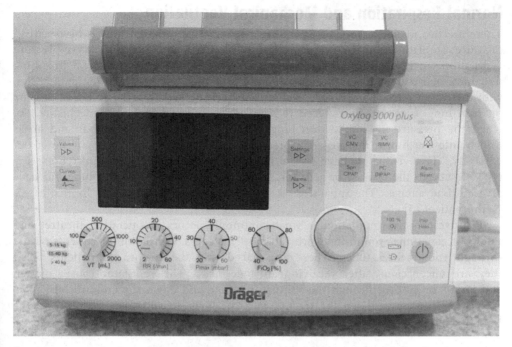

Figure 13.1 Example of a transport ventilator (Dräger Oxylog® 3000 plus)

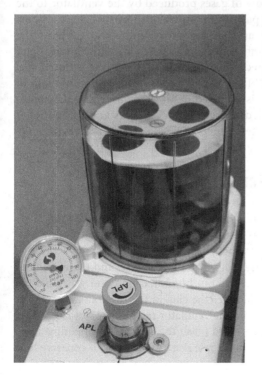

Figure 13.2 Ventilator component of an anaesthetic machine (with pressure gauge and adjustable pressure-limiting (APL) valve). The bellows can be seen to move up and down with each ventilatory breath. In many modern ventilators, the bellows are hidden inside the machine.

Normal Respiration and Mechanical Ventilation

There are two main methods of providing mechanical ventilation; one is by negative-pressure ventilation and the other by positive-pressure ventilation. Negative-pressure ventilation, an example of which is the 'iron lung', simulates the natural breathing dynamics of a patient. The ventilators consist of a large box in which the patient lies, with their head outside and a tight seal around their neck. The pressure inside the box or 'iron lung' is repeatedly reduced to simulate the normal breathing mechanics. So, when the pressure inside the iron lung is reduced, the ribcage expands and air is drawn into the lungs. The negative pressure is then removed and the air flows out passively. These ventilators have several advantages as the patient does not require any type of tube in the trachea or sedation to be used. However, the iron lung did have several disadvantages. The apparatus was large, bulky, cumbersome, and limited access to the patient [5].

Positive-pressure ventilation is what commonly occurs in operating theatres and intensive care units around the world. In most instances, ventilation of patients occurs through endotracheal tubes. These are placed into the trachea of patients when they are unconscious, after receiving an anaesthetic. The ventilator causes oxygen and air to be pushed through the ventilator tubing and down the endotracheal tube. The gases then move down the trachea into the lungs to allow gas exchange in the lung alveoli.

Anaesthetic Breathing Systems

The anaesthetic breathing system links the flow of gases produced by the ventilator to the endotracheal tube placed in the trachea of the patient. In theatre settings, this is usually part of a circle system with an inspiratory limb and an expiratory limb. The gas exits the anaesthetic machine down the inspiratory limb and the gas passes through the heat and moisture exchange (HME) filter, which is joined via connection tubing to the endotracheal tube. The expired gas flows through the HME filter and back down the expiratory limb to the anaesthetic machine. The carbon dioxide is removed by the soda lime and the anaesthetic gases and oxygen remaining are recycled, thereby reducing costs and waste. Other anaesthetic breathing systems may be encountered such as a Bain circuit, where gases are not recycled.

Heat and Moisture Exchange Filter

The HME filter is a vital part of the anaesthetic circuit. It acts in two main ways to mimic the normal physiology of the upper airway, which is bypassed by using an endotracheal tube. The HME filter acts first to heat and humidify the anaesthetic gases used to ventilate the patient. The upper airway, especially the nasal cavity, acts to both heat and humidify the air we breathe. When a patient is intubated, the gas entering the lungs bypasses the nose and therefore does not benefit from being warmed and humidified. Without humidification and warming, the lungs are subjected to cold and dry air, which damages the cilia in the respiratory tract. The HME filter also acts to protect both the patient and the ventilator from microscopic particles and microorganisms (bacteria and viruses) which could infect the patient or contaminate the ventilator [6]. The use of low-flow anaesthesia within circle systems also acts to conserve heat and moisture. The use of soda lime to absorb carbon dioxide generates heat and water during the chemical reaction, which also aids the delivery of warm, moist gases to the patient.

Measurement of Humidity

Humidification is an important concept in the theatre environment. Humidity is the amount of water in the air per unit volume of air. It is important to control the humidity of the theatre environment to maintain safety (an increased risk of static electricity if air too dry, an increased risk of spreading infection if atmosphere too humid), and for the comfort of the personnel working. In modern theatre complexes, it is controlled along with the temperature of the theatre environment.

Humidity is measured using a hygrometer. Hygrometers can be classified as either electrical or non-electrical (analogue) devices. Common analogue hygrometers use two thermometers, one with a wet bulb and one with a dry bulb. The latent heat of evaporation causes the wet bulb to cool more quickly than the dry bulb (like becoming cold more quickly when getting out of a swimming pool). The humidity can then be determined from the difference in temperature between the two thermometers. Theatres use electrical hygrometers, and they measure the change in resistance or capacitance in an electrical circuit. Both the absolute and relative humidity can be measured. The absolute humidity is the amount of water vapour held in a cubic unit of air. The relative humidity is the proportion of water vapour held in the air, compared to the maximum amount of water that volume of air can hold, expressed as a percentage.

Important Ventilator Parameters

Certain parameters are always seen on ventilators, and these help the anaesthetist or intensivist to individualise the ventilation strategy for each patient. Table 13.1 highlights important ventilatory parameters which are commonly seen on all ventilators.

Modes of Ventilation

Controlled Mechanical Ventilation

Controlled mechanical ventilation can be thought of as basic IPPV when the patient is paralysed and making no respiratory effort. Parameters must be selected for the patient based upon age and weight, and they are the responsibility of the anaesthetist.

Pressure-Controlled and Volume-Controlled Ventilation

Tidal volume and respiratory rate are the parameters used to determine the minute ventilation (respiratory rate multiplied by tidal volume). Either the tidal volume or the peak inspiratory pressures are controlled by the doctor caring for the patient. The tidal volume may be pre-set directly by a volume-control mode, where gases are pushed into the patient airways until a set volume is achieved. The tidal volume is variable when a pressure-control mode is utilised. In this mode, a set upper pressure limit is set, and the ventilator pushes air into the patient airways until the set pressure is reached. As the patient chest compliance (stretchiness) changes, the tidal volume achieved with each breath on a pressure-control mode will change.

Table 13.1 Common ventilator parameters

Parameter	Units of measurement	Meaning of abbreviation	Need for parameter
iO_2	Fraction, e.g., 0.5 or percentage, e.g., 50%	Inspired proportion of oxygen	To control the proportion of oxygen the patient is breathing (as high proportions of oxygen can be toxic)
eO_2	As above	Expired proportion of oxygen	To monitor the oxygen proportion used by the patient
$ETCO_2$	mmHg or cmH_2O	End-tidal carbon dioxide levels	To monitor the adequacy of ventilation and maintain normal carbon dioxide and blood pH levels
V_T or TV	mL	Tidal volume	To monitor the ventilation strategy and prevent volutrauma
RR	Respirations per minute	Respiratory rate	To monitor the adequacy of the ventilation strategy
MV	mL/min	Minute volume	The amount of air moved into or out of the lungs in one minute (respiratory rate multiplied by tidal volume)
P_{INSP} or P_{IP}	mmHg or cmH_2O	Peak inspiratory pressure	The highest pressure measured inside the patient airways during inspiration, monitored to prevent barotrauma
PEEP	mmHg or cmH_2O	Positive end expiratory pressure	Added to prevent the collapse of small airways at the end of an expiratory breath

Positive End-Expiratory Pressure

Positive end-expiratory pressure (PEEP) is not a mode of ventilation but an increase in the pressure of the small airways at the end of expiration or a breathing cycle. It is used to keep the alveoli and small airways open and can benefit patients by increasing oxygenation. All patients can have PEEP added to the anaesthetic circuit even if they are breathing spontaneously. In this respect, it is usually termed as CPAP – continuous positive-airway pressure – and is utilised in home breathing masks for patients with conditions such as obstructive sleep apnoea.

Specialist Ventilation

High-Frequency Oscillatory Ventilation

High-frequency oscillatory ventilators are used in paediatric practice and occasionally in adult intensive care when standard ventilation methods are failing to oxygenate the patient. These ventilators hold the lungs open using high PEEP but using tiny tidal volumes. Carbon dioxide is still cleared, and the improved lung recruitment allows for improved oxygenation.

Extra Corporeal Membrane Oxygenation

This is not a type of ventilator but another method of oxygenating the blood. During extra corporeal membrane oxygenation, blood leaves the body and is pumped through an oxygenator and then back to the body. It is similar to a heart–lung bypass machine. It may be used after certain cardiac operations or in severe respiratory failure that does not respond to routine treatments.

Prone Ventilation

In patients with severe lung conditions, prone positioning may be utilised to help improve oxygenation. This occurs because in the prone position ventilation of the lung bases is improved, where lung perfusion is optimal. Hence, the ventilation–perfusion match in the lungs is improved and oxygenation increases.

Jet Ventilation

Jet ventilation may be utilised in specialist settings such as thoracic surgery and, occasionally, throat surgery. A 'jet' of oxygen is released into a rigid bronchoscope to oxygenate the patient during procedures on the trachea. During this technique, anaesthesia must be maintained by total intravenous anaesthesia, as the oxygen comes from the auxiliary outlet and does not pass through the vaporizer.

The Systemic Effects of Mechanical Ventilation

Respiratory Effects

Changing the ventilation mechanics from the physiological negative-pressure to positive-pressure ventilation affects the relationship between blood flow and ventilation within the lung. During normal physiological breathing the lower lobes of the lungs get most of the blood flow as they expand most with normal breathing. However, during IPPV, the more compliant upper lobes stretch more during inspiration and therefore receive a greater proportion of oxygen and anaesthetic gases. However, the upper lobes are less well perfused, so there becomes a ventilation–perfusion mismatch (also known as V:Q mismatch). This can be overcome by using a higher concentration of inspired oxygen and PEEP to help open the lower lobes.

Expiration of gas remains a passive process even with IPPV and is due to the elastic recoil of the lungs. Care must be taken in some patients to avoid gas trapping and the risk of pneumothorax (e.g., asthma and chronic obstructive pulmonary disease).

Cardiovascular Effects

An increase in mean intra-thoracic pressure (as occurs during IPPV) will increase the pressure in the right atrium and will therefore impede venous return. This will in turn lead to reduced cardiac output. These changes in intra-thoracic pressure, along with the cardiac depressant action of anaesthetic drugs and gases, can lead to reductions in coronary and brain blood flow, which can lead to myocardial ischaemia or stroke [7].

Central Nervous System Effects

The blood flow in the brain is dependent upon the difference between the mean arterial pressure and the intracranial pressure (the pressure inside the brain). Mechanical ventilation, and the use of PEEP, increases intra-thoracic pressure and in turn obstructs the venous return from the jugular veins, increasing the intracranial pressure. Reduced cardiac output leads to reduced mean arterial pressure. Autoregulation promotes healthy brain perfusion. Caution in the use of PEEP should be noted for patients with brain pathology such as traumatic brain injuries, where mechanical ventilation is required.

Other Systems

Kidney

Positive-pressure ventilation causes reduced renal water and sodium excretion. This is because the reduction in mean arterial pressure is sensed by baroreceptors, which increases sympathetic activity by the autonomic nervous system and leads to increased vasopressin levels, reducing urine output. The reduced renal perfusion activates the renin–angiotensin system which leads to angiotensin II formation. This stimulates aldosterone production and further reabsorption of sodium and water by the kidney. Reduced venous return and hence decreased stretch of the right atrium causes reduced atrial naturietic peptide release, which results in further sodium and water reabsorption. Healthy individuals can adapt to these changes, but pre-existing kidney pathology may be worsened by mechanical ventilation.

Liver

Hepatic blood flow comprises blood from the hepatic artery and blood from the gut: the portal circulation. The reduced cardiac output associated with mechanical ventilation will reduce blood flow to the liver. The liver may also become congested, as blood flow out of the liver is impeded by the raised intra-thoracic pressure (as it is a low-pressure system).

Ventilatory Consideration for Specific Medical Conditions

Asthma and Chronic Obstructive Pulmonary Disease

Asthma is an acute obstructive airway disorder characterised by wheeze and bronchospasm, caused by hyper-reactive airways. Chronic obstructive pulmonary disease (COPD) is usually a slowly progressive disease and is mostly linked to cigarette smoking. There is lung-tissue destruction over time and the chest becomes hyperinflated. Expiration, which is usually a passive process, becomes an active process and causes premature closure of the small airways, leading to gas trapping. This gas trapping causes intrinsic PEEP. Inspiration then becomes more active to overcome this intrinsic PEEP and gas trapping.

Ventilation strategies are similar for asthma and COPD. High tidal volumes need to be avoided to reduce the risk of barotrauma (injury to the lungs caused by high pressure). The expiratory time also needs to be sufficiently long to minimise gas trapping. COPD exacerbations may be managed with CPAP or BiPAP (bi-level support) on the wards. This technique can reduce the need for intubation and ventilation in COPD patients.

Adult Respiratory Distress Syndrome

Adult respiratory distress syndrome (ARDS) is a severe respiratory condition. It is characterised by increased permeability of the cells in the lungs, leading to increased fluid in the lungs. It is defined by poor lung oxygenation, characteristic X-ray (plain radiograph) changes, no evidence of heart failure, and a recognised cause of ARDS. To prevent further damage to the lung tissue, ventilation strategies include high respiratory rates with small tidal volumes to prevent volutrauma (injury to the lungs caused by high volumes) and prone positioning to improve oxygenation.

Neurological Injury

Neurological injury can be in the form of external trauma resulting from a fall, a blow to the head, or intra-cranial pathology such as an intracerebral bleed. Anaesthesia and artificial ventilation in this setting aims to prevent further injury to the brain tissue, which is called secondary brain injury (primary brain injury causes the initial damage). This involves deep sedation and muscle relaxation, adequate oxygenation, with careful control of the end-tidal carbon dioxide and blood pressure control.

In addition to controlling the end-tidal carbon dioxide levels, regulation of ventilation also controls the pH of the blood and thereby controls the blood volume within the brain. Hypocapnia (overventilation) causes respiratory alkalosis, while hypercapnia (underventilation) causes respiratory acidosis. Hypocapnia causes vasoconstriction and reduces the cerebral pressure but also limits blood flow.

Hypercapnia, in contrast, causes vasodilation and increased blood flow. Cerebral perfusion pressure (calculated by mean arterial pressure minus jugular venous pressure) is also affected by the IPPV and PEEP.

The Ideal Ventilator

The ideal ventilator has several key characteristics. These include being:

- easy to set up and control;
- easy to clean and decontaminate;
- robust and easily portable;
- able to ventilate a wide range of patients (although it is common to need separate ventilators for neonates and infants); and
- rechargeable with a long battery life.

References

1. G. L. Sternbach, J. Varon, R. E. Fromm, et al. Galen and the origins of artificial ventilation, the arteries and the pulse. *Resuscitation* 2001; **49**: 119–122.

2. W. A. Tossach. A man dead in appearance, recovered by distending the lungs with air.

Medical Essays and Observations of the Royal Society of Edinburgh 1744; **5**: 605–608.

3. C. M. Ball and P. J. Featherstone. The early history of cardiac massage. *Anaesthesia and Intensive Care* 2018; **46**: 251–253.

4. J. D. Young and M. K. Sykes. Artificial ventilation: history, equipment and techniques. *Thorax* 1990; **45**: 753–758.

5. A. Thomson. The role of negative pressure ventilation. *Archives of Disease in Childhood* 1997; **77**: 454–458.

6. A. R. Wilkes. Heat and moisture exchangers and breathing system filters: their use in anaesthesia and intensive care. Part 2: practical use, including problems, and their use with paediatric patients. *Anaesthesia* 2011; **66**: 40–51.

7. A. Corp, C. Thomas, and M. Adlam. The cardiovascular effects of positive pressure ventilation. *BJA Education* 2021; **21**: 202–209.

<table>
<tr><td>Chapter</td></tr>
<tr><td>14</td></tr>
</table>

Management of Perioperative Medical Emergencies

Nathan Gamble

Introduction

Even the most routine surgery includes disturbances to normal human physiology – such as general anaesthesia, the surgical procedure or intervention, and the administration of blood products and intravenous fluids. These interventions have the potential to cause new problems or compound pre-existing ones. Patients who undergo anaesthesia and surgery in a precarious state (e.g., trauma or acute heart failure) are particularly at risk. Thus, it is important that all healthcare professionals involved in perioperative care are aware of common perioperative medical emergencies, in order that they can be recognised and treated promptly.

Adverse Drug Reactions

Anaphylaxis

Allergic anaphylaxis is a severe hypersensitivity reaction, typically caused when a type of antibody (immunoglobulin E (IgE)) recognises and binds to an allergen (e.g., latex or penicillin) [1, 2]. The IgE–allergen complex then triggers the release of histamine and cytokines from basophils and mast cells (parts of the immune systems), causing rapid vasodilation, hives, skin redness/swelling, bronchial spasm, abdominal discomfort, and diarrhea/vomiting [1–5]. Some substances, such as opioids and contrast medium, can directly cause this degranulation from mast cells and basophils without IgE.

In surgical patients who are being anaesthetised – both pre and post induction – sudden hypotension or bronchospasm may be the most easily observed symptoms and should prompt consideration of anaphylaxis [6]. Some of the most high-risk medications for anaphylaxis include blood products, antibiotics (especially penicillins and cephalosporins), contrast dye, and neuromuscular blocking agents (e.g., rocuronium and suxamethonium) [3]. Anaphylaxis can be distinguished from more benign allergic reactions by hypotension or respiratory compromise.

Treatment

The following steps are recommended:

- Cease administration of the suspected anaphylaxis trigger and position the patient to optimise breathing [5, 7].
- Administer 500 micrograms of intramuscular adrenaline (alternatively, 50 micrograms by the intravenous route). This will help reverse vasodilation/hypotension and

bronchospasm [2, 5, 7]. Multiple doses or an infusion (in a monitored setting) may be required [2, 5, 7].

- Rapidly infuse 500–1,000 mL crystalloid intravenous fluid to help manage hypotension [7].
- Provide supplementary oxygen to the patient until stabilised and consider nebulised adrenaline (5 mg) [2, 5, 7].
- If airway challenges persist despite supplementary oxygen and adrenaline, a secure airway may be required [7].

While many clinicians also administer antihistamines, inhaled bronchodilators, and gluco-corticoids, the clinical evidence supporting them is relatively poor and they are not priorities in a resuscitation for anaphylaxis [2, 4, 5, 8].

Suxamethonium Apnoea

Suxamethonium is a depolarizing muscle relaxant, often selected in anaesthesia because of its rapid onset and relatively brief duration (e.g., in rapid sequence intubation) [9–11]. Under normal circumstances, suxamethonium is rapidly broken down by an enzyme – plasma cholinesterase [9, 11]. However, in patients with defective or deficient plasma cholinesterase (typically the result of genetic defects, but liver failure, pregnancy, severe illness, and malnutrition can also play a role), the effect of suxamethonium can be extended by minutes to hours [9, 12].

Typically, suxamethonium is eliminated within five minutes, long before the end of a surgical case. Thus, if a patient fails to spontaneously breathe but shows signs of awareness after the general anaesthetic is removed (i.e., hypertension, tachycardia, sweating), cholin-esterase deficiency ('suxamethonium apnoea') should be strongly considered. The initial diagnosis is clinical. Suspicion may be aroused earlier if nerve stimulation is used during the case and muscle twitches are absent or may exhibit fade [11].

Treatment

The following steps are recommended:

- Provide assisted ventilation until suxamethonium wears off and the patient can breathe independently.
- Sedate the patient – being paralysed and ventilated is distressing for awake patients.
- Lighten sedation when nerve stimulation testing is normal.
- Extubate the patient when they demonstrate muscle strength on command – such as raising their head off the bed and firmly squeezing a hand.
- Inform the patient of the incident, especially as they may remember the period of alertness while still paralysed.
- Investigate the cause of the suxamethonium apnoea and avoid suxamethonium in future procedures [10, 12].

Malignant Hyperthermia

Malignant hyperthermia (MH) is a life-threatening hypermetabolic state triggered by suxamethonium and volatile anaesthetic gases in genetically susceptible individuals [13]. MH and its treatment is covered in detail in Chapters 21 and 28. In brief, its chief hallmarks include an uncontrolled rise in temperature, the administration of a known trigger (usually within an hour of symptom onset), mixed respiratory and metabolic acidosis, hypercapnia, increased oxygen consumption, hyperthermia/diaphoresis, unstable blood pressure, tachycardia/arrhythmias, and rhabdomyolysis [13].

Local Anaesthetic Systemic Toxicity

Local anaesthetic systemic toxicity (LAST) is more thoroughly discussed in Chapter 18. Local anaesthetic agents are very commonly used in the operating room and chiefly exert their effect by blocking voltage-gated sodium channels [14]. In peripheral nerves, this prevents the transmission of pain signals to the cerebral cortex. If sufficient doses are delivered systemically, local anaesthetic agents can alter the function of sodium channels in the heart and thalamocortical neurons [15, 16]. Delivery of toxic doses is not infrequently the result of inadvertent intravascular injection or a dosing error, although even selecting a safe dose within proposed limits is not without challenges [15]. Predisposing factors include renal, cardiac, and hepatic dysfunction, pregnancy, administration to areas of high absorption, and extremes of age [15]. While highly variable, the clinical presentation can include visual changes, tinnitus, slurred speech, perioral numbness, metallic taste, mental status changes, and tachycardiac and hypertension that can progress to bradycardia and hypotension [13, 15]. Severe complications include conduction blocks, ventricular arrhythmias, and seizures. The occurrence of any of these after local anaesthetic administration should prompt consideration of LAST [15], as early recognition is important.

Treatment

The following steps are recommended:

- Discontinue the responsible agent.
- Manage the patient's airway and administer 100% oxygen.
- Administer lipid rescue therapy (which will bind local anaesthetic) if there is concern for cardiac or neurological compromise [14, 15].
- Treat seizures with benzodiazepines and arrhythmias with amiodarone [15].
- Once stabilised, transfer the patient to a unit with capacity for close neurological and cardiac monitoring [17].
- Cardiopulmonary bypass may be considered for very severe cases [15].

Neurological Emergencies

Seizures

Epilepsy is a relatively common condition, affecting 0.5–1% of the population [18]. The perioperative period almost inevitably involves common epileptic triggers, such as changes in sleep cycle, food consumption, and drug intake schedules (including alcohol abstinence, possibly leading to withdrawal) [18]. Approximately 3.5% of patients with epilepsy will have a seizure in the perioperative period, with many neurosurgical procedures seeing higher incidences [18]. A common trigger is sub-therapeutic antiepileptic drug (AED) levels [18], a risk that can be mitigated by careful planning regarding AED administration. If a seizure occurs, metabolic triggers should be thoroughly investigated, such as hyponatraemia, hypocalcaemia, and acidosis [19]. While many anaesthetic agents suppress seizures (e.g., propofol), some volatile gases such as sevoflurane and enflurane have been reported to make seizures more likely [20, 21].

Treatment

The following steps are recommended:

- Administer a quick-acting parenteral benzodiazepine (e.g., 2–4 mg of lorazepam, repeated every 3–5 minutes up to 0.1 mg/kg) [19].
- Treat any hypoglycaemia with parenteral glucose, proceeded by 100 mg of parenteral thiamine to prevent Wernicke's encephalopathy (especially seen in patients with thiamine deficiency from alcohol abuse) [19].
- Reverse any significant metabolic derangements identified by investigations (e.g., consider treating hyponatraemia with 100 mL of 3% saline) [19].
- Consult critical care and neurology for status epilepticus if the seizure is not terminated in the first 3–5 minutes (or if a second seizure occurs before the patient returns to baseline).
- The cause of all new seizures should be investigated – not automatically regarded as an anaesthetic side effect.

Stroke (Cerebrovascular Accident)

Perioperative strokes are a relatively rare but serious surgical complications (occurring in approximately 0.1–9.5%, depending on risk factors), with the majority representing embolic phenomena [22]. Strokes are far more likely after cardiac and vascular procedures than general surgery [22].

Treatment

The following steps are recommended:

- Investigate any new focal neurological deficit with an emergency non-contrast CT scan.
- Consider stroke in a patient with delayed recovery from anaesthesia.
- Notify the stroke team for management, including consideration of thrombolysis and mechanical thrombectomy (both of which may be contraindicated by surgical factors) [22].
- Check for hypoglycaemia, which can mimic stroke.

Pulmonary Emergencies

Pulmonary Embolisms

A pulmonary embolism (PE) occurs when a substance obstructs a pulmonary artery or one of its branches. While surgical issues may lead to emboli from fat (e.g., trauma and major orthopaedic surgery), air (e.g., central line placement), and amniotic fluid (e.g., obstetrical scenarios), this chapter focuses on emboli from venous thrombotic events, which are more common [23], especially in immobility and postoperatively. The incidence of PEs varies significantly by type of surgery and underlying risk factors, with estimates ranging from 20% in untreated trauma surgery patients [16] to much less than 1% in minor plastic surgeries [17]. Validated measures (e.g., the UK Department of Health and Social Care's venous thromboembolism (VTE) risk assessment tool) can help predict a patient's risk of a thromboembolic event [24].

PEs often clinically manifest with pleuritic chest pain, dyspnoea, bloody coughing, and calf pain and swelling (suggesting a blood clot in the leg) [25, 26]. A physical examination may additionally reveal tachycardia, tachypnoea, rales (coarse crackles), and jugular venous distension [25, 26]. Some of these signs and symptoms may be masked by anaesthesia or mistaken for other surgical issues and complications [25, 26]. The simplified Well's score can help clinically assess the likelihood of a PE in a symptomatic patient [27].

ECGs may show a right heart strain pattern (also observable on echocardiogram) but more frequently are unremarkable or show sinus tachycardia [26, 28]. Chest X-rays often demonstrate no acute abnormalities, but are useful for excluding alternative causes of hypoxia [26, 28]. An arterial blood gas may reveal a respiratory alkalosis (from tachypnoea) along with hypoxaemia [25]. While a negative D-dimer (a marker of clot breakdown) can essentially exclude a PE if the pre-test probability is low to moderate, a positive D-dimer has a wide differential, is not diagnostic for a PE, and should prompt imaging [28]. If there is a high pre-test probability of a PE, clinicians should proceed directly to CT pulmonary angiography to diagnose or exclude a PE (or a V/Q scan if the CT pulmonary angiogram is contraindicated – e.g., poor renal function) [26, 28].

Treatment

The risk of bleeding presents a significant challenge to treating a PE in the perioperative setting [25]. Numerous variables will influence the management: the anatomy of the PE, haemodynamic stability, whether the PE occurred before, after, or in-between surgeries, the type of surgery, contraindications to certain therapies (e.g., heparin-induced-thrombocytopaenia), etc. Treatment will only be discussed here in broad terms (see Table 14.1). It is advisable to consult an expert in thrombosis medicine for complicated scenarios involving a perioperative PE. Relatively little high-quality research has addressed perioperative management of acute PEs [25].

Gastric Aspiration

Approximately one in 2,000–3,000 patients undergoing surgery experiences an aspiration event related to the procedure (higher in unplanned and emergency procedures), generally during intubation or extubation [31–33]. About half of such patients develop aspiration pneumonia or pneumonitis [32]. According to data from the Royal College of Anaesthetists 4th National Audit Project (NAP4), aspiration accounted for more deaths than failure to intubate or ventilate [34]. When gastric contents (which are acidic) come into contact with lung parenchyma, they cause direct epithelial damage and increase fluid permeability, and also trigger an inflammatory and immune response, magnifying alveolar capillary leak [35, 36]. With as little as 20 mL of regurgitated gastric contents, pneumonitis may become clinically apparent. If large particles are aspirated, airway obstruction may also occur. While usually sterile, the damage inflicted by gastric contents can compromise the lung's infection defences, increasing the chances of pneumonia as a sequelae (a pathological condition that arises from previous injury or disease) [36].

The diagnosis of aspiration pneumonitis is made clinically, taking into account the course of the patient's signs and symptoms and risk factors: general anaesthesia, unprotected airway, obesity, gastrointestinal obstruction, Caesarean section, oesophageal structural abnormalities,

Table 14.1 Management of common PE scenarios

PE scenario	Treatment	Possible treatments if high bleeding risk
Haemodynamic instability	Systemic thrombolysis: tissue-type plasminogen activator (tPA) [29]. Recent surgery may make the risk of bleeding from tPA more serious than the PE itself [25].	Surgical or endovascular clot removal (i.e., embolectomy) or catheter-directed thrombolysis [25, 30]. Embolectomy may also be considered if tPA fails.
Haemodynamic stability	Anticoagulation [29] – unfractionated heparin is generally preferred perioperatively, as its short half-life allows therapy to be promptly ended if further procedures are needed or if significant bleeding occurs. Anticoagulation, unlike thrombolysis, does not eliminate a PE but prevents further thrombotic events while the body breaks down the clot.	Inferior vena cava filter [29].
Hypoxia	Supplemental oxygen: failure necessitates critical care consultation and consideration of intubation and ventilation.	
Hypotension	Intravenous fluids (cardiac output with significant PEs significantly depends on adequate filling of the ventricles (preload)): failure necessitates critical care consultation and consideration of inotropes [28].	

and medications that decrease lower oesophageal sphincter tone (e.g., opioids) [37–39]. Sudden-onset hypoxaemia, coughing, and dyspnoea (if the patient is independently breathing) are typical features of pneumonitis, along with focal crackles and wheezes on auscultation [36]. While an unremarkable chest X-ray does not exclude aspiration, a chest X-ray with new infiltrates or consolidations in gravity-dependent lung segments supports the diagnosis, which typically appear within hours and resolve after 2–3 days [35, 39].

Treatment

The treatment of pulmonary aspiration of gastric aspiration is supportive and includes administering supplementary oxygen and ensuring that the patient's airway is protected.

- Suction any visible possible aspirate from the oropharynx [37].
- Position the patient in a left lateral decubitus position and consider head down to help minimise further aspiration [37].
- Intubate any patient who deteriorates or cannot protect their airway [36]. Approximately 10–20% develop subsequent acute respiratory distress syndrome, typically requiring assisted ventilation [33, 40].

- If large particulate matter is aspirated, consider bronchoscopy to suction the obstructions.
- Treat bronchospasm (which can worsen hypoxaemia) with bronchodilators (e.g., salbutamol).

Routine antibiotics for aspiration pneumonitis do not appear to improve outcomes [41]. Antibiotics are only to be considered in severe cases or if the patient has a gastrointestinal obstruction, as the bacterial load of this aspirate will be high [36, 39]. Immediately apparent fever, leukocytosis, and consolidation are typically direct sequelae of damage from the acidic gastric contents, not bacteria [36]. A few studies have explored the use of steroids in patients with aspiration pneumonitis [42, 43]. None has demonstrated clear benefit.

Tension Pneumothorax

A pneumothorax occurs when air enters the pleural cavity from the external environment (e.g., in penetrating trauma), a break in the lung tissue (e.g., ruptured bleb), or – rarely – from gas-producing organisms in the pleural space [44, 45]. If sufficient pressure builds up in the affected chest cavity via a one-way valve mechanism in which air enters but cannot leave, the elevated intra-thoracic pressure compromises blood return to the heart. A tension pneumothorax results [45]. While a pneumothorax can occur spontaneously as a result of underlying lung disease, genetic defects, or structural abnormalities, traumatic and iatrogenic (e.g., from central line placement) are typically seen more commonly in surgical settings [45].

If the patient is awake, they may experience severe dyspnoea and chest pain. Haemodynamic compromise – hypotension, tachypnoea, tachycardia, and hypoxia – strongly suggests a tension pneumothorax [45, 46]. A physical examination typically reveals absent air entry, poor/no lung expansion, and hyper-resonance to percussion on the affected side, along with possible tracheal deviation away from the affected side and pronounced neck veins [45, 46]. If clinically suspected, the treatment team should not wait for a chest X-ray to initiate management [45], although immediately available point-of-care ultrasound may supplement the physical examination.

Treatment

The following steps are recommended:

- Perform needle decompression: insert a 14–16-gauge needle into the mid clavicular line of the second intercostal space, or the mid-axillary line of fourth to fifth intercostal space, if anatomic considerations prohibit the first location [44, 45]. A sudden rush of air from the cannula confirms the diagnosis and placement.
- Place a chest drain with underwater seal for further management [45].
- Remove the decompression cannula once bubbling is confirmed in the underwater seal system attached to the chest tube, indicating proper function of the system [45].
- If improvement is not seen on subsequent chest X-rays, consult a team with expertise in chest drains (e.g., trauma or thoracic surgery).
- Refer any pneumothorax without an obvious cause to a pulmonary specialist to evaluate for underlying lung conditions.

Cardiovascular Emergencies

Myocardial Infarction

Major cardiac complications occur in approximately 2% of patients undergoing non-cardiac surgery [47], with half of these experiencing a myocardial infarction (MI) [47]. It is often challenging to diagnose an MI perioperatively. Anaesthesia and postoperative analgesia may also mask the most notable symptoms: chest pain/tightness (with possible radiation to the neck, arms, and back) worsened by exertion and improved by rest/nitroglycerine, epigastric discomfort, nausea and vomiting, dyspnoea, and diaphoresis [48–50]. Additionally, surgical teams may interpret some symptoms as effects of the surgery or a surgical issue.

There are typically two types of MIs that can affect patients undergoing non-cardiac surgery. Type 1 myocardial infarction (T1MI) involves the rupture of a coronary plaque, leading to a clot, coronary artery obstruction, and cardiac ischaemia [48]. Surgical factors – emotional/physiological stress, disturbed inflammatory and coagulation cascades, and tachycardia/hypertensin (possibly causing shear stress on plaques) may promote a T1MI [50].

Type 2 myocardial infarction (T2MI) occurs when there is insufficient oxygen delivery to meet cardiac demand [48]. Such a scenario is more likely with atherosclerotic narrowing of coronary arteries, anaemia, hypovolaemia, and prolonged tachycardia [48].

Various guidelines (not addressed here) have been written regarding preoperative management of patients with high cardiac risks and screening tests to detect silent ischaemia post-surgery [47, 51–53]. If an MI is suspected, blood should be taken for the following tests and sent immediately: serial troponins and ECGs, full blood count (FBC), electrolytes (including magnesium and calcium), arterial blood gas, glucose, and creatinine. An acute troponin change (with one value above the 99th percentile of the reference range) and dynamic ECG changes (i.e., ST-segment and T-wave changes or new bundle branch blocks) are consistent with an MI, especially if the patient is alert and describes MI symptoms [48].

Treatment

The majority of perioperative MIs are T2MI [50]. Troponin elevations in patients who are asymptomatic, haemodynamically stable, and who have low-risk ECGs are generally managed conservatively with judicious use of beta blockers, fluid replacement if hypovolaemic, oxygen if hypoxaemic, reversal of metabolic derangements, and pain control [50]. There is evidence to support transfusions of packed red blood cells for haemoglobin levels below 80 g/L [54]. If antiplatelet agents were withheld for surgery, they should be restarted as soon as the bleeding risk is tolerable. Beta blockers should not be held for surgery, but – if held – should be judiciously restarted. Patients who have not had a recent cardiac assessment but in whom there is suspicion of cardiac disease should be considered for further evaluation and management, such as non-urgent referral to cardiology and initiation of medications to mitigate cardiac risk (e.g., beta blockers and statins).

If high-risk features are seen on the ECG (e.g., a new left bundle branch block and territorial ST-segment deviations), the cardiology team should be consulted urgently for further evaluation and management, which may include coronary angioplasty (opening the clot with a wire-guided balloon), thrombolysis (powerful clot-destroying drugs), and supportive medical care – such as antiplatelets, anticoagulation, and beta blockers [50].

It is important to recognise that the differential for a troponin elevation includes problems aside from acute heart damage (e.g., renal failure) [48].

Shock

Shock is a state of tissue and cellular hypoxia, which results from inadequate oxygen delivery and/or impaired oxygen consumption. Without intervention – and sometimes even with treatment – shock leads to multiorgan failure and death. The causes of shock are diverse but can be broken down into four categories: hypovolaemic, distributive, obstructive, and cardiogenic. Patients may have more than one type of shock, which can result in more complicated management (e.g., septic shock and critical aortic stenosis).

Hypovolaemic Shock

Tissue hypoxia in hypovolaemic shock results from inadequate blood volume, which impairs oxygen delivery. Hypovolaemic shock further consists of non-haemorrhagic causes – such as gastrointestinal losses (e.g., vomiting and diarrhea), renal losses (e.g., high doses of diuretics), skin (e.g., burns and environmental exposure), fluid leaks into 'third spaces' (e.g., pancreatitis), and haemorrhagic causes. In addition to symptoms specific to each of these causes, patients may also experience pre-syncope, fatigue, and thirst. A patient with hypovolaemic shock may show evidence of low intravascular volume (e.g., dry axilla and low jugular venous pressure) in addition to tachycardia and hypotension.

Treatment

The following steps are recommended:
- Identify and treat the underlying cause (e.g., ruptured abdominal aortic aneurysm).
- Rapidly infuse 500–1,000-mL boluses of crystalloid fluid, frequently re-evaluating their volume status and vitals. There is some evidence to favour balanced solutions (e.g., Hartmann's solution) over normal saline [55, 56]. Colloid fluids (e.g., albumin and gelatin) are more costly but provide no additional benefit [57].
- If the patient os haemodynamically unstable after adequate fluid resuscitation, consider vasoactive medications.

Significant haemorrhage may be so rapid that extravascular fluid does not have time to shift and restore intravascular volume (which would dilute/lower the haemoglobin). Thus, a normal or mildly low haemoglobin does not necessarily exclude blood loss [58]. If the patient is bleeding:
- Send an FBC, group and crossmatch, and coagulation parameters (including fibrinogen) [59].
- If blood loss is significant (100% in 24 hours, 50% in 3 hours, or 150 mL/min) or the patient is unstable (systolic blood pressure < 90 mmHg or heart rate > 110 beats per minute), initiate a massive haemorrhage protocol [59]. This typically releases universal donor blood products for immediate use and mobilises further products (if needed) [59].
- In more stable patients, transfuse packed red blood cells to maintain haemoglobin above 70 g/L [60].

Distributive Shock

Distributive shock occurs when there is insufficient vascular tone to maintain the blood pressure. The most common cause is sepsis, but anaphylaxis and neurogenic shock also fall into the category. Anaphylaxis is addressed elsewhere in this chapter.

Sepsis

Septic shock is caused by an inappropriate inflammatory and immune response to infection, leading to blood vessel dilation, hypotension, impaired oxygen consumption, and organ dysfunction [61]. Sepsis is diagnosed on the basis of infection and an increase of two points from baseline on the Sequential Organ Failure Assessment (SOFA) score [61]. The following treatment steps are recommended [62, 63]:

- Immediately administer antibiotics (sufficient to cover likely pathogens) and provide adequate resuscitation with a balanced crystalloid fluid (e.g., Ringer's lactate) [64–68].
- If possible, take blood cultures before administering empiric antibiotics (to help guide their prompt de-escalation).
- Send investigations to identify the source of the infection and possible complications (e.g., organ failure). Address any suspected source as quickly as possible (e.g., urinary catheter).
- If vasoactive medications are needed to maintain a mean arterial pressure of 65 mmHg, start promptly with norepinephrine as the first-line choice [69, 70].

Neurogenic Shock

Neurogenic shock [71] is caused when nervous system signals required to constrict blood vessels are lost and resting/parasympathetic tone is unopposed. This typically occurs after spinal cord injury. Recommended treatments are as follows:

- Diagnose and manage the underlying cause.
- Administer a bolus of crystalloid fluid.
- Add vasoactive medications if unresponsive to fluids or if hypotension is severe.
- Monitor respiratory status, as nerves that control breathing may also have been damaged.
- Avoid hypoxia and take extreme care with endobronchial suction, which may stimulate parasympathetic tone and further destabilise the patient.

Obstructive Shock

Obstructive shock occurs when the circulatory system is partially or completely blocked, either entering or exiting the heart. There are four main causes: a massive PE, a tension pneumothorax, cardiac tamponade, and critical aortic stenosis (AS). While supportive measures may temporarily mitigate circulatory collapse, the only meaningful treatment is relieving the obstruction. Pes and tension pneumothoraxes are addressed earlier in this chapter.

Cardiac tamponade occurs when fluid becomes trapped in the pericardium, preventing adequate filling of the ventricles [72]. Acute tamponade may be iatrogenic, related to aortic dissection, or secondary to free wall rupture. More chronic causes include inflammatory conditions, malignancy, and infection. A diagnosis is made clinically but is greatly aided by echocardiography [72]. Blood in the pericardium must be drained surgically, whereas other fluid can often be drained percutaneously [72].

AS, which is the most common valvular heart disease in Europe, is caused by chronic calcific degeneration of the valve, made more likely by congenital defects [73, 74]. In AS, the narrowed aortic valve limits blood exiting the left ventricle, often leading to ventricular hypertrophy and impaired function [73]. Due to the blood flow limitation, a patient with AS may be unable to increase their cardiac output and adequately respond if their peripheral vascular resistance decreases (i.e., the arteries dilate) – possibly resulting in severe hypotension, poor coronary perfusion of the hypertrophied ventricle, and myocardial ischaemia [75, 76]. Many anaesthetic techniques induce this loss of vascular tone, making surgery risky in AS [75, 76].

Careful consideration should be given to whether the benefits of non-cardiac surgery outweigh the dangers posed by AS [76]. In patients with symptomatic AS, the valve should be treated before elective procedures; vital non-cardiac surgery may be performed in patients with symptomatic AS, but only with invasive haemodynamic monitoring [77, 78]. In patients with asymptomatic AS, low- to intermediate-risk surgery may be feasible with careful preoperative assessment and planning (usually including a recent echocardiogram) [78]. Care must be given to avoid hyper- and hypovolaemia, as this can result in heart failure and low blood pressure, respectively. As noted above, the anaesthetic strategy should mitigate the risk of hypotension; techniques and drugs that are prone to decrease peripheral vascular resistance are typically avoided (e.g., spinal anaesthesia) [79]. When hypotension is encountered, vasoactive medications are crucial for restoring the blood and coronary perfusion pressures [75].

The cardiac output in AS relies on good left-ventricular filling, which can be impaired by tachyarrhythmias [75]. Anaesthetic agents that cause tachycardia (e.g., ketamine) may not be tolerated [76]. Atrial fibrillation is of particular concern because it not only causes tachycardia (reducing diastole – the time when the ventricle fills and coronary arteries perfuse the heart) but also prohibits the left atrium from effectively squeezing blood into the left ventricle [75, 79]. Tachyarrhythmias, especially atrial fibrillation, need to be promptly addressed [79].

Cardiogenic Shock

Cardiogenic shock is defined by laboratory and clinical evidence of hypoperfusion in the context of insufficient cardiac output [80], either from inadequate contraction (i.e., compromised muscle), insufficient preload (i.e., inadequate filling), excessive afterload (i.e., resistance to blood moving out of the heart), or flow in the wrong direction (i.e., valvular insufficiency). Most cases of cardiogenic shock are due to ischaemia [80]. Other causes include infiltrative processes (e.g., amyloidosis), valvular pathology (e.g., aortic insufficiency), abnormal rhythms, and acute structural defects (e.g., ruptured ventricular septum).

A clinician should examine for volume overload, pulmonary oedema, abnormalities of the normal heart sounds, extra heart sounds, murmurs, and compromised peripheral perfusion, which will inform diagnosis and management [80]. T1MI must always be excluded (see the section on MI). B-type natriuretic peptide (BNP) above 400–500 pg/mL supports a diagnosis of heart failure and a value of below 50 pg/mL virtually excludes it – but levels can be influenced by factors such as obesity (BNP lowered) and renal failure (BNP increased) [81, 82]. A trans-thoracic echocardiogram can help clarify the cause of the cardiogenic shock (tamponade, wall motion abnormalities, valvular defects, etc.). More advanced imaging, such as angiogram or cardiac MRI, may be helpful.

Treatment

The fundamental objectives in cardiogenic shock are to improve cardiac output while maintaining a sufficient perfusion pressure [83] and to carefully address hypervolemia [84]. This requires thorough familiarity with cardiac pathologies and vasoactive medications, as inappropriate vasoactive medications may worsen the pathology. The heart rate, contractility, preload, and afterload should be manipulated to inimize forward flow [80, 83]. Dopamine and vasopressin should be avoided [85], as the former promotes arrythmias and the latter selectively worsens afterload. Intravenous diuretics are preferred for the treatment of volume overload (oral diuretics may not be absorbed by an oedematous gastrointestinal tract) [80]. Electrolytes and organ function should be monitored for abnormalities [83].

Arrythmias

Please refer to Chapter 9 regarding the diagnosis and management of arrythmias.

Metabolic Emergencies

Diabetic Ketoacidosis

Diabetic ketoacidosis (DKA) is a life-threatening emergency typically seen in type 1 diabetes, as well as severe, ketone-prone type 2 diabetes. It is caused by relative or absolute insulin deficiency, which prevents sufficient absorption and metabolism of glucose intracellularly, leading to fatty acid consumption as an alternative energy source, ketone production, and a drop in serum pH [86, 87]. Dehydration, acidemia, and inadequate insulin can also result in fatal electrolyte disturbances [88]. DKA is often triggered by physiological stresses common to acute surgical patients – such as trauma, infections, ischaemia, or even surgery itself – which elevate endogenous hormones (e.g., cortisol) that increase insulin resistance [86].

Missed or inadequate insulin doses may also lead to DKA, and type 1 diabetics should receive insulin and glucose infusions while NPO (nothing by mouth) perioperatively. Positive ketones (e.g., beta-hydroxybutyrate), low bicarbonate, and a wide anion gap metabolic acidosis are central laboratory features, with polydipsia/dehydration, polyuria, abdominal pain (may be misdiagnosed as an acute abdomen), and confusion being common clinical signs and symptoms [86].

While serum glucose is generally high in DKA, marked hyperglycaemia is not required [86, 88]. Euglycaemic DKA is a well-established phenomenon, particularly among patients with minimal food intake and type 2 diabetics on sodium glucose co-transporter (SGLT2 inhibitors; e.g., canagliflozin, empagliflozin) [88, 89]. Due to the complexity of DKA treatment, the Joint British Diabetes Societies recommend that treatment teams with expertise in diabetes should be consulted for management and follow-up [90].

Treatment

The following treatments are recommended [86, 88, 90, 91]:

- Send investigations for common DKA triggers (e.g., infections, MI, stroke, and pancreatitis). Treat any identified cause.
- Infuse crystalloid boluses of 500–1,000 mL until the patient's dehydration is fully corrected, and then continue at an adequate maintenance rate (typically with 20–40 mmol/L of potassium, depending on serum potassium levels).
- Administer intravenous insulin, initially at 0.1 unit/kg per hour. Titrate as needed to achieve a decrease in ketones of at least 0.5 mmol/L per hour and a decrease in glucose of 3–5 mmol/L per hour.
- Continue the patient's long-acting subcutaneous insulin, if previously prescribed.
- Along with ketones and glucose, frequently check (hourly at first) and address the patient's potassium and sodium – which can be disturbed by the administration of large doses of insulin and crystalloid intravenous fluids.
- Consider bicarbonate if the serum pH is < 6.9.

The clinical target of DKA management is not restoration of euglycaemia but resolution of ketosis (< 0.6 mmol/L) and a pH over 7.3 [86]. As a result, supplementary glucose is required once serum glucose falls below 14 mmol/L so that sufficient insulin can be administered to achieve the above objectives. Once these targets are met and the patient is eating, restart the patient's rapid-acting insulin before breakfast or lunch (when the transition period can be easily monitored) and stop the insulin infusion one hour later [86, 91].

Treating DKA in patients with advanced renal or heart failure is more nuanced and beyond the scope of this chapter.

Hypoglycaemia

Hypoglycaemia is a common problem (glucose <4.0 mmol/L; severe hypoglycaemia is defined by the need for third-party treatment) [92], occurring in approximately 7–18% of admitted patients [92–95]. Hypoglycaemia is associated with increased morbidity and mortality, longer hospital stays, and higher hospital costs [95–97]. Risks for hypoglycaemia include previous hypoglycaemia, hypoglycaemic unawareness, aggressive glycaemic therapy, and lower haemoglobin A1c levels, old age, and organ failure [98, 99]. Hypoglycaemia is more common among type 1 than type 2 diabetics [92].

The physiological regulation of glucose levels is intricate, involving a series of regulatory and counter-regulatory hormones. Insulin – a pancreatic hormone – is critical and functions by signalling tissues to absorb glucose and the liver to stop creating and releasing glucose [100]. Other hormones (e.g., cortisol and adrenalin) dampen the sensitivity of tissues to insulin. Glucagon counters the effect of insulin by instructing the liver to create as well as release glucose (stored as glycogen) into the blood release [100]. Thus, glucose metabolism can be dysregulated not only by poor oral intake and inappropriate insulin levels, but by significant stress and illness, liver failure, renal failure, altered metabolic states (e.g., infection), and medications that impact insulin sensitivity (e.g., beta blockers and steroids).

Under normal circumstances, hypoglycaemia activates the sympathetic nervous system in an attempt to prompt glucose consumption, resulting in palpitations, diaphoresis, hunger, and shaking [92]. The direct effect of low serum glucose can also cause neurological symptoms: fatigue/malaise, altered mental status, speech difficulties, focal neurological deficits, and seizures [92]. However, many of these signs and symptoms can be masked with sedative medications and general anaesthesia, necessitating regular glucose checks during surgery [101]. Moreover, in some patients with chronic diabetes (especially type 1) and multiple previous hypoglycaemic episodes, the normal physiological response to low plasma glucose may be blunted and fail to produce typical symptoms [99].

Hypoglycaemia in a non-diabetic – which is only diagnosed if accompanied by relevant symptoms or if critically low (< 2.2 mmol/L) – should prompt evaluation from an experienced clinician in order to determine the cause.

Treatment

The following treatments are recommended [92]:

- If able to tolerate oral intake, instruct the patient to consume 15–20 grams of carbohydrates, approximately five glucose tablets, or 200 mL of fruit juice.
- If oral intake not possible, administer 20 g of intravenous glucose – ideally in a 10–20% glucose solution, as higher concentrations carry a greater risk of extravasation injury.
- If intravenous access is unavailable, intramuscularly inject 1 mg of glucagon to cause hepatic glucose release (this takes at least 15 minutes to work and intravenous access should be attempted in the interim).
- Closely monitor glucose levels until they are consistently and comfortably within the normal range. Hypoglycaemia secondary to oral agents and long-acting insulin has a higher chance of recurring [92].
- Especially if the patient has type 1 diabetes, do not withhold the patient's insulin (see section on DKA), although dosages should be re-evaluated.

Haematological Emergencies

Acute Disseminated Intravascular Coagulopathy

Acute disseminated intravascular coagulopathy (DIC) is a life-threatening dysregulation of both clot formation and breakdown, resulting in bleeding, thrombotic events, and consequent multiorgan damage [102]. The pathophysiology of DIC is complex but always involves a trigger that disrupts the intricate system responsible for preventing both bleeding and clot formation in blood vessels [102, 103]. The most common triggers include trauma, sepsis, malignancy, and obstetric complications (e.g., amniotic embolism and preeclampsia) [102].

The diagnosis of DIC is based on both clinical and laboratory information. DIC can present with bleeding (operating theatre teams are often alerted to DIC by prominent 'oozing' from surgical sites and drains), thromboembolism, and central nervous system, renal, hepatic, and respiratory dysfunction [102]. Abnormalities may also be seen in laboratory tests, such as the prothrombin time (prolonged), platelet count (low), fibrinogen, and D-dimer (high) – all of which should be sent for testing if DIC is suspected, along with a peripheral blood smear to examine for fragmented blood cells [102, 103]. Fibrinogen is typically elevated in malignancy, sepsis, and inflammatory conditions; thus, fibrinogen within the 'normal range' may actually be low and in keeping with DIC [103].

While no laboratory finding is particularly sensitive or specific for DIC, a validated algorithm published by the International Society on Thrombosis and Haemostasis (ISTH) can help assess the compatibility of the above investigations with DIC [103, 104]. A clinical interpretation of the overall presentation is always necessary for diagnosis [103].

Treatment

The fundamental treatment for DIC is reversing the trigger [102, 105]. Other interventions directed at clotting and bleeding specifically are essentially supportive and only to be used in specific settings. Given generally weak evidence for interventions in DIC, it is particularly important to carefully examine the clinical situation as treatment decisions are made [106].

Anticoagulation

- Administer prophylactic anticoagulation for all non-bleeding DIC patients with critical illness [103, 107].
- The British Society for Haematology and the ISTH recommends full anticoagulation with unfractionated or low-molecular-weight heparin if the patient has substantial blood clots and no significant bleeding [103, 105, 108]. However, randomised control trials (RCTs) have not demonstrated clear clinical benefit from therapeutic anticoagulation [103, 105].

Blood Products

There is limited high-quality evidence to inform practice regarding blood product administration in DIC, and the only RCTs – examining platelet and fresh frozen plasma (FFP) – failed to show survival benefit [106]. However, an international consensus paper and guidelines from Britain, Japan, Italy, and the ISTH have proposed essentially uniform treatment recommendations based on available data [106, 109].

If actively bleeding, replace depleted components in the clotting process:

- Administer FFP for low fibrinogen (<1.5 g/L) or prolonged prothrombin time/partial thromboplastin time (1.5 times normal). Consider cryoprecipitate if FFP is unavailable [103, 105, 106].
- If fibrinogen remains low despite FFP, consider fibrinogen concentrates [103, 105].
- Transfuse platelets if counts are less that 50,000 per microlitre (or there is a high bleeding risk and counts of less than 20,000 per microlitre) [103, 105, 106].
- If surgery is required (e.g., to achieve source control for an infection), consult haematology regarding bleeding and blood product administration.
- Monitor for and treat hypovolaemia and blood loss.

The goal of blood product administration in DIC is not to reverse laboratory abnormalities but to stop the bleeding [103]. Several other blood product interventions have been explored but are not currently supported by strong evidence [110, 111].

Transfusion Reactions

Transfusion reactions and their management are addressed in depth in Chapter 30. While the most common transfusion reactions are essentially benign (i.e., minor allergic and febrile non-haemolytic reactions), significant disturbances of a patient's vital signs in the context of recent blood products should always prompt consideration of serious complications [112, 113]. Any transfusion still running should be stopped and re-evaluated [113].

Transfusion reactions may also present clinically as back and chest pain, dyspnoea, chills, nausea, red/cola-coloured urine, and low urine output [112, 113].

References

1. J. Soar. Emergency treatment of anaphylaxis in adults: concise guidance. *Clinical Medicine* 2009; **9**: 181.

2. H. A. Sampson, A. Muñoz-Furlong, R. L. Campbell, et al. Second Symposium on the Definition and Management of Anaphylaxis: summary report – Second National Institute of Allergy and Infectious Disease/Food Allergy and Anaphylaxis Network Symposium. *Journal of Allergy and Clinical Immunology* 2006; **117**: 391–397.

3. D. L. Hepner and M. C. Castells. Anaphylaxis during the perioperative period. *Anesthesia and Analgesia* 2003; **97**: 1381–1395.

4. A. Sheikh, Y. Shehata, S. Brown, and F. Simons. Adrenaline for the treatment of anaphylaxis: Cochrane Systematic Review. *Allergy* 2009; **64**: 204–212.

5. J. Soar, R. Pumphrey, A. Cant, et al. Emergency treatment of anaphylactic reactions: guidelines for healthcare providers. *Resuscitation* 2008; **77**: 157–169.

6. P. Dewachter, C. Mouton-Faivre, and D. L Hepner. Perioperative anaphylaxis: what should be known? *Current Allergy and Asthma Reports* 2015; **15**: 21.

7. Working Group of Resuscitation Council UK. *Emergency Treatment of Anaphylaxis: Guidelines for Healthcare Providers.* London: Resuscitation Council UK, 2021.

8. R. Y. Lin, A. Curry, G. R. Pesola, et al. Improved outcomes in patients with acute allergic syndromes who are treated with combined H_1 and H_2 antagonists. *Annals of Emergency Medicine* 2000; **36**: 462–468.

9. M. Andersson, A. Møller, and K. Wildgaard. Butyrylcholinesterase deficiency and its clinical importance in anaesthesia: a systematic review. *Anaesthesia* 2019; **74**: 518–528.

10. S. L. Orebaugh. Succinylcholine: adverse effects and alternatives in emergency medicine. *The American Journal of Emergency Medicine* 1999; **17**: 715–721.

11. Royal College of Anaesthetists. Suxamethonium apnoea (succinylcholine or scoline apnoea) (SA), 2018. Available from: www.rcoa.ac.uk/sites/default/files/documents/2019-11/Factsheet-Suxapnoeaweb.pdf.

12. H. M. Rubinstein, M. K. Rosenberg, J. H. Bolgla, and B. M. Cohen. Prolonged apnea after administration of succinylcholine. *New England Journal of Medicine* 1960; **262**: 1107–1111.

13. K. Glahn, F. Ellis, P. Halsall, et al. Recognizing and managing a malignant hyperthermia crisis: guidelines from the European Malignant Hyperthermia Group. *British Journal of Anaesthesia* 2010; **105**: 417–420.

14. K. El-Boghdadly, A. Pawa, and K. J. Chin Local anesthetic systemic toxicity: current perspectives. *Local and Regional Anesthesia* 2018; **11**: 35.

15. L. E. Christie, J. Picard, and G. L. Weinberg. Local anaesthetic systemic toxicity. *BJA Education* 2015; **15**: 136–142.

16. L. M. Barrera, P. Perel, K. Ker, et al. Thromboprophylaxis for trauma patients. *Cochrane Database of Systematic Reviews* 2013; **3**: CD008303.

17. S. P. Davison, M. L. Venturi, C. E. Attinger, S. B., Baker, and S. L. Spear. Prevention of venous thromboembolism in the plastic surgery patient. *Plastic and Reconstructive Surgery* 2004; **114**: 43e–51e.

18. A. D. Niesen, A. K. Jacob, L. E. Aho, et al. Perioperative seizures in patients with a history of a seizure disorder. *Anesthesia and Analgesia* 2010; **111**: 729–735.

19. S. Knake, H. M. Hamer, and F. Rosenow. Status epilepticus: a critical review. *Epilepsy and Behavior* 2009; **15**: 10–14.

20. W. A. Kofke. Anesthetic management of the patient with epilepsy or prior seizures.

Current Opinion in Anesthesiology 2010; **23**: 391–399.

21. A. Perks, S. Cheema, and R. Mohanraj. Anaesthesia and epilepsy. *British Journal of Anaesthesia* 2012; **108**: 562–571.

22. M. Selim. Perioperative stroke. *New England Journal of Medicine* 2007; **356**: 706–713.

23. P. Jorens, E. Van Marck, A. Snoeckx, and P. Parizel. Nonthrombotic pulmonary embolism. *European Respiratory Journal* 2009; **34**: 452–474.

24. G. Stansby and I. Donald. Reducing the risk of hospital-acquired deep vein thrombosis or pulmonary embolism in medical inpatients. *Clinical Medicine* 2019; **19**: 100.

25. D. M. Ruohoniemi, A. K. Sista, C. F. Doany, and P. M. Heerdt. Perioperative pulmonary thromboembolism: current concepts and treatment options. *Current Opinion in Anaesthesiology* 2018; **31**: 75–82.

26. G. Piazza and S. Z. Goldhaber. Acute pulmonary embolism, part I: epidemiology and diagnosis. *Circulation* 2006; **114**: e28–e32.

27. N. Van Es, N. Kraaijpoel, F. A. Klok, et al. The original and simplified Wells rules and age-adjusted D-dimer testing to rule out pulmonary embolism: an individual patient data meta-analysis. *Journal of Thrombosis and Haemostasis* 2017; **15**: 678–684.

28. J. Bělohlávek, V. Dytrych, and A. Linhart. Pulmonary embolism, part I: epidemiology, risk factors and risk stratification, pathophysiology, clinical presentation, diagnosis and nonthrombotic pulmonary embolism. *Experimental and Clinical Cardiology* 2013; **18**: 129.

29. S. Schulman, S. Konstantinides, Y. Hu, and L. V. Tang. Venous thromboembolic diseases: diagnosis, management and thrombophilia testing. Observations on NICE guideline [NG158]. *Thrombosis and Haemostasis* 2020; **120**: 1143–1146.

30. V. A. Kumar, O. Qaqi, C. Mclendon, et al. Ultrasound enhanced catheter directed thrombolysis for patients with massive and submassive pulmonary embolism presenting to the emergency department. *Circulation* 2016; **134**(suppl._1): A17801.

31. J. Mellin-Olsen, S. Fasting, and S. Gisvold. Routine preoperative gastric emptying is seldom indicated. A study of 85 594 anaesthetics with special focus on aspiration pneumonia. *Acta Anaesthesiologica Scandinavica* 1996; **40**: 1184–1188.

32. G. Olsson, B. Hallen, and K. Hambraeus-Jonzon. Aspiration during anaesthesia: a computer-aided study of 185 358 anaesthetics. *Acta Anaesthesiologica Scandinavica* 1986; **30**: 84–92.

33. M. A. Warner, M. E. Warner, and J. G. Weber. Clinical significance of pulmonary aspiration during the perioperative period. *Anesthesiology: The Journal of the American Society of Anesthesiologists* 1993; **78**: 56–62.

34. M. Robinson and A. Davidson. Aspiration under anaesthesia: risk assessment and decision-making. *Continuing Education in Anaesthesia Critical Care and Pain* 2014; **14**: 171–175.

35. T. Engelhardt and N. Webster. Pulmonary aspiration of gastric contents in anaesthesia. *British Journal of Anaesthesia* 1999; **83**: 453–460.

36. P. E. Marik. Pulmonary aspiration syndromes. *Current Opinion in Pulmonary Medicine* 2011; **17**: 148–154.

37. K. S. Nason. Acute intraoperative pulmonary aspiration. *Thoracic Surgery Clinics* 2015; **25**: 301–307.

38. K. Jenkins and A. B. Baker. Consent and anaesthetic risk. *Anaesthesia* 2003; **58**: 962–984.

39. L. A. Mandell and M. S. Niederman. Aspiration pneumonia. *New England Journal of Medicine* 2019; **380**: 651–663.

40. L. J. Bynum and A. K. Pierce. Pulmonary aspiration of gastric contents. *American Review of Respiratory Disease* 1976; **114**: 1129–1136.

41. V. Dragan, Y. Wei, M. Elligsen, et al. Prophylactic antimicrobial therapy for

acute aspiration pneumonitis. *Clinical Infectious Diseases* 2018; **67**: 513–518.

42. J. E. Wolfe, R. C. Bone, and W. E. Ruth. Effects of corticosteroids in the treatment of patients with gastric aspiration. *The American Journal of Medicine* 1977; **63**: 719–722.

43. M. Sukumaran, M. Granada, H. Berger, M. Lee, and T. Reilly. Evaluation of corticosteroid treatment in aspiration of gastric contents: a controlled clinical trial. *The Mount Sinai Journal of Medicine* 1980; **47**: 335.

44. L. Yarmus and D. Feller-Kopman. Pneumothorax in the critically ill patient. *Chest* 2012; **141**: 1098–1105.

45. A. Macduff, A. Arnold, and J. Harvey. Management of spontaneous pneumothorax: British Thoracic Society Pleural Disease Guideline 2010. *Thorax* 2010; **65**(suppl. 2): ii18–ii31.

46. A. Sharma and P. Jindal. Principles of diagnosis and management of traumatic pneumothorax. *Journal of Emergencies, Trauma and Shock* 2008; **1**: 34.

47. T. H. Lee, E. R. Marcantonio, C. M. Mangione, et al. Derivation and prospective validation of a simple index for prediction of cardiac risk of major noncardiac surgery. *Circulation* 1999; **100**: 1043–1049.

48. K. Thygesen, J. S. Alpert, A. S. Jaffe, et al. Fourth universal definition of myocardial infarction (2018). *Journal of the American College of Cardiology* 2018; **72**: 2231–2264.

49. A. V. Ferry, A. Anand, F. E. Strachan, et al. Presenting symptoms in men and women diagnosed with myocardial infarction using sex-specific criteria. *Journal of the American Heart Association* 2019; **8**: e012307.

50. G. Landesberg, W. S. Beattie, M. Mosseri, A. S. Jaffe, and J. S. Alpert. Perioperative myocardial infarction. *Circulation* 2009; **119**: 2936–2944.

51. E. Duceppe, J. Parlow, and P. Macdonald, et al. Canadian Cardiovascular Society guidelines on perioperative cardiac risk assessment and management for patients who undergo noncardiac surgery. *Canadian Journal of Cardiology* 2017; **33**: 17–32.

52. L. A. Fleisher, K. E. Fleischmann, A. D. Auerbach, et al. 2014 ACC/AHA guideline on perioperative cardiovascular evaluation and management of patients undergoing noncardiac surgery: a report of the American College of Cardiology/American Heart Association Task Force on Practice Guidelines. *Circulation* 2014; **130**: e278–e333.

53. S. De Hert, S. Staender, G. Fritsch, et al. Pre-operative evaluation of adults undergoing elective noncardiac surgery. *European Journal of Anaesthesiology* 2018; **35**: 407–465.

54. J. L. Carson, G. Guyatt, N. M. Heddle, et al. Clinical practice guidelines from the AABB: red blood cell transfusion thresholds and storage. *Journal of the American Medical Association* 2016; **316**: 2025–2035.

55. M. W. Semler, W. H. Self, J. P. Wanderer, et al. Balanced crystalloids versus saline in critically ill adults. *New England Journal of Medicine* 2018; **378**: 829–839.

56. W. H. Self, M. W. Semler, J. P. Wanderer, et al. Balanced crystalloids versus saline in noncritically ill adults. *New England Journal of Medicine* 2018; **378**: 819–828.

57. P. Perel and I. Roberts. Colloids versus crystalloids for fluid resuscitation in critically ill patients. *Cochrane Database of Systematic Reviews* 2012; **6**: CD000567.

58. L. Alder and A. Tambe. Acute anemia. In *Statpearls [Internet]*. Treasure Island, FL: StatPearls Publishing, 2019.

59. D. Norfolk. Transfusion management of major haemorrhage. In D. Norfolk (ed.), *Handbook of Transfusion Medicine*, 5th ed. London: United Kingdom Blood Services, 2014, pp. 82–87.

60. National Institute for Health and Care Excellence. Blood transfusion: NICE guideline NG24. Available from: www.nice.org.uk/guidance/ng24.

61. M. Singer, C. S. Deutschman, C. W. Seymour, et al. The Third International Consensus definitions for

sepsis and septic shock (Sepsis-3). *Journal of the American Medical Association* 2016; **315**: 801–810.

62. M. D. Howell and A. M. Davis. Management of sepsis and septic shock. *Journal of the American Medical Association* 2017; **317**: 847–848.

63. M. M. Levy, L. E. Evans, and A. Rhodes. The Surviving Sepsis Campaign bundle: 2018 update. *Intensive Care Medicine* 2018; **44**: 925–928.

64. R. Ferrer, I. Martin-Loeches, G. Phillips, et al. Empiric antibiotic treatment reduces mortality in severe sepsis and septic shock from the first hour: results from a guideline-based performance improvement program. *Critical Care Medicine* 2014; **42**: 1749–1755.

65. V. X. Liu, V. Fielding-Singh, J. D. Greene, et al. The timing of early antibiotics and hospital mortality in sepsis. *American Journal of Respiratory and Critical Care Medicine* 2017; **196**: 856–863.

66. P. R. Mouncey, T. M. Osborn, G. S. Power, et al. Trial of early, goal-directed resuscitation for septic shock. *New England Journal of Medicine* 2015; **372**: 1301–1311.

67. E. Rivers, B. Nguyen, S. Havstad, et al. Early goal-directed therapy in the treatment of severe sepsis and septic shock. *New England Journal of Medicine* 2001; **345**: 1368–1377.

68. M. Sethi, C. G. Owyang, C. Meyers, et al. Choice of resuscitative fluids and mortality in emergency department patients with sepsis. *The American Journal of Emergency Medicine* 2018; **36**: 625–629.

69. T. S. Vasu, R. Cavallazzi, A. Hirani, et al. Norepinephrine or dopamine for septic shock: systematic review of randomized clinical trials. *Journal of Intensive Care Medicine* 2012; **27**: 172–178.

70. D. De Backer, H. Aldecoa Njimi, and J.-L. Vincent. Dopamine versus norepinephrine in the treatment of septic shock: a meta-analysis. *Critical Care Medicine* 2012; **40**: 725–730.

71. H. Guly, O. Bouamra, and F. Lecky. The incidence of neurogenic shock in patients with isolated spinal cord injury in the emergency department. *Resuscitation* 2008; **76**: 57–62.

72. J. K. Jensen, S. H. Poulsen, and H. Mølgaard. Cardiac tamponade: a clinical challenge. *E-Journal of Cardiology Practice* 2017; **15**; 27 September.

73. B. R. Lindman, R. O. Bonow, and C. M. Otto. Current management of calcific aortic stenosis. *Circulation Research* 2013; **113**: 223–237.

74. B. R. Lindman, M.-A. Clavel, P. Mathieu, et al. Calcific aortic stenosis. *Nature Reviews Disease Primers* 2016; **2**: 1–28.

75. M. Christ, Y. Sharkova, G. Geldner, and B. Maisch. Preoperative and perioperative care for patients with suspected or established aortic stenosis facing noncardiac surgery. *Chest* 2005; **128**: 2944–2953.

76. A. J. Mittnacht, M. Fanshawe, and S. Konstadt. Anesthetic considerations in the patient with valvular heart disease undergoing noncardiac surgery. *Seminars in Cardiothoracic and Vascular Anesthesia* 2008; **12**: 33–59.

77. A. Vahanian, O. Alfieri, F. Andreotti, et al. Guidelines on the management of valvular heart disease (version 2012): the Joint Task Force on the Management of Valvular Heart Disease of the European Society of Cardiology (ESC) and the European Association for Cardio-Thoracic Surgery (EACTS). *European Heart Journal* 2012; **33**: 2451–2496.

78. S. D. Kristensen J., Knuuti, A. Saraste, et al. ESC/ESA guidelines on non-cardiac surgery – cardiovascular assessment and management. The Joint Task Force on Non-Cardiac Surgery: Cardiovascular Assessment and Management of the European Society of Cardiology (ESC) and the European Society of Anaesthesiology (ESA). *European Heart Journal* 2014; **35**: 2383–2431.

79. J. Brown and N. J. Morgan-Hughes. Aortic stenosis and non-cardiac surgery. *Continuing Education in Anaesthesia Critical Care and Pain* 2005; **5**: 1–4.

80. S. Van Diepen, J. N. Katz, N. M. Albert, et al. Contemporary management of

cardiogenic shock: a scientific statement from the American Heart Association. *Circulation* 2017; **136**: e232–e268.

81. J. Doust, R. Lehman, and P. Glasziou. The role of BNP testing in heart failure. *American Family Physician* 2006; **74**: 1893–1898.

82. D. Korenstein, J. P. Wisnivesky, P. Wyer, et al. The utility of B-type natriuretic peptide in the diagnosis of heart failure in the emergency department: a systematic review. *BMC Emergency Medicine* 2007; **7**: 1–9.

83. P. Squara, S. Hollenberg, and D. Payen. Reconsidering vasopressors for cardiogenic shock: everything should be made as simple as possible, but not simpler. *Chest* 2019; **156**: 392–401.

84. C. Vahdatpour, D. Collins, and S. Goldberg. Cardiogenic shock. *Journal of the American Heart Association* 2019; **8**: e011991.

85. B. Levy, J. Buzon, and A. Kimmoun. Inotropes and vasopressors use in cardiogenic shock: when, which and how much? *Current Opinion in Critical Care* 2019; **25**: 384–390.

86. Joint British Diabetes Societies Inpatient Care Group. *The Management of Diabetic Ketoacidosis in Adults*, 2nd ed. London: Joint British Diabetes Societies Inpatient Care Group for NHS Diabetes, 2014.

87. A. E. Kitabchi, G. E. Umpierrez, J. M. Miles, and J. N. Fisher. Hyperglycemic crises in adult patients with diabetes. *Diabetes Care* 2009; **32**: 1335–1343.

88. M. R. Burge, K. J. Hardy, and D. S. Schade. Short-term fasting is a mechanism for the development of euglycemic ketoacidosis during periods of insulin deficiency. *The Journal of Clinical Endocrinology and Metabolism* 1993; **76**: 1192–1198.

89. H. Qiu, A. Novikov, and V. Vallon. Ketosis and diabetic ketoacidosis in response to SGLT2 inhibitors: basic mechanisms and therapeutic perspectives. *Diabetes/ Metabolism Research and Reviews* 2017; **33**: e2886.

90. K. Kohler and N. Levy. Management of diabetic ketoacidosis: a summary of the 2013 Joint British Diabetes Societies guidelines. *Journal of the Intensive Care Society* 2014; **15**: 222–225.

91. National Institute for Health and Care Excellence. Diabetic ketoacidosis: management. Available from: www .nice.org.uk/guidance/ng17/ifp/chapter/ diabetic-ketoacidosis.

92. D. Stanisstreet, E. Walden, and A. Graveling. *The Hospital Management of Hypoglycaemia in Adults with Diabetes Mellitus.*. London: Joint British Diabetes Societies Inpatient Care Group for NHS Diabetes, 2018.

93. L. Boucai, W. N. Southern, and J. Zonszein. Hypoglycemia-associated mortality is not drug-associated but linked to comorbidities. *The American Journal of Medicine* 2011; **124**: 1028–1035.

94. H. L. Drews III, A. L. Castiglione, S. N. Brentin, et al. Perioperative hypoglycemia in patients with diabetes: incidence after low normal fasting preoperative blood glucose versus after hyperglycemia treated with insulin. *AANA Journal* 2012; **80**: S17–S24.

95. A. Turchin, M. E. Matheny, M. Shubina, et al. Hypoglycemia and clinical outcomes in patients with diabetes hospitalized in the general ward. *Diabetes Care* 2009; **32**: 1153–1157.

96. S. Curkendall, J. Natoli, C. Alexander, et al. Economic and clinical impact of inpatient diabetic hypoglycemia. *Endocrine Practice* 2009; **15**: 302–312.

97. S. Finfer, D. R, Chittock, S. Y-S. Su, et al. Intensive versus conventional glucose control in critically ill patients. *New England Journal of Medicine* 2009; **360**: 1283–1297.

98. American Diabetes Association. Defining and reporting hypoglycemia in diabetes: a report from the American Diabetes Association Workgroup on Hypoglycemia. *Diabetes Care* 2005; **28**: 1245–1249.

99. R. D. Hulkower, R. M. Pollack, and J. Zonszein. Understanding hypoglycemia in

hospitalized patients. *Diabetes Management* 2014; **4**: 165.

100. C. L. Triplitt. Examining the mechanisms of glucose regulation. *American Journal of Managed Care* 2012; **18**: S4.

101. R. Sreedharan and B. Abdelmalak. Diabetes mellitus: preoperative concerns and evaluation. *Anesthesiology Clinics* 2018; **36**: 581–597.

102. S. Gando, M. Levi, and C.-H. Toh. Disseminated intravascular coagulation. *Nature Reviews Disease Primers* 2016; **2**: 1–16.

103. M. Levi, C. Toh, J. Thachil, and H. Watson. Guidelines for the diagnosis and management of disseminated intravascular coagulation. *British Journal of Haematology* 2009; **145**: 24–33.

104. F. B. Taylor, C.-H. Toh, W. K. Hoots, H. Wada, and M. Levi. Towards definition, clinical and laboratory criteria, and a scoring system for disseminated intravascular coagulation. *Thrombosis and Haemostasis* 2001; **86**: 1327–1330.

105. H. Wada, J. Thachil, M. N. Di, et al. Guidance for diagnosis and treatment of DIC from harmonization of the recommendations from three guidelines. *Journal of Thrombosis and Haemostasis* 2013; Feb 4; DOI 10.1111/jth.12155.

106. A. Squizzato, B. J. Hunt, G. T. Kinasewitz, et al. Supportive management strategies for disseminated intravascular coagulation. *Thrombosis and Haemostasis* 2016; **116**: 896–904.

107. S. Gando, A. Sawamura, and M. Hayakawa. Trauma, shock, and disseminated intravascular coagulation: lessons from the classical literature. *Annals of Surgery* 2011; **254**: 10–19.

108. M. K. Gould, D. A. Garcia, S. M. Wren, et al. Prevention of VTE in nonorthopedic surgical patients: antithrombotic therapy and prevention of thrombosis: American College of Chest Physicians evidence-based clinical practice guidelines. *Chest* 2012; **141**: e227S–e277S.

109. H. Wada, T. Matsumoto, and Y. Yamashita. Diagnosis and treatment of disseminated intravascular coagulation (DIC) according to four DIC guidelines. *Journal of Intensive Care* 2014; **2**: 15.

110. A. J. Martí-Carvajal, V. Anand, and I. Sola. Treatment for disseminated intravascular coagulation in patients with acute and chronic leukemia. *Cochrane Database of Systematic Reviews* 2015; **6**: CD008562.

111. A. J. Martí-Carvajal, G. Comunián-Carrasco, and G. E. Peña-Martí. Haematological interventions for treating disseminated intravascular coagulation during pregnancy and postpartum. *Cochrane Database of Systematic Reviews* 2011; **3**: CD00857.

112. M. Delaney, S. Wendel, R. S. Bercovitz, et al. Transfusion reactions: prevention, diagnosis, and treatment. *The Lancet* 2016; **388**: 2825–2836.

113. H. Tinegate, J. Birchall, A. Gray, et al. BCSH Blood Transfusion Task Force. Guideline on the investigation and management of acute transfusion reactions. *British Journal of Haematology* 2012; **159**: 143–153.

Chapter 15

Total Intravenous Anaesthesia

Scott Miller

Introduction

Since initial experiments with nitrous oxide and diethyl ether in the nineteenth century, general anaesthesia has been near synonymous with inhaled agents. However, total intravenous anaesthesia (TIVA) may offer advantages in certain circumstances. TIVA can be defined as the induction and maintenance of general anaesthesia using agents given solely intravenously and in the absence of all inhalational agents including nitrous oxide. It may be necessary when volatile anaesthesia is contraindicated or infeasible or may be chosen for other benefits.

Why Use TIVA?

There are many good reasons and advantages to use TIVA over the traditional volatile anaesthetic agents; these include:

- reduced postoperative nausea and vomiting (PONV) [1];
- reduced atmospheric pollution [2];
- smoother recovery;
- haemodynamic stability due to not changing from intravenous induction to volatile maintenance;
- preservation of hypoxic pulmonary vasoconstriction [3];
- reduction in intracranial pressure [4]; and
- oncological benefits [5].

Moreover, there are specific contraindications to volatile anaesthesia that include:

- patient history of malignant hyperpyrexia [6];
- long QT syndrome [7];
- certain airway procedures where endotracheal ventilation is unsuitable (e.g., rigid bronchoscopy);
- patients requiring intraoperative transfer between environments; and
- history of severe PONV.

How Is TIVA Given?

As with volatile anaesthesia, the triad of anaesthesia applies – analgesia, hypnosis, and relaxation. In TIVA, analgesia is commonly provided by a potent and short-acting opiate such as remifentanil, hypnosis is usually provided by propofol, and muscle relaxation if needed is maintained by a neuromuscular blocking agent. While it is theoretically possible to maintain TIVA using simple repeat boluses or volumetric infusion pumps, the use of

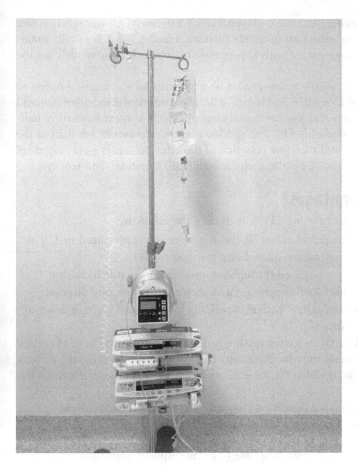

Figure 15.1 TIVA pump with intravenous fluids and warmer

target-controlled infusion (TCI) pumps have revolutionised TIVA and enhanced its popularity, simplifying the administration of drugs while improving safety.

Why Not Just Give Injections?

A single injection of propofol causes a rapid increase in plasma concentration followed by a reduction in concentration as the drug is redistributed to other tissues. Repeated injections give differing results as the drug has not yet been fully eliminated from those other tissues, giving rise to accumulation. Thus, while a large bolus may be required to induce anaesthesia and will clinically wear off in a short time due to redistribution, subsequent doses will have an enhanced effect and take longer to wear off. In other words, the half-life of the drug increases with the infusion duration.

Why Not Just Use a Simple Infusion?

Similarly, while an infusion of several hundred milligrams per hour of propofol may be required to achieve anaesthesia within a clinically useful induction period, that rate would cause a rapid accumulation of drug to toxic and fatal levels. Conversely, a lower infusion rate may be inadequate to provide induction in timely manner. Hence, TIVA is usually maintained by infusion pumps programmed with appropriate pharmacokinetic models for the drugs administered.

Propofol administration is usually accompanied by a potent and short-acting opiate to reduce the quantity of propofol required and improve haemodynamic stability. Remifentanil has become very popular in this role due to its short and relatively context-insensitive half-life. Because remifentanil is metabolised by non-specific plasma esterases rather than in the liver, accumulation is minimal and therefore cessation of the infusion causes a very rapid fall in plasma concentration. Alternative opiates include sufentanil, alfentanil, and fentanyl.

What Are the Disadvantages?

There are several disadvantages in using TIVA, including the following:

- Specialist training may be required as not all clinicians may be experienced in TIVA.
- The risk of pump failure must be considered and planned for.
- Reliable intravenous access is required throughout, precluding volatile induction.
- Increased waste – disposables such as syringes and surplus drugs require disposal.
- Remifentanil-induced hyperalgesia – patients spending long periods on high doses of opiates may develop tolerance [8].
- An increased risk of accidental awareness during general anaesthesia has been suggested due to the inability to measure the concentration of anaesthetic drugs within the patient, unlike volatile anaesthesia in which the patient's end-tidal agent concentration can be monitored [9].
- Propofol infusion syndrome is a condition characterised by metabolic acidosis, rhabdomyolysis, myoglobinuria, lipaemic plasma, enlarged liver, and can cause refractory bradycardia, leading to asystole. It is associated with high-dose propofol infusions (> 4 mg/kg per hour), prolonged use (e.g., intensive therapy unit sedation, especially in children) but has rarely been reported in TIVA cases, where the duration is shorter[10].

How Is TIVA Administered?

As described above, TIVA is usually administered using two infusion pumps suitably programmed with a pharmacokinetic model. In the UK, one will usually be used for propofol and the other for remifentanil. It should be noted at this point that many pharmacokinetic models have proven to be clinically useful and so pumps may vary in the pharmacokinetic model used.

Equipment

The equipment required for TIVA includes the following:

- Two fully charged and serviced infusion pumps with suitable pharmacokinetic software, for example, Diprifusor™, Perfusor™, or Alaris PK™.
- Drugs in suitable form and quantities, for example, propofol 1% or 2% in syringe (specific Diprifusor™ prefilled syringes may be required), remifentanil (50 micrograms/mL commonly).

- An intravenous fluid giving set with a visible drip chamber.
- Awareness monitoring such as the bispectral index (BIS) may be considered. BIS is a simplified electroencephalogram (EEG), which measures the depth of anaesthesia, providing a scale from 0 to 100; 0 would represent no EEG activity and 100 would be awake.
- Reliable intravenous access is essential – ideally, a free-running drip should be attached, and the line and cannula should be clearly visible to allow constant vigilance for failure of the infusion site, for example, extravasation.
- A three-way infusion set to permit the hypnotic agent, analgesic agent, and fluid through the same cannula.
- The gravity-fed intravenous fluid line must include an anti-reflux valve to prevent 'backtracking' [11].
- Anti-siphon valves should be used on the pump driven lines.

Preoperative Considerations

A full history should have been taken from the patient and all relevant information should have been obtained. History taking should include questions on drug and food allergies, noting the potential contraindication for propofol in egg and soya allergies [12]. The patient's height, weight, age, and sex may be required for pharmacokinetic modelling. It should be noted that some pharmacokinetic models are unreliable at extremes of age or weight. All equipment should be checked and lines primed.

Prior to induction after all routine checks, an intravenous cannula of suitable gauge will be sited and secured in a vein which should ideally be visible throughout the procedure. The pumps will be programmed with the patient data and required concentration (usually plasma concentration). The pump pressure limits and alarms should be set appropriately to minimise and detect extravasation. Extravasation describes the unintentional leak of intravenous fluids or drugs from the cannulation site or vein into the surrounding tissue, with the potential to cause injury. After confirming that the patient and all staff are ready to proceed, induction can commence.

Induction

As with volatile anaesthesia, there are many variations in technique. Pre-oxygenation may be used if required, as may depth of anaesthesia monitoring. The intravenous fluid line will be started, and the consistent flow noted. The pumps will then be started to commence induction.

Some clinicians choose to start the pumps at their intended *effect site* concentration (C_e). This may lead to a slow induction in pumps using *plasma* concentration (C_p), so a higher C_p may be set temporarily in order to achieve a quick onset of anaesthesia, similar to the use of 'overpressure' in a volatile induction. Pumps are available which permit the C_e to be set directly, administering a larger initial bolus to ensure rapid onset.

Rapid sequence induction may be achieved by setting a higher C_p until loss of consciousness, but some clinicians may be more comfortable with a manually administered bolus by syringe and then starting the pump for maintenance. Caution must be taken in this case as the pump will have no data relating to this manually administered drug, resulting in a second bolus being administered.

Airway maintenance is broadly similar to a volatile anaesthetic. A neuromuscular blocking agent may be used to facilitate intubation, but some clinicians choose to rely on the airway reflex suppression afforded by remifentanil. Alternatively, a supraglottic airway such as a laryngeal mask airway may be used if it is suitable for the procedure. If spontaneous ventilation is desired then remifentanil may need to be maintained at a lower dose than for mechanical ventilation, with a higher dose of propofol to compensate.

Maintenance

It is essential that the intravenous infusion lines and cannula site are constantly supervised. Any leakage or suspicion of extravasation must be dealt with immediately. The drug concentration settings will be adjusted throughout based on the patient's level of consciousness, as measured by monitoring and clinical signs. Typical drug concentration settings for a young, healthy adult are as follows: with propofol, 4–6 micrograms/mL for spontaneous ventilation; 3–4 micrograms/mL for mechanical ventilation; with remifentanil, 1–3 nanograms/mL for spontaneous ventilation; 5–8 nanograms/mL for mechanical ventilation.

The infusion pumps require constant supervision. Changes in the pump pressure, especially occlusion alarms, raise the suspicion of extravasation or disconnection. It is essential that power is maintained throughout as a pump failure such as a flat battery will result in the complete loss of data, making further pharmacokinetic modelling impossible. As propofol has a vasodilatory effect, its effect is predominantly on blood pressure, and vasopressors may be required to maintain normotension. Remifentanil has strongly cholinergic effects and may cause significant bradycardia so, at high levels, an anticholinergic drug may be required to maintain a normal heart rate.

Emergence

Towards the end of the procedure, postoperative analgesia should be administered as necessary. The potential for postoperative remifentanil-induced hyperalgesia should be included, especially in planning the dosage of any opiates. Neuromuscular blockade should be managed as with any other technique. At the end of the procedure, the patient can be woken by weaning down or stopping the pumps. Many pumps display a predicted time to emergence, which may guide the reduction of drug infusions, but clinical judgement should be paramount.

Postoperative Care

All intravenous lines must be flushed or changed to ensure no anaesthetic agent remains. Among the many claims made for the benefits of TIVA are the subjectively improved emergence and reduced PONV. However, the rapid reduction in remifentanil concentration may require additional attention to postoperative analgesia. The use of remifentanil has been associated with both acute opioid tolerance (desensitisation to opioids) and opioid-induced hyperalgesia (increased sensitivity to painful stimuli) [13].

What Is Awareness?

Accidental awareness during general anaesthesia describes the scenario where a patient becomes conscious when they should be unconscious. This can result in the patient having memories of events in the operating theatre and it can be a distressing experience for some

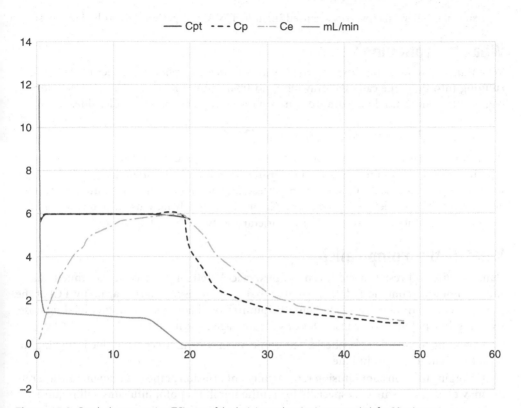

Figure 15.2 Graph demonstrating TCI propofol administered at 6 micrograms/mL for 20 minutes

patients. Whereas volatile agent administration is reliably monitored by end-tidal agent monitoring, the plasma concentration of drugs in TIVA cannot be measured simply, and the only available estimate is based on a model run in the computer of the pump. Therefore, a failure of the model, computer, calculation, or infusion could result in low plasma concentrations and therefore awareness [9]. Additional monitoring such as BIS may reduce this risk.

What Is Backtracking?

When more than one intravenous line is attached to a single cannula, the intention is that all the infusions are delivered to the patient. However, if the system becomes blocked at the cannula, drugs infused by a pump may instead be pushed back up the intravenous fluid line. The infusion pressure alarm on the pump may not detect this, leading to a significant volume of drug being forced up the fluid line.

If the clinician notices this and unblocks or resites the cannula, then the intravenous fluid line will be able to run freely again, releasing a potentially dangerous bolus of the drug into the patient.

Therefore, when a potentially dangerous drug is infused by a pump sharing a cannula with intravenous fluids, it is essential to include an anti-reflux valve on the 'gravity-fed' (intravenous fluid) line.

Examples where such valves are used include TIVA and patient-controlled analgesia.

What Is Syphoning?

When an intravenous line runs freely, it can produce a 'syphoning' effect on other lines running into the same cannula, drawing fluid from those infusions. Thus, a free-running bag of intravenous fluid may draw down propofol or opiate from the other line.

What Is a Pharmacokinetic Model?

A pharmacokinetic model is a mathematical simulation predicting drug concentrations in a patient. They use multiple calculations using several patient parameters, including age, weight, height, and sex. All models are imperfect, and no model will be absolutely correct for any patient. The model may predict the C_p or C_e values. It may use a publicly available protocol (e.g., Marsh for propofol) or proprietary software (e.g., Diprifusor™).

What If the Pump Fails?

Pump failure will result in the loss of all pharmacokinetic data, making continued anaesthesia somewhat complicated. It is essential that propofol is not started again by TCI at the previous concentration. This is because the pump would administer another loading dose, resulting in a potential overdose. Options for management include:

- Changing to volatile anaesthesia. The clinician may be more comfortable returning to a tried-and-tested technique.
- Changing to a constant infusion rate. A constant infusion at the last known infusion rate may be a good estimate, especially for remifentanil. Propofol infusions will require repeated adjustments to consider accumulation over time.

References

1. G. Kumar, C. Stendall, R. Mistry, et al. A comparison of total intravenous anaesthesia using propofol with sevoflurane or desflurane in ambulatory surgery: systematic review and meta-analysis. *Anaesthesia* 2014; **69**: 1138–1150.

2. M. Charlesworth and F. Swinton. Anaesthetic gases, climate change, and sustainable practice. *Lancet Planet Health* 2017; **1**: e216–e217.

3. A. B. Lumb and P. Slinger. Hypoxic pulmonary vasoconstriction: physiology and anesthetic implications. *Anesthesiology* 2015; **122**: 932–946.

4. J. Preethi, P. U. Bidkar, A. Cherian, et al. Comparison of total intravenous anesthesia vs. inhalational anesthesia on brain relaxation, intracranial pressure, and hemodynamics in patients with acute subdural hematoma undergoing emergency craniotomy: a randomized control trial. *European Journal of Trauma and Emergency Surgery* 2021; **47**: 831–837.

5. T. J. Wigmore, K. Mohammed, and S. Jhanji. Long-term survival for patients undergoing volatile versus IV anesthesia for cancer surgery: a retrospective analysis. *Anesthesiology* 2016; **124**: 69–79.

6. P. K. Gupta and P. M. Hopkins. Diagnosis and management of malignant hyperthermia. *BJA Education* 2017; **17**: 249–254.

7. P. D. Booker, S. D. Whyte, and E. J. Ladusans. Long QT syndrome and anaesthesia. *British Journal of Anaesthesia* 2003; **90**: 349–366.

8. C. Santonocito, A. Noto, C. Crimi, et al. Remifentanil-induced postoperative hyperalgesia: current perspectives on mechanisms and therapeutic strategies.

Local and Regional Anesthesia 2018; **11**:15–23.

9. J. J. Pandit, J. Andrade, D. G. Bogod, et al. 5th National Audit Project (NAP5) on accidental awareness during general anaesthesia: summary of main findings and risk factors. *British Journal of Anaesthesia* 2014; **113**: 549–559.

10. J. M. Wong. Propofol infusion syndrome. *American Journal of Therapeutics* 2010; **17**: 487–491.

11. Medicines and Healthcare products Regulatory Agency. Intravenous (IV) extension sets with multiple ports: risk of backtracking. Available from: www.gov .uk/drug-device-alerts/medical-device- alert-intravenous-iv-extension-sets-with- multiple-ports-risk-of-backtracking.

12. P. M. Mertes, J. M. Malinovsky, L. Jouffroy, et al. Reducing the risk of anaphylaxis during anesthesia: 2011 updated guidelines for clinical practice. *Journal of Investigational Allergology and Clinical Immunology* 2011; **21**: 442–453.

13. E. H. Yu, D. H. Tran, S. W. Lam, and M. G. Irwin. Remifentanil tolerance and hyperalgesia: short-term gain, long-term pain? *Anaesthesia* 2016; **71**: 1347–1362.

Chapter 16

Fundamentals of Basic Patient Monitoring

Victoria Cadman and Efua Hagan

Introduction

Monitoring provides information and feedback on a patient's physiological state in response to any therapeutic interventions or stimuli during anaesthesia and surgery. It is vital that perioperative practitioners understand the underlying principles of basic patient monitoring. This includes understanding how and what is being measured, how the monitoring is assembled, and how to problem solve to ensure optimal functionality and accuracy.

Monitors rarely measure variables directly and generally consist of four key components: an attachment that connects to the patient; a measuring device (usually a transducer) that converts information from the patient into an electrical signal; a filter or amplifier, which may integrate the signal with other variables; and a display to provide the results either as a wave, a numeric, or a combination of the two. This means that readings do not always directly reflect the physiology of the patient and therefore require interpretation. This is one of the reasons why baseline measurements of a patient are important to identify their 'normal' parameters and any factors that can affect the accuracy of the readings. Prior to use, all monitoring equipment should be checked following national and/or local guidelines and should include servicing and calibration at timely intervals.

Monitoring during anaesthesia and surgery reduces the risk of harm to the patient through continuous physiological assessment which allows for the early detection of a deteriorating patient or the consequences of an error [1]. Clinical observation of a patient is still a key aspect of monitoring their condition and reliance on monitoring alone should be avoided. Minimum monitoring should be attached to a patient prior to induction and continued until they have recovered from anaesthesia. However, there may be instances where this is not always possible or appropriate, in which case it should be attached at the earliest opportunity. Such situations include anaesthetising young children, or when treating uncooperative adult patients. In these cases, the explanation of why monitoring was delayed must also be recorded on the anaesthetic chart. In the UK, the proposed minimum requirements of monitoring for a patient undergoing general anaesthesia irrespective of the location are as follows [1]:

- adequate supervision;
- pulse oximetry;
- non-invasive blood pressure (NIBP);
- electrocardiogram (ECG);
- gas analysis (inspired and expired oxygen, carbon dioxide by waveform capnography, nitrous oxide and volatile anaesthetic agents if used);

- airway pressure, tidal volume, and respiratory rate during mechanical ventilation;
- peripheral nerve stimulation if neuromuscular blocking drugs used; and
- temperature, before anaesthesia and every 30 minutes until the end of surgery.

For patients undergoing regional techniques, appropriate monitoring should still include pulse oximetry, NIBP, ECG, and, in cases where sedation is being used, end-tidal carbon dioxide should also be monitored [2]. It is essential that baseline readings are taken prior to commencing anaesthesia.

Pulse Oximetry

Measuring the amount of oxygen circulating within the arterial blood is useful for assessing a patient's condition. Peripheral oxygen saturation (SpO_2) can be measured using a non-invasive pulse oximeter and is used to estimate arterial oxygen saturation (SaO_2), which can also be measured directly by blood gas analysis. A single red blood cell can contain 200–300 million haemoglobin molecules. Each haemoglobin molecule can transport up to four oxygen molecules at which point it can be described as 'saturated' with oxygen; when all the binding sites are full with oxygen, the haemoglobin is 100% saturated.

A pulse oximeter usually takes the form of a probe that can be placed on an extremity of the patient such as the finger, toe, or earlobe, where there is an adequate peripheral pulse. For neonates and infants, such probes are often too large and risk providing an inaccurate reading and pressure damage to the skin; a disposable adhesive oximeter is more appropriate. The site of the saturation probe should be changed at 2-hour intervals to preserve skin integrity and should be assessed at the end of the procedure. During anaesthesia, SpO_2 should lie between 95% and 100%; a value below 94% indicates hypoxia and should be treated quickly, and below 90% should be regarded as a clinical emergency [3]. The monitoring of SpO_2 is such a significant indicator of a patient's condition that it is included on the World Health Organization's Safer Surgery Checklist [4].

Pulse oximetry utilises the differing electromagnetic spectra (one of the ranges of radiation) of oxygenated haemoglobin (HbO_2) and deoxygenated haemoglobin (Hb) to detect changes and generate a reading. The visual difference between arterial and venous blood is usually obvious and is caused by HbO_2 appearing redder, whereas Hb appears bluer. The electromagnetic spectrum for each is different, except at 660 nm, at which point they are the same. Pulse oximeters work by transmitting alternating beams of red and infrared light from a pair of light-emitting diodes (LEDs) through the tissue (at frequencies of 660 nm and 940 nm) in a sequence at a rate of 30 times per second (see Figure 16.1). The

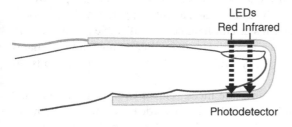

LEDs
Red Infrared

Photodetector

Figure 16.1 Pulse oximeter (reprinted from C. Vacanti, S. Segal, P. Sikka, and R. Urman (eds.), *Essential Clinical Anesthesia*. Cambridge: Cambridge University Press, 2011)

tissues, including blood vessels, absorb some of this light and a photodiode at the opposite side detects how much of the light remains as it emerges from the body. The result of this at 660 nm provides a reference point that represents background tissue absorption as the absorption spectra are the same for both HbO_2 and Hb at this frequency. This can then be compared with the result obtained at 940 nm as a reference point and subsequently detects changes that are due to the variation in haemoglobin saturation. This is done through electronically eliminating background activity and the use of a complex algorithm, with results averaged out over a few seconds as per the Beer–Lambert law of absorbance, thus excluding readings from stationary tissue, venous, and capillary blood, and resulting in a value being determined for arterial SpO_2 [5].

Pulse oximetry is not without limitations. There is a time lag of several seconds between what is displayed and the patient's true saturation status. There can be a significant delay in identifying acute desaturation; the response time to desaturation is quicker with an ear probe (<20 seconds) compared to a finger probe (>60 seconds). Oximeters are also unable to detect abnormal haemoglobins and can lead to under- or over-reading. Carboxyhaemoglobin (HbCO), present in those who have been exposed to carbon monoxide, can over-read at 1% for every 1% of HbCO, so a CO-oximeter should be used where carbon monoxide poisoning is suspected. Some more recent pulse oximeter designs utilise multiple wavelengths to avoid providing a false saturation reading due to the presence of carboxyhaemoglobin.

As the pulse oximeter only detects pulsatile flow, when blood pressure is low such as in hypovolaemic shock, low cardiac output, or if the patient has an arrhythmia, the pulse may be weak and so difficult for the oximeter to detect a signal. This is also the case if the patient is cold, as peripheral vessels become vasoconstricted leading to reduced blood flow, resulting in a poor signal. Other factors that can affect readings are patient movement, including shivering, and a bright light on the sensor. Nail polish has previously been considered to interfere with readings; however, the most recent evidence shows that in most cases any reduction, if seen, fell within the usual margin of error of accuracy of the oximeter and therefore is not clinically significant [6].

Non-invasive Blood Pressure

Blood pressure is a measurement of the circulating blood volume on the blood vessel walls. Blood pressure is measured in millimetres of mercury (mmHg), which is a manometric unit of pressure. A typical adult blood pressure may be 110 mmHg when the heart beats (systolic) and 70 mmHg when the heart relaxes (diastolic). Blood pressure can vary with age, disease, patient positioning, stress, and because of the drugs that have been administered. NIBP monitoring is undertaken using a sphygmomanometer. To obtain a reading, a pneumatic cuff of the appropriate size is placed, usually around the patient's upper arm. Cuffs should have a width approximately 40% of the arm's circumference, the inflatable bladder within should encompass half of the arm [7]. This is essential to maintain accuracy as a cuff that is too small will overestimate blood pressure, while one that is too large leads to underestimation.

The cuff is connected to a meter, recording the measurement in mmHg. If a manual sphygmomanometer is used, then the cuff is first inflated to occlude the blood vessels and so restrict blood flow. The cuff is then slowly released until stage 1 Korotkoff sounds (named after Dr Nikolai Korotkoff who discovered them) are heard with a stethoscope overlying the artery; these are 'whooshing' sounds that signify the return of blood flow through the brachial artery. This denotes the systolic blood pressure. The cuff is then further released until the pressure falls to the point at which no sounds can be heard once more (stage 5); this value is recorded as the diastolic pressure [8].

During surgery, it would be impractical to conduct NIBP monitoring using the manual method, which relies on auscultation of the brachial artery as the cuff is inflated and deflated, and so a digital meter is employed. Such meters utilise a microprocessor pressure transducer to detect oscillometric measurements from arterial pulsations in place of auscultation to calculate values to provide a reading. Systolic pressure corresponds to rapidly increasing oscillations, with diastolic pressure corresponding to rapidly decreasing oscillations. Mean arterial pressure is denoted by the maximum oscillation at the lowest cuff pressure.

There are additional considerations to acquiring NIBP measurements during surgery. Placement of the cuff should typically be on the opposite arm to the site of intravenous access to avoid intermittent obstruction of the flow of intravenous fluids and/or medication, as well as the backflow of blood into the cannula and intravenous giving set. If only one arm is available for both monitoring and infusion, then a one-way anti-reflux valve should be used on any intravenous giving set to prevent backflow, or other options for placing the cuff could be considered, such as the calf. Such instances include upper limb surgery or in conditions like lymphoedema. NIBP readings are taken regularly throughout the duration of surgery and can be affected by several factors such as any pre-existing diagnosis, medications, and the type and duration of surgery. As NIBP monitoring records only intermittent 'snapshots' of blood pressure it may not provide the level of monitoring required in critical illness or haemodynamic stability, in which case invasive blood pressure monitoring by way of an arterial line should be utilised.

ECG

Although a full 12-lead ECG is used for diagnostic purposes, a three-lead ECG is common for continuous monitoring to permit analysis of the cardiac rhythm perioperatively and can detect arrhythmias arising from cardiac disease, drugs, hypoxia, hypercarbia, and electrolyte imbalance. It is essential that good contact is made with the skin surface for the sticky electrodes to minimise interference. Damp skin and the presence of hair are both common problems which can reduce the adherence and quality of the electrical contact of the electrodes.

Normal cardiac rhythm is referred to as sinus rhythm, but it is possible for patients to have abnormal rhythms and to be asymptomatic [9]. The ECG can be used to monitor the heart rhythm and rate in the pre-, intra-, and postoperative phases of care. Though this is the main technique used, it also presents some limitations, such as electrical interference due to mechanical activity or diathermy limiting its efficacy. Surgical or patient factors may alter the sites available for electrode placement and can also have a bearing on the traces displayed.

Figure 16.2 shows an electrocardiogram depicting sinus rhythm. Each feature of the trace can be summarised as follows:

P wave: This shows atrial contraction after the initiation of the conduction process by the sinoatrial (SA) node. The shape of the P wave may be altered by abnormal activity such as atrial hypertrophy.

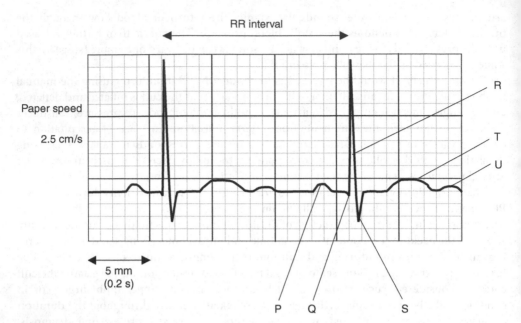

Figure 16.2 Sample electrocardiogram trace (reprinted from T. Smith, C. Pinnock, and T. Lin (eds.). *Fundamentals of Anaesthesia*, 3rd ed. Cambridge: Cambridge University Press, 2009, p. 274)

PR interval: This represents the time taken for the electrical impulse to travel from the SA node and to pass the atrioventricular (AV) node. Measurement starts from the P wave to the beginning of the QRS complex. Normal timing is considered as 0.12–0.20 seconds and tells us that the impulse has travelled through the conduction system in the correct manner.

QRS complex: This is measured after the PR interval and represents the conductivity pathway during the ventricular contraction. There are three distinct waves within this segment – Q, R, and S. The Q wave precedes the R wave and may be deeper or wider than normal in myocardial infarction, but the QRS complex is usually considered as a single entity with a normal duration of 0.08–0.10 seconds). A longer QRS duration or wider complex is caused by a longer time for the impulse to travel through the ventricles. Examples of causes are ventricular arrhythmias and bundle branch block.

ST segment: This represents when the heart has a brief resting state after ventricular depolarisation. This may be lower in myocardial ischaemia (ST depression) or elevated in myocardial infarction (ST elevation).

T wave: This is usually rounded and upright, representing ventricular repolarisation. Abnormalities can occur due to ischaemia, hyperkalaemia, and myocardial infarction.

QT interval: This represents the start of ventricular depolarisation and the end of ventricular repolarisation and is one of the most important aspects of the ECG. The interval is measured from the beginning of the QRS complex to the end of the T wave. The time varies depending on an individual's heart rate, with the average being 0.35–0.42 seconds. The QT interval varies with heart rate so a 'corrected' value of QT_c is calculated.

Airway Gas Analysis

The monitoring of airway gases is important to ensure the patient is anaesthetised appropriately. Carbon dioxide, nitrous oxide, and anaesthetic vapours absorb infrared radiation at different wavelengths, and this is utilised in monitoring equipment to detect gas levels in expired gases [10]. Capnography is the measurement of carbon dioxide against time, and it produces a capnography trace, which is a graphical plot of the partial pressure of expired carbon dioxide, confirming that ventilation is taking place (see Figure 16.3). Expired carbon dioxide is measured in kPa or mmHg; normal values are 4.0–5.7 kPa or 35–45 mmHg and should be continuously monitored when a patient is being ventilated. If no waveform trace is present following an intubation attempt it should be assumed that the endotracheal tube is in the wrong place such as the oesophagus.

Airway Pressure

Airway pressure monitoring should always be used whenever positive-pressure ventilation is being used as excessive pressures can lead to barotrauma (damage to the lungs) [7]. Pressure monitors are now incorporated into ventilators and so separate pressure monitors are rarely used. Maximum pressures can be set on ventilators to help protect the patient; however, these measure the pressure within the monitor rather than within the airway itself [10].

Peripheral Nerve Stimulation

Peripheral nerve stimulation is typically used towards the end of a surgical procedure to assess whether neuromuscular blockade from the use of muscle relaxants has reduced adequately for the reversal of anaesthesia. This is done through transcutaneous stimulation of a peripheral nerve with a current of approximately 50 mA via two electrodes, and either observing, feeling, or measuring the response. An example commonly used is stimulation of the ulnar nerve at the wrist and monitoring the contraction of the adductor pollicis, the muscle that adducts the thumb. The most used stimulation consists of four stimuli and is often referred to as a 'train-of-four' (TOF) stimulation. This assesses the degree of

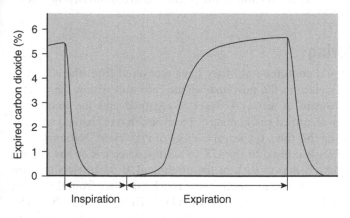

Figure 16.3 Capnograph trace (reprinted from T. Smith, C Pinnock, and T. Lin (eds.). *Fundamentals of Anaesthesia*, 3rd ed. Cambridge: Cambridge University Press, 2009, p. 813)

neuromuscular blockade by comparing the strength of the fourth 'twitch' to that of the first. Other sequences are the double-burst stimulation, tetanic stimulus, and post-tetanic count (PTC). A PTC is used in cases where a TOF stimulation is unsuccessful to assess profound neuromuscular blockade [11].

Temperature Monitoring

The maintenance of body temperature, normothermia, is a key aspect of patient safety given the many factors within perioperative care that can cumulatively lower the body temperature significantly, leading to hypothermia. These include the cooler theatre environment, the body being exposed, open wounds, blood loss, the use of anaesthetic gases, and muscle relaxants which prevent the action of shivering. This is exacerbated further in particular groups of patients: the elderly, the very young, burns patients, and those who are vascularly compromised. The UK's National Institute for Health and Care Excellence guidance on the prevention and management of hypothermia in adults having surgery [12] states that patients should have a temperature of 36 °C or above before induction of anaesthesia is commenced unless clinical urgency requires surgery to be expedited. During surgery, the following should be undertaken to reduce heat loss and maintain body temperature [12]:

- The patient should remain covered and not exposed until surgical preparation.
- 500 mL or more of intravenous fluids and blood products should be warmed to 37 °C using a fluid warming device.
- A forced air warming device should be used for surgeries longer than 30 minutes, or when patients are at higher risk of inadvertent hypothermia.
- Intraoperative irrigation fluids should be warmed in a thermostatic warming cabinet to 38–40 °C prior to use.
- Temperature should be monitored for patients to ensure that a core body temperature of between 36.5 °C and 37.5 °C is maintained, and is essential during procedures expected to take longer than 30 minutes.
- Temperature monitoring can be carried out intermittently using a tympanic thermometer. Continuous monitoring should be used for procedures longer than 60 minutes using an invasive temperature probe placed in the nasopharynx, or the oesophagus below the level of the bifurcation of the trachea to avoid interference from gas flow.

Postoperative Monitoring

Monitoring of the patient should continue until they have recovered from the effects of anaesthesia. Initially, this takes place in the post-anaesthetic care unit within the theatre department itself while full control of airway reflexes is regained and the immediate postoperative complications are identified and managed. To ensure that the patient remains physiologically stable [13] during this time, the Royal College of Physicians' National Early Warning Score System (NEWS2) is utilised in the UK to aid the detection of any patient deterioration. This system assigns scores to each of the physiological parameters that are routinely taken during patient monitoring to identify how much they vary from the norm, with the aggregate score identifying when action is required [14]. These readings should be recorded on a NEWS2 chart to enable comparisons to previous recordings and are continued on the ward or day surgery unit once the patient is transferred and care handed over from theatre staff to the ward or similar.

References

1. A. A. Klein, T. Meek, E. Allcock, et al. Recommendations for standards of monitoring during anaesthesia and recovery: guideline from the Association of Anaesthetists. *Anaesthesia* 2021; **76**: 1212–1223.

2. J. Kim and J. Gadsden. Monitoring and sedation in regional anesthesia. In A. D. Kaye, R.D. Urman, and N. Vadivelu (eds.), *Essentials of Regional Anaesthesia*, 2nd ed. Cham, Cham Springer International Publishing, 2018, pp. 107–120.

3. World Health Organization. *Pulse Oximetry Training Manual.* Geneva: WHO, 2011.

4. A. B. Haynes, T. G. Weiser, W. R. Berry, et al. A surgical safety checklist to reduce morbidity and mortality in a global population. *The New England Journal of Medicine* 2009; **360**: 491–499.

5. E. D. Chan, M. M. Chan, and M. M. Chan. Pulse oximetry: understanding its basic principles facilitates appreciation of its limitations. *Respiratory Medicine* 2013; **107**: 789–799.

6. S. Ballesteros-Peña, I. Fernández-Aedo, A. Picón, et al. Influence of nail polish on pulse oximeter readings of oxygen saturation: a systematic review. *Emergencias* 2015; **27**: 325–331.

7. M. Gwinnut and C. L. Gwinnut. *Clinical Anaesthesia*, 5th ed. Oxford: John Wiley & Sons. 2016.

8. R. Hammond and H. Spurgeon. Observations. In L. Dougherty and S. Lister (eds.), *The Royal Marsden Manual of Clinical Nursing Procedures*, 9th ed. Hoboken, NJ: John Wiley & Sons 2015, pp. 595–674.

9. J. R. C. Hampton. *The ECG Made Easy*, 8th ed. Edinburgh: Churchill Livingstone, 2013.

10. S. Scott. Clinical measurement and monitoring. In A. R. Aitkenhead and J. P. Thompson (eds.), *Smith and Aitkenhead's Textbook of Anaesthesia*, 6th ed. London: Elsevier 2013, pp. 312–356.

11. H. Kennedy and M. Wilson. Monitoring techniques: neuromuscular blockade and depth of anaesthesia. *Anaesthesia and Intensive Care Medicine* 2020; **21**: 373–378.

12. National Institute for Health and Care Excellence. Hypothermia: prevention and management in adults having surgery clinical guideline [CG65]. Available from: www.nice.org.uk/guidance/cg65.

13. N. Preston and M. Gregory. Patient recovery and post-anaesthesia care unit (PACU). *Anaesthesia and Intensive Care Medicine* 2015; **16**: 443–445.

14. Royal College of Physicians *National Early Warning Score (NEWS)2: Standardising the Assessment of Acute-Illness Severity in the NHS.* Updated report of a working party. London: RCP, 2017.

Haemodynamic Monitoring

Michael Donnellon

Introduction

Haemodynamic monitoring describes the measurement of the cardiovascular stability of the patient. Invasive blood pressure monitoring and central venous pressure monitoring provide a 'real-time' measurement of the patient's haemodynamic status and better allows clinicians to pre-emptively treat a patient before a more serious problem arises. Although invasive blood pressure monitoring has several advantages compared to non-invasive blood pressure monitoring, it is not without risk. Central venous pressure monitoring is similarly beneficial in that it supports the clinical decision making regarding a patient's fluid status [1] but also comes with additional risks, such as accidental arterial punctures, haematomas, and infection.

Arterial Cannulation and Invasive Blood Pressure Monitoring

Arterial cannulation enables the measurement of invasive blood pressure and access for repeated arterial blood sampling. Although the procedure is not without its hazards and complications, the direct measurement of arterial pressure using an indwelling cannula or catheter is the most accurate and real-time method of monitoring beat-to-beat blood pressure [2].

Once only witnessed in intensive care units and cardiac operating theatres, invasive blood pressure monitoring is now far more routine. Direct measurement of arterial pressure is indicated where rapid fluctuations in pressure are anticipated, where accurate control of blood pressure is required, and for repeated sampling of blood gases [3]. Invasive blood pressure monitoring would also be indicated for those patients receiving vasoactive drugs.

Contraindications

Arterial cannulation is contraindicated for those patients experiencing uncontrolled coagulopathy and where local infection may prohibit the choice of puncture site. As with any invasive technique, there are complications associated with arterial cannulation. These include infection, line disconnection and bleeding, thrombosis, embolisation (air or blood), tissue necrosis, injury to nearby nerves, retained guidewire (Seldinger technique), accidental drug administration, and dampened waveforms leading to misinterpretation of invasive blood pressure readings.

Sites for Cannulation

Common sites for cannulation insertion include the radial, ulnar, brachial femoral, and dorsalis pedis arteries. Table 17.1 identifies the clinical points of interest of each insertion

Table 17.1 Equipment required for arterial cannulation

Cannulation site	Clinical points of interest
Radial artery	Good accessibility Position of the wrist can cause overdamping
Ulnar artery	Primary source of blood flow to the hand
Brachial artery	Median nerve damage is a potential hazard
Femoral artery	Accurate Increased risk of infection Catheter required
Dorsalis pedis artery	Favoured in neonates Difficult to cannulate

site. The radial artery is the most common site for cannulation due to its accessibility and the presence of a collateral blood supply [4]. The radial artery is connected to the ulnar artery through the palmar arch in 25% of patients. An Allen's test can be used to determine the collateral blood flow in the hand and is performed by compressing both the radial and ulnar arteries while the patient clenches their fist. Observing for skin colour changes while sequentially releasing pressure on each artery indicates the dominant artery supplying blood to the hand. However, the value of the Allen's test in predicting potential ischaemic injury after radial artery cannulation is controversial [5].

The equipment required for arterial cannulation includes:

- a monitor;
- an interface cable;
- an arterial cannula or catheter;
- a pressure monitoring set including transducer;
- a solution to maintain pressure monitoring set patency;
- a pressure infusion bag;
- a 2% chlorhexidine gluconate and 70% isopropyl alcohol skin preparation; and
- a transparent dressing.

Arterial Cannulation Insertion Techniques

Three insertion techniques are associated with arterial cannulation; direct threading, trans-fixation–withdrawal, and the Seldinger technique. Typically, when cannulating the radial artery using the direct-threading technique, the cannula is inserted at a 30° angle with the wrist in dorsiflexion. The Seldinger technique is beneficial where difficulty in cannulation insertion is expected. However, the disadvantage of this technique is the increased risk of infection due to handling of the guidewire and the possibility of blood loss.

Most commonly, an arterial cannula is used for insertion into the artery. The arterial cannula (Figure 17.1) is suitable for radial artery placement with a size of 20 g for an adult and 22 g for paediatrics. The cannula is made of polytetrafluoroethene (Teflon) and has parallel walls (over the needle) [6]. If a three-way tap is attached to the arterial cannula, for safety purposes this should be coloured coded with a red peg to prevent inadvertent drug

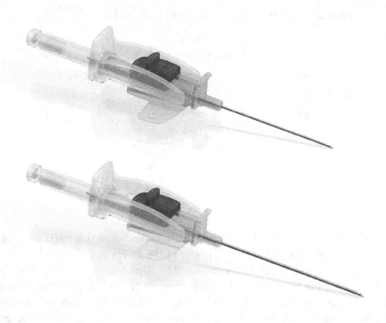

Figure 17.1 Arterial SWITCH™ (courtesy of Greiner Bio-One Ltd)

administration. After successful placement, the arterial cannula should be secured with a transparent peripheral intravenous catheter dressing. Some anaesthetists may prefer to suture the cannula in place for additional security.

Pressure Monitoring Set and Transducer

Connected to the arterial cannula or catheter is the fluid-filled pressure monitoring set, incorporating a transducer and flushing device (Figure 17.2). The tubing of the pressure monitoring set (and any extension tubing connected to this) should be non-compliant to ensure passage of the waveform. Maintenance of the arterial cannula or catheter is essential in order to prevent clotting. The pressure monitoring set is kept patent by the use of a flush solution infused under pressure. This solution can be either a 500-mL bag sodium chloride 0.9% or 500 mL of heparinised (1,000 iu/L) sodium chloride 0.9%. The use of heparinised sodium chloride 0.9% is associated with several risks including thrombocytopaenia and haemorrhage [7].

Blood sampling from a heparinised arterial cannula or catheter may give clinically misleading information because of contamination with small amounts of heparin. However, the use of heparinised sodium chloride 0.9% is associated with a significant reduction in the incidence of arterial catheter occlusion and thrombosis together with an increased lifespan of the arterial cannula or catheter [8]. Once primed, the 500-mL bag is pressurised to 300 mmHg to prevent backflow through the cannula/catheter. Although national advice in the UK has been published identifying that sodium chloride 0.9% solution without heparin should be used as the flush solution [9], there is a suggestion that the

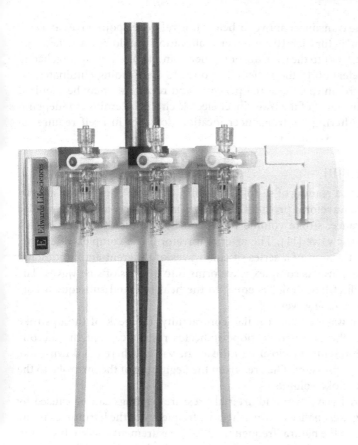

Figure 17.2 TruWave™ pressure transducers and TruClip™ holder (courtesy of Edwards Lifesciences Corporation)

guidance should be reviewed given the higher incidence of blockage when using sodium chloride 0.9% solution without heparin [7]. Furthermore, critically ill patients with COVID-19 have been noticed to experience high rates of arterial cannula thrombosis, and some centres suggest that heparinised saline should therefore be used when managing this condition [10]. The flushing device within the pressure monitoring set allows a basal flow of 2–4 mL per hour of solution, and manual flushing is also possible.

The pressure in the artery is transmitted to a transducer, which in turn converts the pulsatile pressure to an electrical signal; this is then amplified and displayed in a monitor. A diaphragm acts as an interface between the transducer and the fluid-filled tubing of the pressure monitoring set. Most transducers contain four bonded wire strain gauges. Pulsatile pressure causes a small movement of the diaphragm, which in turn alters the length of the strain gauge wires and electrical resistance/current flow. The four strain gauges are configured as four resistors of a Wheatstone bridge circuit, which uses a null-deflection galvanometer system. Changes in resistance and current are measured and displayed as systolic, diastolic, and mean arterial pressure (MAP).

The transducer should be positioned at the level of the right atrium/mid-axillary line and the fourth intercostal space as this provides a reference point (known as the phlebostatic axis). Raising or lowering the transducer above or below this reference point gives an error reading equivalent to 7.5 mmHg for each 10 cm. A zero calibration should be undertaken by turning the three-way tap adjacent to the transducer (rather than a three-way tap attached to the arterial cannula or catheter) off to the patient and open to air. Zeroing eliminates the effect of atmospheric pressure on the measured pressure and re-zeroing may be required periodically to prevent baseline drift of the transducer electric circuits. Zeroing is independent of the reference point. Altering the transducer location does not in itself require re-zeroing as atmospheric pressure is constant.

Arterial Pressure Waveform

The monitor not only displays a reading of systolic, diastolic, and MAP, but also an arterial waveform (Figure 17.3). The waveform provides additional information including cardiac contractility, vascular resistance, stroke volume together with the dicrotic notch, which represents closure of the aortic valve [11]. The arterial waveform is a complex sine wave, which can be deemed to be the sum of a series of sine waves of different amplitudes and frequencies. Fourier analysis converts complex waveforms into a series of sine waves. The fundamental frequency (or first harmonic) is equal to the heat rate and subsequent harmonics (up to 10) contribute to the waveform.

The upstroke part of the wave reflects cardiac contractility, the peak of the upstroke represents systolic pressure, the downstroke slope indicates resistance, and the dicrotic notch on the downstroke represents the closure of the aortic valve. Where the downstroke flattens, this indicates diastolic pressure. The area from the beginning of the upstroke to the dicrotic notch estimates the stroke volume.

Inaccuracies of the arterial waveform and arterial pressure readings can be caused by either resonance or damping. Resonance occurs when the frequency of the harmonics in the pressure waveform is similar to the natural frequency of the measurement system. Increased resonance will elevate the systolic blood pressure reading and a lowering of the diastolic blood pressure reading. Inaccuracy due to resonance can be avoided by using components

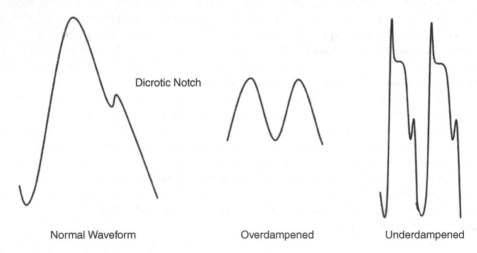

Figure 17.3 Arterial waveforms

with a natural frequency dissimilar to arterial pressure waves. In practice, this involves using stiff, short, and wide tubing.

Damping is the loss of energy and the reduced amplitude of oscillations due to frictional forces. Overdamping underestimates systolic blood pressure and overestimates diastolic blood pressure, with loss of detail in the arterial waveform. Causes of over overdamping include clots, air bubbles, or kinks within the pressure monitoring set. When using the radial artery as a cannulation site, the position of the wrist can also cause overdamping. Underdamping overestimates systolic blood pressure and underestimates diastolic blood pressure, with an exaggerated or spiking of the arterial waveform.

It is important to maintain an optimally dampened arterial waveform otherwise there is a risk of inaccurate blood pressure readings, and treatment options could have an adverse effect on the safety of the patient. In both resonance and damping, the MAP remains constant and therefore many departments choose to include recordings of MAP on their anaesthetic charts [12].

In the hypovolaemic patient, the arterial waveform can be narrow with a low dicrotic notch and a systolic peak pressure which varies with the respiratory cycle. This is sometimes referred to as respiratory swing and can be analysed electronically to guide fluid therapy.

Removal of the Arterial Cannula

Removal of the arterial cannula or catheter is performed using an aseptic technique, and the dressing should be removed and the cannula or catheter gently withdrawn while applying pressure on the insertion site, which should then be maintained for five minutes. The integrity of the cannula or catheter should be checked before disposing of it, and a gauze dressing should then be applied over the insertion site.

Arterial Blood Gas Analysis

Arterial blood gas (ABG) analysis is an important diagnostic tool to assess the adequacy of ventilation, perfusion of the tissues and acid-base balance. ABG analysis primarily measures five key parameters, these are: hydrogen ion concentration (pH), partial pressure of oxygen (PaO_2), partial pressure of carbon dioxide ($PaCO_2$), bicarbonate ($HCO3^-$), and base excess (BE) (see Table 17.2).

The results of the ABG analysis will also provide information on:

- lactate (0.5–2.0 mmol/L);
- potassium (K^+) (3.5–5.0 mmol/L);
- sodium (Na^+) (136–145 mmol/L);
- chloride (Cl^-) (98–106 mmol/L);
- glucose (3.6–5.3 mmol/L);
- haemoglobin (Hb) (1–17g/dL);
- methaemoglobin (MetHb) (0–1.5%); and
- arterial oxygen saturation (SaO_2) (>95%).

There are many published guides available to aid in the interpretation of an ABG using a step-by-step process. Despite there being some variation in the order, a common approach is:

(1) Review the patient.

Table 17.2 Normal arterial blood gas ranges

pH	7.35–7.45
$PaCO_2$	4.67–6 kPa
PaO_2	10.67–13.33 kPa
HCO_3^-	22–26 mmol/L
BE	−2 to +2

(2) Assess the pH for the presence of acidosis (pH < 7.35) or alkalosis (pH > 7.45).

(3) Assess the $PaCO_2$.

(4) Assess the bicarbonate.

(5) Match either the $PaCO_2$ or the HCO_3 with the pH.

(6) Determine whether the $PaCO_2$ or the HCO_3 go in the opposite direction of the pH.

(7) Assess the PaO_2 and SaO_2 for hypoxaemia.

Central Venous Cannulation and Measurement of Central Venous Pressure

Central venous cannulation is the insertion of a catheter into a large vein such as the internal jugular, subclavian, or femoral vein. Indications for central venous cannulation include the measurement of central venous pressure (CVP), access for continuing infusions, access for venotoxic drugs which require high blood flow to dilute the drug, such as vasopressors, inotropes, and total parenteral nutrition [13]. Additionally, cannulation permits large venous access during massive haemorrhage, facilitation of transvenous cardiac pacing, and haemofiltration. The procedure is not without risk with reports of catheter-related bloodstream infections arising from central venous cannulation being at 5–26% and patients suffering mechanical complications (e.g., dysrhythmias, nerve injury during cannulation, pneumothorax) at 5–19% [14].

CVP represents right atrial pressure, which in turn equals right-ventricular end-diastolic (filling) pressure. The normal range of CVP during spontaneous respiration is 3–6 mmHg [15]. Measurement of CVP should not be interpreted in isolation but in conjunction with heart rate, blood pressure, and urine output. Although absolute values of CVP can be measured, its trend is more informative [16]. Originally, measurement was determined using the hydrostatic method (commonly a drum cartridge inserted into the antecubital vein and attached to a manometer) and measurement was in cmH_2O. A transducer system is now used and measurement is in mmHg.

Sites for Cannulation

The most common insertion sites for central venous cannulation include the internal jugular vein and the subclavian vein. The femoral vein, the antecubital vein, and the external jugular can also be used. Both the subclavian and the internal jugular veins carry a risk of pneumothorax; however, the subclavian vein is perhaps more comfortable postoperatively for the patient. The internal jugular vein carries a high rate of successful insertion, but occlusion can occur with head movement.

Central venous catheters (Figure 17.4) can be manufactured with several lumina (1 to 7) with sizes ranging from 12 g to 16 g; paediatric sizes are also available. Catheter lengths range from 12.5 cm to 20 cm. Catheters are often coated with an antimicrobial agent to reduce the risk of catheter-related bloodstream infections, with many manufacturers using silver based active ingredients to achieve this. Each lumen of the catheter leads to an individual aperture along the distal section of the catheter. The catheter is inserted under sterile conditions using the Seldinger approach. Initially, a cannula or needle is inserted into the vein and a J-shaped soft-tip guidewire is advanced through into the vein. The cannula can then be removed. The J-shape tip is designed to minimise trauma to the vein's endothelium [17]. A small incision in the skin is then made and a dilator is introduced over the guidewire in order to ease insertion of the catheter through the skin and subcutaneous tissue. The dilator is withdrawn and the catheter is 'railroaded' over the guidewire into its final position. The guidewire is then withdrawn, and the catheter is sutured into place and covered with a sterile, semi-permeable, transparent dressing. A chest X-ray should be undertaken for subclavian and internal jugular vein cannulations.

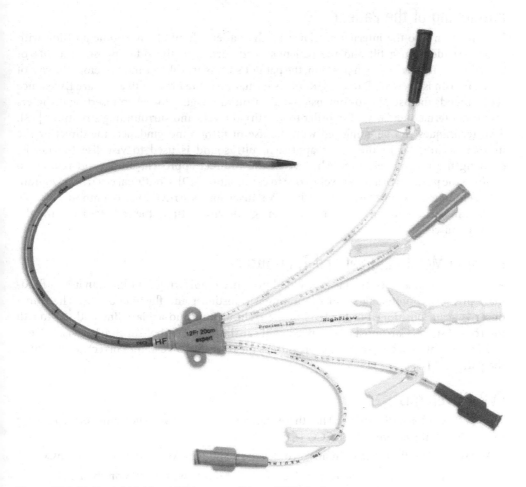

Figure 17.4 Multicath 5 Highflow UP™ (courtesy of Vygon UK Limited)

Equipment Required for Central Venous Cannulation

The equipment required for central venous cannulation includes:

- a monitor;
- an interface cable;
- a central venous cannula;
- three-way taps (one for each lumen);
- pressure monitoring set including transducer;
- a solution to maintain pressure monitoring set patency;
- a pressure infusion bag;
- a 2% chlorhexidine gluconate and 70% isopropyl alcohol skin preparation or povidine iodine solution;
- two-dimensional ultrasound imaging; and
- a transparent dressing.

Positioning of the Patient

For insertion into the internal jugular vein, the patient should be in supine position with slight Trendelenburg tilt and the patient's head turned to the side opposite the site of insertion. In this head-down position, the patient's veins are dilated and therefore the risk of air embolism is decreased. In the UK, the National Institute for Health and Care Excellence recommends the use of two-dimensional ultrasound imaging for when inserting catheters into the internal jugular vein in order to identify the vein and surrounding structures [18]. Two techniques can be employed with the use of ultrasound guidance, the direct or the indirect technique. In the direct approach, ultrasound is used to visualise the needle entering the vein in real time whereas, in the indirect approach, ultrasound is used to confirm the position of a patent vein prior to cannulation [19]. Continual electrocardiogram (ECG) monitoring must be in use during CVP insertion as arrhythmias (commonly ectopic beats) can occur, commonly attributed to the guidewire or tip of the catheter irritating the cardiac muscle.

Pressure Monitoring Set and Transducer

A similar system as used for invasive blood pressure monitoring is utilised, that is, a fluid-filled pressure monitoring set incorporating a transducer and flushing device. The transducer is again positioned at the level of the right atrium/mid-axillary line and the fourth intercostal space. Care must be taken to avoid causing an air embolism and, because CVP is low, it is essential to ensure that the pressure is measured relative to the correct zero point of the patient [11].

CVP Waveforms

The CVP waveform (Figure 17.5) has three characteristic positive deflections corresponding to the electrical elements of the ECG [15]:

A wave: This reflects the right atrial contraction and follows the P wave on the ECG.

C wave: This represents tricuspid valve closure and follows the QRS on the ECG.

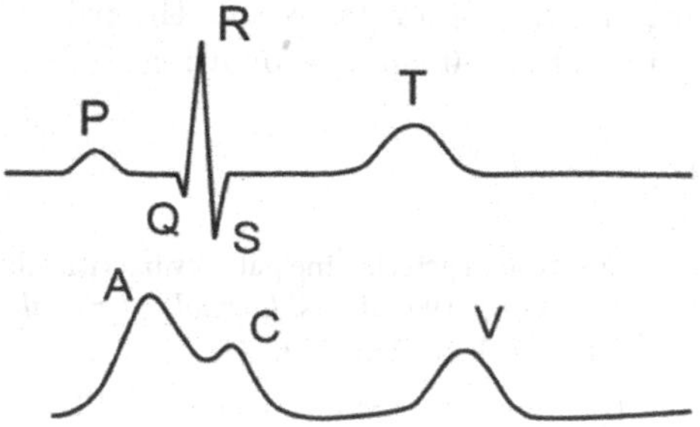

Figure 17.5 A CVP waveform

V wave: This represents the pressure generated to the right atrium by the contracting right ventricle and corresponds to the latter half of the T wave on the ECG.

Factors Affecting CVP Measurement

CVP can be raised due to an increase in intra-thoracic pressure such as intermittent positive-pressure ventilation. This is particularly significant when high levels of positive end-expiratory pressure are used [14]. Other causes include hypervoleamia, right-sided heart failure, and superior vena cava obstruction. CVP is lowered due to major haemorrhage, hypovolaemia leading to reduced venous return, reduced right atrial pressure, and reduced intra-thoracic pressure. A fluid challenge can be given in the presence of a low CVP measurement. In this circumstance, a rapid infusion of fluid is given and the CVP is measured. In the hypovolaemic patient, the CVP increases briefly and then falls to approximately the previous reading. In the euvolaemic patient, the CVP will show a greater and more sustained rise [16].

Complications Relating to Central Venous Cannulation

Cannula misplacement can result in the puncturing of the carotid artery, the subclavian artery, and the aortic arch. Misplacement may also cause a pneumothorax or haemothorax; unintended proximal direction is also possible. Arrhythmias are due to stimulation of the sinoatrial node, and a puncture of the endocardium can lead to a tamponade. Other complications include air embolism, occlusion, retained wire and infection.

Removal of the Central Venous Cannula

Central venous catheters should be removed when they are no longer required or when complications (e.g., occlusion, infection) are suspected. At the time of removal and in order to reduce the risk of an air embolism, the patient should lie flat and, if their condition allows, a head-down tilt should be applied at an angle of 10–20 degrees. If the patient is breathing spontaneously, they should be asked to take in and hold a deep breath. The catheter is then withdrawn and firm pressure should be applied to the site followed by the application of a transparent occlusive dressing. If the patient is unable to lie flat, they should undertake the Valsalva manoeuvre during catheter removal. In the ventilated patient, the catheter should be removed at the end of inspiration to minimise the risk of air embolism. The patient should subsequently remain in the supine position for at least 30 minutes following removal of central venous access [20].

References

1. B. Hill. Role of central venous pressure monitoring in critical care settings. *Nursing Standard* 2018; **32**: 41–48.

2. G. Thomas and D. Rees. Monitoring arterial blood pressure. *Anaesthesia and Intensive Care Medicine* 2018; **19**: 194–197.

3. C. Watson and M. Wilkinson. Monitoring central venous pressure, arterial pressure and pulmonary wedge pressure. *Anaesthesia and Intensive Care Medicine* 2011; **13**: 116–120.

4. P. Barash, B. Cullen, R. Stoelting, et al. *Clinical Anesthesia*, 7th ed. Philadelphia, PA: Lippincott Williams and Wilkins, 2013.

5. S. Wilson, I. Grunstein, E. Hirvela, and D. Price. Ultrasound-guided radial artery catheterisation and the modified Allen's test. *Journal of Emergency Medicine* 2010; **38**: 354–358.

6. Vygon. *Vigmed Switch Product Leaflet-v1.* Swindon: Vygon, 2018.

7. M. Everson, L. Webber, C. Penfold, S. Smith, and D. Freshwater-Turner. Finding a solution: heparinised saline versus normal saline in the maintenance of invasive arterial lines in intensive care *Journal of Intensive Care Society* 2016; **17**: 284–289.

8. R. Tully, B. McGrath, J. Moore, J. Rigg, and P. Alexander. Observational study of the effect of heparin-containing flush solutions on the incidence of arterial catheter occlusion. *Journal of Intensive Care Society* 2014; **15**: 213–215.

9. National Patient Safety Agency. *Rapid Response Report NPSA/2008/RRR002: Risks with Intravenous Heparin Solutions.* London: National Patient Safety Agency, 2008.

10. L. R. Maurer, C. M. Luckhurst, A. Hamidi, et al. A low dose heparinized saline protocol is associated with improved duration of arterial line patency in critically ill COVID-19 patients. *Journal of Critical Care* 2020; **60**: 253–259.

11. J. Thompson, I. Moppett, and M. Wiles. *Smith and Aitkenhead's Textbook of Anaesthesia*, 7th ed. London: Elsevier, 2019.

12. C. Goodman and G Kitchen. Monitoring arterial blood pressure. *Anaesthesia and Intensive Care Medicine* 2020; **22**: 49–53.

13. P. Williamson and C. Cattlin. Central venous cannulation. *Anaesthesia and Intensive Care Medicine* 2018; **19**: 627–628.

14. M. Gilbert Central venous pressure and pulmonary artery pressure monitoring. *Anaesthesia and Intensive Care Medicine* 2018; **19**: 189–193.

15. S. Adam, S. Osborne, and J. Welch. *Critical Care Nursing*, 3rd ed. Oxford: Oxford University Press, 2017.

16. M. Gwinutt and C. Gwinnutt. *Clinical Anaesthesia: Lecture Notes*, 7th ed. Chichester: John Wiley & Sons, 2017.

17. B. Al-Shaikh and S. Stacey. *Essentials of Equipment in Anaesthesia, Critical Care and Peri-Operative Medicine*, 5th ed. London: Elsevier, 2019.

18. National Institute for Health and Care Excellence. *Guidance on the Use of Ultrasound Locating Devices for Placing Central Venous Catheters.* London: National Institute for Health and Care Excellence, 2002.

19. S. Flood and A. Bodenham. Central venous cannulation: ultrasound techniques. *Anaesthesia and Intensive Care Medicine* 2015; **17**: 5–8.

20. C. J. McCarthy, S. Behravesh, S. G. Naidu, and R. Oklu. Air embolism: practical tips for prevention and treatment. *Journal of Clinical Medicine* 2016; **5**: 93.

Chapter 18

Fundamentals of Regional Anaesthesia

Will Angus and Karim Mukhtar

Introduction

Regional anaesthesia is the use of local anaesthetic drugs to block sensations of pain from a large area of the body. It is used to allow surgery to proceed either without general anaesthesia or combined with general anaesthesia to provide superior pain relief than can be achieved with analgesic drugs alone. Neuraxial blocks involve injection of local anaesthetic close to the spinal cord, and there are two broad categories – spinal and epidural. Peripheral nerve blocks involve injection of local anaesthetic near peripheral nerves or plexuses. This can be performed either using a landmark technique, a nerve stimulator, or with ultrasound guidance depending on the chosen block.

There are many advantages to the use of regional anaesthesia. Patients who have received regional anaesthesia tend to have superior postoperative analgesia, reduced side effects related to opioid analgesics, and increased overall satisfaction [1]. The ability to minimise the use of opioid analgesics and therefore expose patients to fewer side effects of these drugs may increase patient satisfaction by reducing postoperative nausea and vomiting and by causing less postoperative sedation, allowing earlier interaction with family. In patients at high risk of postoperative nausea and vomiting, it is advised to consider a regional technique in consensus guidelines [2].

There are other advantages besides reducing pain and improving patient satisfaction. Regional anaesthesia can reduce pulmonary complications such as pneumonia when compared to general anaesthesia [3]. It has been demonstrated to reduce cardiovascular complications and decrease mortality in certain patient populations [4], although careful patient selection and avoidance of complications of some regional techniques (such as hypotension) are critical. Regional anaesthesia has also been shown to reduce blood loss in major surgery – particularly lower limb surgery, though the mechanisms of this are not entirely clear [3]. As with all anaesthetic techniques, regional anaesthesia requires careful patient selection, correct preparation, and high standards to minimise risk and improve patient care.

Local Anaesthetic Toxicity

Local anaesthetic toxicity is a rare and life-threatening complication caused by systemic toxicity secondary to the injection of local anaesthetic drugs, primarily consisting of neurological and cardiovascular complications. Neurological signs may be disorientation, perioral tingling, tinnitus, and slurred speech progressing to generalised tonic–clonic seizures and coma. Cardiovascular signs may consist of hypotension and cardiac arrhythmias, which can be a wide array of conduction blocks, bradycardias, or ventricular tachyarrhythmias, or they may present with a sudden cardiac arrest with ventricular fibrillation or

191

asystole. Advanced life support must be initiated immediately with cessation of injection of any local anaesthetic. A lipid emulsion (such as Intralipid) must be administered and prolonged resuscitation of several hours should be considered. Those involved with caring for patients who have received regional anaesthesia should familiarise themselves with where lipid emulsion is stored and the emergency protocols for the management of local anaesthetic systemic toxicity, such as that provided by the Association of Anaesthetists [5], which is commonly available in areas where blocks are performed.

Central Neuraxial Blockade

Neuraxial blockade involves injection of local anaesthetic near to the spinal cord and central nerve roots within the spinal column. There are three neuraxial techniques in common use (see Figure 18.1). A subarachnoid block or 'spinal' involves injection of local anaesthetic in the subarachnoid space into the cerebrospinal fluid that surrounds the spinal cord. An epidural involves placement of a catheter in the epidural space via a Tuohy needle to allow continued infusion of local anaesthetic for more prolonged regional anaesthesia.

A caudal is less widely used in adult practice but involves injecting local anaesthetic into the caudal canal, allowing blockade of sacral nerve roots for 6–8 hours (see Figure 18.2). Caudal anaesthesia is frequently used in paediatric patients undergoing procedures such as inguinal and umbilical hernia repair, orchidopexy, and hypospadias surgery.

Preparation

Fully informed consent must be gained by the anaesthetist in the preoperative visit. Adequate intravenous access must be secured with intravenous fluids connected. Full monitoring as per the Association of Anaesthetists must be used (continuous ECG monitoring, pulse oximetry, and blood pressure). The procedure must be performed with sterile technique, requiring adequate skin preparation commonly using chlorhexidine 0.5% solution and a full surgical scrub undertaken by the anaesthetist who should then wear a hat, mask, sterile gown, and sterile gloves. Commonly, the block is performed with the patient sitting up and leaning slightly forwards to reduce lumbar lordosis and allow easier access between bony landmarks. Occasionally, for example for hip-fracture surgery, the block will be performed with the patient lying on the side and may require analgesia or mild sedation. Contraindications to central neuraxial blockade and potential complications are listed in Tables 18.1 and 18.2.

Spinal Anaesthesia

Injection of local anaesthetic into the subarachnoid space causes blockade of neural transmission within the spinal cord. This causes profound motor block (complete inability to move the legs) and sensory block (loss of sensation and pain). Hyperbaric ('heavy') bupivacaine, which contains bupivacaine (commonly 0.5% or 5 mg/mL) and glucose (80 mg/mL) is the most common local anaesthetic used. This results in an increased density, allowing it to flow with the aid of gravity to the desired spinal region depending on patient position. Often, the local anaesthetic will be combined with an opiate for longer-lasting analgesia, such as diamorphine or fentanyl. The dose and volume selected by the anaesthetist will be determined by the height of the block required and the duration of surgery.

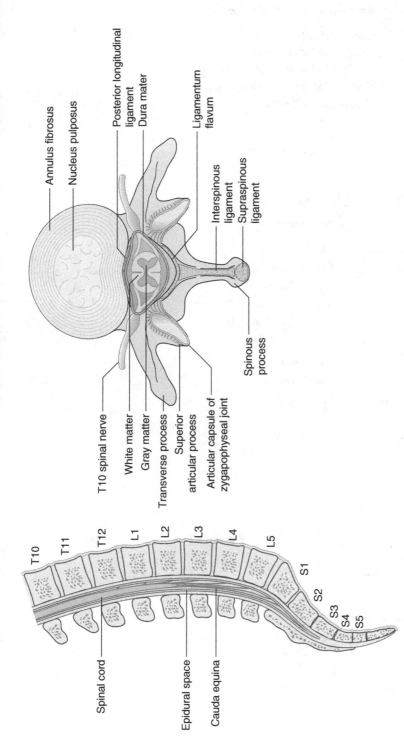

Figure 18.1 To perform a spinal, a needle is passed through the dura mater into the subarachnoid space; to perform an epidural, a needle is passed through the ligamentum flavum into the epidural space, without piercing the dura

Table 18.1 Contraindications to central neuraxial blockade

Absolute contraindications	Patient refusal Local anaesthetic allergy Active infection at injection site
Relative contraindications	Coagulopathy or thrombocytopaenia Anticoagulant medications Systemic sepsis Severe cardiac disease such as aortic stenosis Raised intracranial pressure

Table 18.2 Complications of central neuraxial blockade [6]

Complication	Occurrence
Significant hypotension	1 in 50
Post-dural puncture headache (PDPH)	1 in 100 (epidural) 1 in 500 (spinal)
Nerve damage	Temporary – 1 in 1,000 Permanent – 1 in 13,000
Epidural abscess	1 in 50,000
Meningitis	1 in 100,000
Epidural haematoma	1 in 170,000
Total spinal (accidental unconsciousness)	1 in 100,000
Severe nerve injury/ paralysis	1 in 250,000

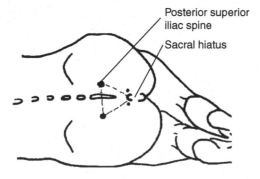

Posterior superior iliac spine

Sacral hiatus

Figure 18.2 Patient position for caudal anaesthesia

Indications

Spinal anaesthesia can provide anaesthesia for around 2 hours and analgesia for up to 12 hours depending on the drugs selected. It is commonly used in obstetrics for Caesarean section, lower limb surgery such as hip or knee arthroplasty, and urological surgery such as transurethral resection of the prostate.

Equipment

The following equipment is used:

- a 25-gauge (25 G) spinal needle (Sprotte, Whitacre, or Quinke) with an introducer;
- a sterile drape;
- a small sterile dressing;
- non-luer spinal syringes are increasingly used to prevent accidental connection of syringes containing drugs not intended for intrathecal injection; and
- 0.5% 'heavy' bupivacaine.

There are various types of spinal needles, largely separated into those with a conventional point and those with a 'pencil point'. Examples of pencil-point needles are the Sprotte and Whitacre, whereas an example of a conventional needle is the Quinke. A conventional needle has a sharp tip designed to cut through tissue with a distal opening for injection. A pencil-point needle has a blunt cone-shaped tip designed to be atraumatic as it passes through tissue, reducing the likelihood of post-dural puncture headache, a complication that presents 24–48 hours following dural puncture due to a cerebrospinal fluid leak characterised by post-dural headache, which is relieved by lying flat. Conservative management includes rest, regular pain relief, and staying hydrated until the headache resolves, which can be up to 10 days. If this does not work, then a blood patch might be indicated. This involves injecting 20–30 mL of the patient's own blood into the epidural space to seal the hole in the dura and relieve the post-dural headache.

Performing the Block

The patient can be positioned in either sitting or lateral position (see Figure 18.3), curled forwards to allow easier palpation of the lumbar spinous processes and easier passage of the needle between them. Often this will require an assistant standing in front of the patient to support their position and to offer reassurance. The procedure is performed using full sterile technique, with skin preparation, for example using 0.5% chlorhexidine and a full surgical scrub, wearing a sterile gown, gloves, and mask, by the anaesthetist. Higher concentrations of chlorhexidine solutions (e.g., 2%) is avoided due to the clear evidence of neurotoxicity [7].

The block is usually performed using landmark technique, commonly at the L2/3 or L3/4 interspace. This is identified by palpating the iliac crests and then locating a suitable space between spinous processes. If difficulty is encountered locating the landmarks, ultrasound may be used. Local anaesthetic (such as lignocaine) is injected to the skin and subcutaneous tissues to reduce discomfort during the procedure. The spinal needle is inserted until cerebrospinal fluid is seen and then the chosen local anaesthetic mixture injected. Any pain felt by the patient, such as pain down one leg, may indicate proximity to a nerve root and should be reported to the anaesthetist to allow redirection of the needle. Following injection, the patient should be laid flat to allow correct spread of the local anaesthetic.

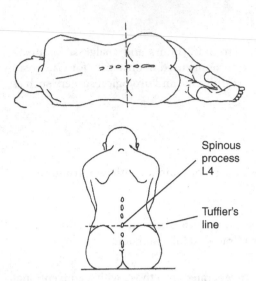

Figure 18.3 Patient positions for spinal anaesthesia

Spinous
process
L4

Tuffier's
line

There are other variants of this spinal technique, for example higher spinal injection to produce a 'segmental' spinal block, but these are beyond the scope of routine practice.

Monitoring

Blood pressure, continuous ECG, and pulse oximetry must be monitored. The height of the block is assessed by the presence and extent of the motor block and the sensory level. Sensation is commonly assessed using loss of cold sensation, for example with ethyl chloride spray.

Complications

Blood pressure must be monitored frequently as spinal anaesthesia can cause hypotension. The block may rise too high, causing the sensation of shortness of breath as the intercostal muscles become anaesthetised. Often this can be managed by simple reassurance. The anaesthetist must be vigilant for respiratory distress and be prepared to manage this. Rarely, a total spinal may occur. This is the result of anaesthesia of the brain stem, caused by a very high block, and presents with unconsciousness, apnoea, and bradycardia. This will require the airway to be secured by intubation and general anaesthesia commenced with support of the cardiovascular system, then allowing time for the block to recede adequately before the patient is allowed to wake and be extubated. Local anaesthetic toxicity is rare due to the small dosages used in spinal anaesthesia; however, close monitoring for this must always be undertaken.

Epidural Anaesthesia

Injection of local anaesthetic into the epidural space allows diffusion into the spinal cord and nerve roots. The epidural space describes the space between the dura mater and the spinal canal. Using a continuous infusion of local anaesthetic via an epidural catheter allows more prolonged anaesthesia and analgesia. The area affected will depend on the dose and volume of local anaesthetic, as well as the location of insertion of the epidural catheter.

Indications

Epidural anaesthesia is commonly used to provide analgesia via continuous infusion for 48–72 hours postoperatively, after which the catheter should be removed to reduce the risk of infection. Local guidelines should be followed regarding the timing of epidural removal in relation to timing of thromboprophylaxis, anticoagulant, or antiplatelet medications. Epidurals are commonly used in obstetrics for labour analgesia and can also be used during major abdominal, vascular, and thoracic procedures.

Equipment

The following equipment is used:

- a 16 G or 18 G Tuohy needle with a loss-of-resistance syringe containing normal saline;
- an epidural catheter and filter connection;
- a sterile drape;
- a clear occlusive dressing and fixation tape/dressing to secure the catheter; and
- correct labelling of the catheter to ensure that only the epidural solution is connected

Performing the Block

The location to which the epidural is sited is determined by the desired area to be anaesthetised; for example, a lumbar epidural for labour analgesia or a thoracic epidural for thoracic or abdominal surgery. The site of injection is identified via the landmark technique. If difficulty is encountered locating the landmarks, ultrasound may be used.

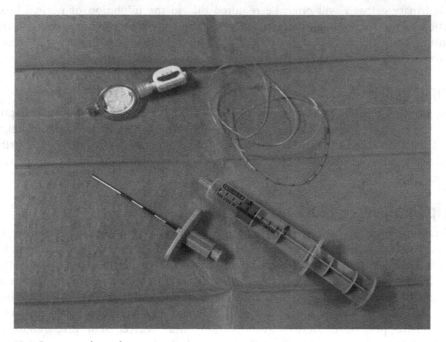

Figure 18.4 Equipment for performing epidural insertion: Tuohy needle and epidural catheter with filter for connection to the giving set

Local anaesthetic (such as lignocaine) is injected into the skin and subcutaneous tissues to reduce discomfort during the procedure. The Tuohy needle is advanced while connected to a loss-of-resistance syringe containing saline (although air may also be used). When loss of resistance is felt, implying entry into the epidural space (there is a negative pressure in this space), the epidural catheter is inserted to the desired depth. Care must be taken to observe for the presence of cerebrospinal fluid or blood in the catheter, indicating incorrect placement. Any pain felt by the patient, such as pain down one leg, may indicate proximity to a nerve root and should be reported to the anaesthetist to allow redirection of the needle. A test dose of a small amount of bupivacaine is administered to ensure the epidural catheter is not in the subarachnoid space (inadvertent subarachnoid spinal placement), before the epidural infusion, commonly after a loading dose of local anaesthetic.

The epidural catheter must be secured to prevent displacement during use, most commonly using a sterile transparent adhesive dressing over the puncture site and adhesive tape to secure the catheter up the back of the patient. The catheter must be secured such that is accessible during surgery and postoperatively, for example, over the shoulder of the patient. A transparent sterile dressing is used over the puncture site to allow monitoring for the presence of bleeding, signs of a fluid leak that may imply displacement, or erythema that may imply infection.

Monitoring

Blood pressure, continuous ECG, and pulse oximetry must be monitored. The height of the block is assessed by the presence and extent of the motor block and the sensory level. Sensation is commonly assessed using loss of cold sensation, for example with ethyl chloride spray. Motor block is less dense than that experienced with spinal anaesthesia.

A urinary catheter will often be required due to the inhibition of normal bladder function by the epidural and patients without a urinary catheter may experience urinary retention. This risk must be balanced with the risk of catheter-related urinary-tract infection and the decision will depend on the nature of the surgery being performed.

Complications

Blood pressure must be monitored frequently as epidural anaesthesia can cause hypotension. The risk of a high block and associated shortness of breath is less than that with spinal anaesthesia but still must be monitored for. Vigilance for signs of local anaesthetic toxicity caused by inadvertent intravascular placement of the epidural catheter is also important.

Peripheral Nerve Blockade

Infiltration of local anaesthetic around a specific nerve can be used as a sole technique, as an adjunct to general anaesthesia, or combined with a central neuraxial block. A nerve block using a single injection can be expected to provide analgesia for up to 8–16 hours [8]. For some blocks, an indwelling catheter can be left in or close to the wound to allow a more prolonged infusion of local anaesthetic and longer-lasting analgesia. They can be performed by the landmark technique, with ultrasound guidance, or using a nerve stimulator. As with any invasive procedure, sterility is important, with correct skin preparation using a chlorhexidine-based solution and sterile gloves required.

Indications

There is a wide range of peripheral nerve blocks. These can be divided into upper limb, lower limb, and truncal/abdominal blocks. The choice of the block will be determined by the site of surgery and the area of the body that analgesia is required for. Commonly performed blocks include fascia iliaca compartment block for hip-fracture surgery, transversus abdominis plane blocks for abdominal surgery, supraclavicular/interscalene blocks for arm and shoulder surgery, and femoral/sciatic blocks for lower limb surgery.

Equipment

The following equipment is used:

- a suitable peripheral nerve block needle (e.g., ultrasound visible needle, nerve stimulator connection needle);
- an ultrasound machine;
- a nerve stimulator if required; and
- a sterile drape.

Preparation

The most commonly used local anaesthetic for peripheral nerve blocks is levobupivacaine, which is available in 0.5% and 0.25% preparations. The final dose, concentration, and volume of the local anaesthetic will be decided upon by the anaesthetist depending

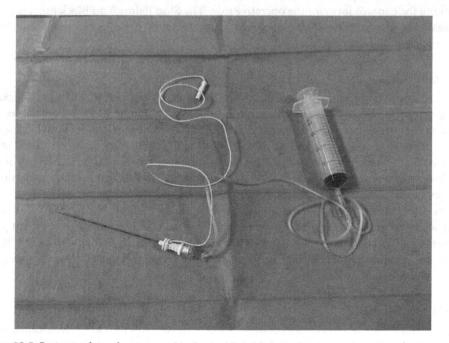

Figure 18.5 Equipment for performing peripheral nerve block: block needle connected to syringe for injection, for use with ultrasound or nerve-stimulator guidance (white cable connection)

on the block or blocks being performed. These should be drawn up in specially designed local anaesthetic syringes compatible with the needles being used and correctly labelled. The ultrasound machine should be available in the room. The patient must have given their informed consent for the regional block procedure as a part of the anaesthetic preoperative assessment. This may involve written or verbal consent depending on local practice.

The position of the patient will depend on the block being performed. Many blocks can be performed in the supine position, but some will require different positions. For example, a paravertebral block requires the patient to be in the lateral position and a sciatic block may require the leg to be lifted, or the patient to be turned lateral or prone depending on technique. The required position should be discussed with the anaesthetist as part of the team brief prior to the case.

Stop Before You Block

Performing a peripheral nerve block on the wrong side is a 'never event' [9] and can lead to a delay in or cancellation of surgery, prolonged hospital stays due to reduced mobility from bilateral blocks, risk of toxicity from repeated blocks, or even wrong-site surgery if the mistake is carried forwards unnoticed. Everyone involved in the anaesthetic care of the patient has a responsibility to ensure this does not occur. The 'Stop Before You Block' campaign is a national patient safety initiative aiming to reduce the incidence of inadvertent wrong-sided nerve blocks during regional anaesthesia [10].

Immediately before needle insertion a Stop moment occurs, and the correct block site is confirmed again. This involves visualising the surgical site marking that indicates the side of surgery, asking the patient to confirm the correct side of surgery if awake and double checking the consent form for the operative side. The Stop Before You Block process can be instigated by any member of the anaesthetic team. Only once the correct side is confirmed does the needle insertion occur.

Ultrasound

There are two important skills to the use of ultrasound for peripheral nerve blockade: imaging of the relevant anatomy to locate the desired nerve or plane for injection; and guiding the needle to the desired location. It is important that the needle is visualised on the screen throughout insertion and manipulation to avoid accidental damage to local structures of inadvertent vascular puncture. A high-frequency linear probe (10 MHz or more) produces a higher-resolution image, at the expense of depth of ultrasound penetration. Nerves appear as round hypoechoic structures surrounded by echogenic connective tissue, which diminish in size as they are followed distally (see Figure 18.6). Groups of these fascicles together often resemble a 'honeycomb' appearance. It is important to distinguish nerves from blood vessels, which can be achieved using the colour Doppler mode. A sterile technique remains important when using ultrasound; commonly, a probe cover or sheath is used to maintain asepsis.

Nerve Stimulator

A nerve stimulator is a device that delivers a low-intensity (up to 5 mA) electrical stimulus for a short duration (0.5 to 1 ms) at a repetition of 1–2 Hz to cause a muscle twitch, to locate

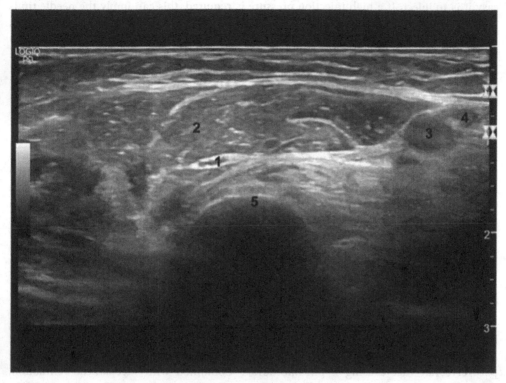

Figure 18.6 Ultrasound image of a musculocutaneous nerve in the arm, demonstrating ultrasound appearances of nerve (1), muscle (2), artery (3), vein (4), and bone (5)

a peripheral nerve or plexus. The desired muscle-twitch response will depend on the nerve being targeted by the block. This can be uncomfortable and is usually performed with the patient anaesthetised. The nerve stimulator is connected to an insulated needle; this needle is inserted using the landmark technique until the desired muscular response is seen, indicating close proximity to the nerve or plexus. The current required to elicit a muscle twitch gives some indication of the proximity of the needle to the nerve. A large current (e.g., 1 mA) indicates that the needle tip may still be too far from the nerve, whereas a very low current (e.g., 0.2 mA) suggests placement within the nerve itself. After negative aspiration is confirmed, the local anaesthetic is injected at which point the muscle-twitch response will cease. If injection is difficult, this may imply that the needle tip is incorrectly positioned, risking intraneural injection and nerve damage. If this is encountered, then the needle should be repositioned, and negative aspiration confirmed again before further injection.

Performing the Block

The needle is correctly positioned using ultrasound or nerve-stimulator guidance. Prior to injection of local anaesthetic, the syringe is aspirated to ensure no blood is present. If blood is aspirated, this indicates intravascular placement of the needle tip. In this instance, the local anaesthetic must not be injected, and the needle must be repositioned. If there is negative aspiration and the local anaesthetic is injected, close attention must be paid to how easy it is to inject. If a high injection pressure is required, this can imply the needle tip is incorrectly positioned and injection should not continue. The needle tip may be in a muscle, in which case the block will not be effective, or in the worst case it may be in the nerve itself. Direct injection of local anaesthetic into a nerve can cause permanent damage resulting in loss of sensation and motor function of the affected area. If the local anaesthetic does not inject easily, the needle tip must be repositioned and negative aspiration confirmed again before further injection.

Monitoring

Blood pressure, continuous ECG, and pulse oximetry must be monitored. Close attention to early symptoms of local anaesthetic toxicity (if awake, perioral tingling, agitation, altered level of consciousness) and clinical signs such as cardiac arrhythmia or hypotension must be observed. If there are any concerns about the presence of these signs, intravascular injection must be suspected, and the patient should be managed as per local anaesthetic systemic toxicity guidance [5].

Complications

Peripheral nerve blocks can have different complications depending on the site of injection. Local bleeding can usually be managed with simple direct pressure until the bleeding stops. If there is concern about damage to large vascular structures, demonstrated by ongoing bleeding or signs of hypoperfusion in the affected limb, urgent vascular surgical review must be sought. Blocks performed in the neck (e.g., interscalene, supraclavicular) or chest (e.g., paravertebral) risk causing a pneumothorax. Combined with mechanical ventilation, a simple pneumothorax can transform into a tension pneumothorax, presenting with life-threatening cardiovascular collapse. This requires urgent decompression and the insertion of an intercostal chest drain. To avoid this, vigilance for the possibility of a pneumothorax is crucial. Early signs may be falling oxygen saturations or rising oxygen requirements, increasing ventilatory pressures, or tachypnoea if the patient is spontaneously breathing.

References

1. C. L. Wu, M. Naqibuddin, and L. A. Fleisher. Measurement of patient satisfaction as an outcome of regional anesthesia and analgesia: a systematic review. *Regional Anesthesia and Pain Medicine* 2001; **26**: 196–208.

2. T. J. Gan, P. Diemunsch, A. Habib, et al. Consensus guidelines for the management of postoperative nausea and vomiting. *Anesthesia and Analgesia* 2014; **118**: 85–113.

3. L. M. Smith, C. Cozowicz, Y. Uda, et al. Neuraxial and combined neuraxial/general anesthesia compared to general anesthesia for major truncal and lower limb surgery: a systematic review and meta-analysis. *Anesthesia and Analgesia* 2017; **125**: 1931–1945.

4. S. G. Memtsoudis, X. Sun, and Y. L. Chiu, et al. Perioperative comparative effectiveness of anesthetic technique in orthopedic patients. *Anesthesiology* 2013; **118**: 1046–1058.

5. The Association of Anaesthetists. Guidelines for the management of severe local anaesthetic toxicity. Available from: https://anaesthetists.org/Home/Resources-publications/Guidelines/Management-of-severe-local-anaesthetic-toxicity.

6. Obstetric Anaesthetists Association. Epidural information card. Available from: www.oaa-anaes.ac.uk/assets/_managed/editor/File/Info%20for%20Mothers/EIC/2008_eic_english.pdf.

7. J. P. Campbell, F. Plaat, M. R. Checketts, et al. Safety guideline: skin antisepsis for central neuraxial blockade. *Anaesthesia* 2014; **69**: 1279–1286.

8. N. Desai, E. Albrecht, and K. El-Boghdadly. Perineural adjuncts for peripheral nerve block. *BJA Education* 2019; **19**: 272–282.

9. NHS Improvement. Never events policy and framework, 2018. Available from: www.england.nhs.uk/publication/never-events/.

10. Regional Anaesthesia United Kingdom. Stop Before you Block. www.ra-uk.org/index.php/stop-before-you-block.

Chapter 19

Fundamentals of the Anaesthetic Machine

Daniel Rodger

Introduction

The primary purpose of the anaesthetic machine is to deliver oxygen, other gases, and volatile agents (if used) safely to the patient – helping to maintain a suitable level of anaesthesia and analgesia for surgery or other intervention [1]. It is vital that any clinician checking and using an anaesthetic machine is familiar with the type of machine they are intending to use and possess a detailed knowledge of how it operates. Machines must be rigorously checked and tested by a suitably trained person before use and a breathing circuit check should take place between each patient [2].

Modern machines commonly house patient monitors (or include an integrated monitor), are easier to decontaminate, and contain drawers, shelves, and additional space for customisation [3]. Some companies have subsequently developed machines that are portable and can easily be transported to remote areas, while others have modifications that allow them to be utilised during magnetic resonance imaging. Although different types and brands of machines can look different, they all have several standardised features in common, ensured by safety specifications in the UK [1]. Even with considerable development and technological advances, the basic design and essential features of the anaesthetic machine have changed very little since the early Boyle's machine. This chapter is intended as an introduction to the anaesthetic machine, highlighting the main components and features that are essential to maintaining user and patient safety.

Background

The first successful public demonstration of diethyl ether anaesthesia was performed by W. T. G. Morton on 16 October 1846 so that the surgeon, J. C. Warren, could remove a tumour from his patient Gilbert Abbott's jaw [4]. It was not until 1917 that H. E. G. Boyle first designed his own machine to deliver anaesthesia. Boyle's machine was a modification of J. T. Gwathmey's lesser-known machine from 1912. Boyle identified some serious mechanical flaws following the prolonged use of the Gwathmey machine – nevertheless, he incorporated several of its main concepts into his own machine design [5].

The Anaesthetic Machine

Modern anaesthetic machines still incorporate many of the features that were present on the early Boyle's machine, such as flowmeters, vaporisers, pressure-reducing valves, and a breathing system [6, 7]. Modern electronically controlled machines frequently use software and an electric motor which drives a piston ventilator that can deliver more precise and stable tidal volumes. Other modern features include disposable carbon dioxide absorbers

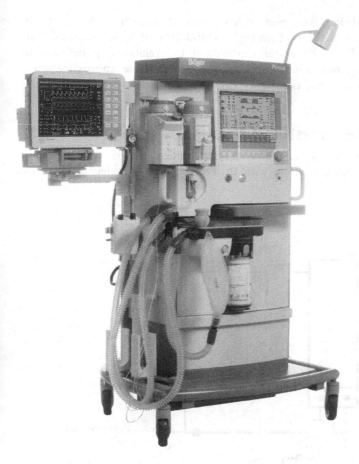

Figure 19.1 Machines such as the Dräger Primus incorporate an automated self-check function

that allow for less disruptive changeovers, electronic flowmeters, automated record keeping, advanced ventilation modes, and an automatic self-check when the machine is first switched on (see, for example, Figure 19.1). However, performing just the automated machine self-check is not sufficient to establish the safety of the machine for patient use.

Electronically controlled machines have several advantages over conventional pneumatic machines, though they can involve a degree of compromise in other areas. Electronically controlled machines depend more heavily on a continuous supply of electricity and therefore have a more limited backup power supply than conventional machines. For instance, all Dräger electronically controlled machines have at least 30 minutes of backup power following a mains power failure, after which time the piston ventilator will cease to function. However, manual, and spontaneous ventilation with anaesthetic gas delivery can continue after that time, although alarms and monitors will no longer be functional [8].

Units of Pressure

Despite attempts at standardisation, a range of different units of pressure continue to be used, which can cause confusion. The gas pressure within the anaesthetic machine is measured in kilopascals (kPa). However, other units of pressure relevant to the machine are millimetres of mercury (mmHg), centimetres of water (cmH$_2$O) and pounds per square inch (psi). To better understand the relationship between the different units of pressure, one atmosphere or one bar (a close approximation of atmospheric pressure at sea level), is roughly equal to: 101 kPa, 15 psi, 760 mmHg, or 1020 cmH$_2$O [9].

Basic Features of the Anaesthetic Machine

Irrespective of the type of anaesthetic machine being used, there are several essential components that must be present, along with their corresponding safety features (see Figure 19.2). These are:

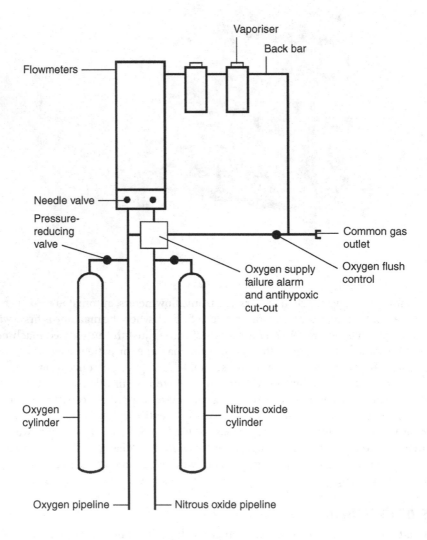

Figure 19.2 Basic components of an anaesthetic machine (reprinted from T. Smith, C. Pinnock, and T. Lin (eds.), *Fundamentals of Anaesthesia*, 3rd ed. Cambridge: Cambridge University Press, p. 834)

- a metal frame;
- pipeline gas circuitry;
- connections for gas cylinders and pressure gauges;
- pressure regulators;
- needle valves or computer-controlled pressure and flow devices;
- rotameters or digital equivalent;
- a back bar;
- vaporisers;
- a common gas outlet and auxiliary gas outlets; and
- scavenging and suction circuitry.

Gas Supply

Gases to the anaesthetic machine are provided through two primary means: piped supply and cylinders, which have been attached directly to the anaesthetic machine.

Piped Gas Supply

Piped gases are provided to the anaesthetic machine via a central source in the form of a liquid tank or a bank of large cylinders, or both. Oxygen originates from a liquid oxygen supply, which is stored in large vessels known as vacuum-insulated evaporators (VIEs), which are usually situated away from the main hospital building. The VIE helps to maintain a temperature of −150 °C to −170 °C at a pressure of approximately 10.5 bar [10]. The size of the VIE will depend on the hospital demand and usually contains enough oxygen for 10 days' use and is refilled on a weekly basis.

Nitrous oxide and medical air are provided using a cylinder manifold, which usually consists of two banks of four to six size J cylinders. When the available gas in the first bank has been exhausted, the supply is then automatically transferred to the second bank of reserve cylinders by a pressure-sensitive control device that links both banks. From these central sources, the gases are distributed through a network of colour-coded pipelines, made from high-quality copper, to a self-closing terminal outlet (Schrader valves), which are distinguished by size, shape, and colour. The Schrader valves ensure that the gas flow is shut off until the appropriate Schrader probe is inserted. In the operating department, the outlets for oxygen, nitrous oxide, medical air, and suction are grouped together.

Flexible Pipeline Hoses

Flexible pipeline hoses connect the piped supply from the terminal outlets to the anaesthetic machine. Pressure-reducing valves ensure that gases are supplied at a pressure of 4 bar (400 kPa). Each individual gas pipeline hose is colour-coded, has a non-interchangeable Schrader probe made to a specific diameter for each gas, and at the anaesthetic machine end has a fixed gas-specific non-interchangeable screw thread, which consists of a nut and probe, a specific diameter shoulder with an O-ring seal, and a specific diameter forward shaft (see Table 19.1) [10]. Importantly, these pipelines should only ever be changed by someone certified to do so. The utilisation of a one-way valve ensures the unidirectional flow of gases between the gas outlets and the anaesthetic machine. These safety features help to minimise the risk of a hypoxic gas mixture being mistakenly delivered to a patient.

Table 19.1 Gas pipeline details

Pipeline	Schrader valve colour (UK)	Hose colour (UK)	Supply pressure
Oxygen	White	White	400 kPa
Nitrous oxide	Blue	Blue	400 kPa
Medical air	Black and white	Black	400 kPa (anaesthetic machine) and 700 kPa (to drive surgical equipment)
Suction	Yellow	Yellow	−53 kPa (−400 mmHg)

Cylinder Gas Supply

Cylinders provide a backup gas supply in the event of a central gas-supply failure or where a pipeline gas supply is not available. The back of the anaesthetic machine commonly has space to accommodate two (older machines may have three) size E cylinders. One of these should always be for oxygen. Each cylinder is made from a lightweight molybdenum steel and contains the following important details: gas chemical symbol, tare weight, hydraulic test date, and a serial number, and is colour-coded by gas contents. Cylinders are produced in several sizes with each denoted a capital letter in ascending order from A to J, marked on each cylinder. The tare weight refers to the empty combined weight of the cylinder and valve for all cylinders. Oxygen and medical air arc stored as a gas whereas nitrous oxide is stored as a liquid and gas. As the nitrous oxide is withdrawn, the number of gaseous molecules decreases and consequently molecules pass from the liquid to the gaseous phase until an equilibrium is re-established. When all the liquid has been converted into gas the internal cylinder pressure will begin to fall in a similar manner to an oxygen cylinder.

Cylinder Safety Features

Cylinders are colour-coded and clearly labelled to identify the correct cylinder more easily and minimise the risk of attempting to attach the wrong one. The gas-specific pin-index system was introduced in 1952 and ensures that an incorrect cylinder cannot be attached to the anaesthetic machine [5]. Pins on the yoke of the anaesthetic machine must align with holes on the valve of the cylinder that conform to British Standard (BS) and equivalent International Standards Organisation (ISO). Each gas has a unique combination of two numbers between one and six, which correspond to a specific space where the yoke and cylinder can meet (see Table 19.2 and Figure 19.3). This significantly reduces the risk of the wrong cylinder being connected to the anaesthetic machine. There must also be a Bodok seal, which is a compressible neoprene washer with a metal periphery that separates the cylinder from the yoke, to form a gas-tight joint, and was first used in 1958 [5, 11]. The thread where the valve screws into the neck of the cylinder is sealed with a material that melts when exposed to intense heat. This reduces the risk of an explosion occurring during a fire by allowing the gas to escape around the threads of the joint.

Table 19.2 Gas-cylinder details

Gas	Physical state in cylinder	Colour (UK)	Capacity (L)	Pin index	Pressure when full
Oxygen	Gas	Body: black Shoulder: white	Size E: 680	2 and 5	13,700 kPa
Nitrous oxide	Gas + liquid	Body: blue Shoulder: blue	Size E: 1800	3 and 5	4,400 kPa
Medical air	Gas	Body: grey Shoulder: white/black	Size E: 680	1 and 5	13,700 kPa

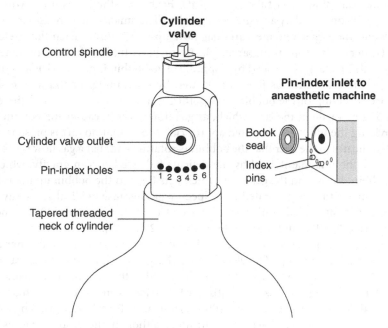

Figure 19.3 Pin-index system for gases and detail of the cylinder head (reprinted from T. Smith, C. Pinnock, and T. Lin (eds.). *Fundamentals of Anaesthesia*, 3rd ed. Cambridge: Cambridge University Press, 2009, p. 831)

Pressure Gauges

Pressure gauges indicate the pressure of pipelines and cylinders being used and must be present on all anaesthetic machines. They are commonly found at the front of the anaesthetic machine. In older machines, Bourdon gauges are used, mainly because they are inexpensive, strong, and able to withstand high pressures. A Bourdon gauge consists of a flexible coiled tube, which is connected to a needle pointer that moves over a dial. The other end of the tube is exposed to the gas supply and pressure causes the tube to uncoil and a gear mechanism to move the calibrated dial, indicating the pressure. However, on newer machines, pressures may be indicated by a digital display figure.

Pressure Regulators

Cylinders supply gases at a variable and much higher pressure than that which it would be safe to deliver to the patient. Primary pressure regulators reduce the cylinder pressure from 13,700 kPa to an operating pressure of less than 420 kPa [1]. These pressures are much more consistent with the pipeline-supplied gases, which are typically around 400 kPa. Secondary pressure regulators reduce the gas supply to a much lower and uniform pressure that can be delivered safely to the patient through a breathing circuit. The pressure that can be safely delivered to the patient should not exceed 3 kPa [12]. These much lower pressures are measured in cmH_2O instead of kPa.

Flowmeters

Flowmeters (or rotameters) measure the flow of gas passing through them, commonly oxygen, nitrous oxide, and air. They are made up of a needle valve, which is situated at the base of the relevant flowmeter tube (valve seat). Each anaesthetic gas uses two flowmeter tubes, which are controlled by a single needle valve. The smaller tube measures gas flow up to 1 L/min and the larger one measures gas flow up to 15 L/min. Each flowmeter tube is a tapered (wider at the top) transparent plastic or glass tube with a lightweight rotating bobbin (or ball) inside it, controlled by a spindle. The bobbin is always visible as it stops at either end of the tube, and gas flow is indicated by it spinning. The flow rate should be measured from the top of the bobbin (midpoint for a ball). The rotation of the bobbin is facilitated by slits made in the rim, which, as gas flows past it, causes the bobbin to rotate freely, providing the tubes are mounted appropriately and that no dirt is present. A dot on the bobbin indicates to the user that the bobbin is rotating and that a gas flow is present. The height of the bobbin is maintained by the delicate balance between gravity, which acts to force the bobbin down, and the gas flow, which acts to push the bobbin up the tube [11].

Each flowmeter tube is calibrated for a specific gas because medical gases have varying densities and viscosities. Calibration takes place at room temperature (20 °C) and atmospheric pressure (101 kPa) and is accurate to about ±2.5% [13]. Tubes are considered leak-proof, using a neoprene washer at either end, and they have an outer and inner antistatic coating to reduce the build-up of an electrostatic charge, which can affect accuracy by up to 35%. Oxygen is added last to the gas mixture, delivered to the back bar in case of damage to the flowmeter, reducing the risk of creating a hypoxic gas mixture. Some machines also provide a basal flow of oxygen (between 100 mL/min and 300 mL/min), which ensures that oxygen flow cannot be completely discontinued, although the amount varies between manufacturers [14]. Flowmeters and the control spindles that control them are colour-coded and labelled clearly to indicate each gas. In the UK, the oxygen spindle is situated on the far left and is commonly larger, with a ridge to make it more distinguishable.

Some newer electronic anaesthetic machines no longer use conventional rotameters; instead, the fresh gas flow is entirely controlled by a microprocessor. On the Dräger Primus, for example, the fresh gas flow is mixed and controlled by electronically controlled valves. They function according to the intended total gas flow and oxygen concentration set by the user. The user chooses the fraction of inspired oxygen and then selects which secondary carrier gas (either nitrous oxide or air) to use [12]. A type of digital rotameter on the display indicates the fresh gas flow and it is likely that this will become the predominant gas mixing system used in all new anaesthetic machines. The digital displays on newer machines are frequently illuminated, which allows them to be more easily identified in a setting that may require low lighting. In the event of a system failure, gas can still be delivered into the circuit by utilising the oxygen safety control (delivering 0–12 L/min), which delivers gas via the vaporiser. The downside to using electronically controlled systems is that they require mains or battery power to function, something that conventional systems do not require.

Back Bar and Vaporisers

The back bar describes a horizontal section of the anaesthetic machine where the vaporisers can be mounted. Part of the fresh has flow enters the vaporiser where it is mixed with the inhalational agent and transported from the back bar to the common gas outlet, by which point the pressure has been reduced so that it can be safely delivered to the patient [10]. Most anaesthetic machines have the capacity to house at least two vaporisers (see Figure 19.4 for examples of a vaporiser). They are seated and can be secured using an interlocking system (e.g., Selectatec), which prevents more than one vaporiser being switched on at a time and avoids inadvertently administering more than one inhalational agent. It also ensures that fresh gas flow can only enter the vaporiser when it has been locked in place and turned on. When two vaporisers are mounted on the back bar and one is switched on, a small pin protrudes out towards the other vaporiser, preventing it from being switched on. Each vaporiser sits on a valve-post with a changeable rubber O-ring that creates a gas-tight seal. A damaged O-ring should be replaced, as this can become the source

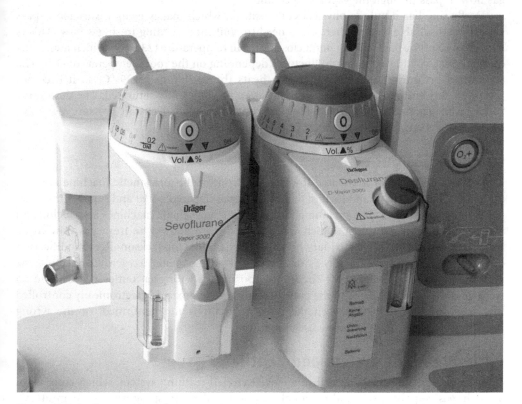

Figure 19.4 Desflurane and sevoflurane vaporisers

of a leak. Also situated on the back bar or further downstream is a non-return pressure relief valve, which opens when pressure in the back bar exceeds 35 kPa [11]. This prevents excess pressure in the back bar damaging the flowmeters and the vaporisers. Other safety features are an anti-spill mechanism, which prevents the wrong agent being introduced into an inappropriate vaporiser and provides a clear indicator of how filled the vaporiser is. Additionally, each specific vaporiser is colour-coded to indicate which volatile agent they contain:

- sevoflurane: yellow;
- isoflurane: purple; and
- desflurane: blue.

The purpose of the vaporiser is to accurately deliver the desired concentration of a volatile inhalational agent. Inhalational agents such as sevoflurane, desflurane, and isoflurane are supplied and stored as liquids. The vaporisers convert the volatile agent from a liquid to a gas, which can be administered to the patient. Each vaporiser is calibrated for use with a specific volatile agent. A vaporiser must be appropriately locked in place on the back bar and turned on (additionally, a desflurane vaporiser must be plugged in) before the fresh gas flow can enter. Most modern vaporisers divide the fresh gas flow into two different streams. The larger stream bypasses the vaporiser and is unaffected, while the smaller stream passes through the vaporiser chamber where it becomes saturated with the volatile agent. By changing the dial on the vaporiser, the ratio of fresh gas flow divided into each stream is modified. Increasing the selected percentage of volatile agent will cause an increase in fresh gas flow to pass through the vaporising chamber.

Desflurane has a unique physical composition, which makes using a variable bypass vaporiser unsuitable, and so there is no need to split the incoming fresh gas flow. This is because desflurane has a boiling point close to room temperature (23.5 °C), which means the output of the volatile agent would fluctuate depending on the room temperature [15]. The specialised pressurised vaporiser therefore heats the desflurane to 39 °C, so it becomes a vapour; this ensures that the fresh gas flow can be sufficiently saturated. The desflurane vapour is then added to the fresh gas flow and controlled by an electronic pressure regulator, sensors, and a variable flow restrictor [2].

Common Gas Outlet

The common gas outlet is situated towards the front of the anaesthetic machine and has a 22-mm male (external) and 15-mm female (external) tapered outlet and supplies the fresh gas flow to the patient via a breathing circuit. Some anaesthetic machines also include an auxiliary common gas outlet, which when switched on allows the fresh gas flow to be redirected for the use of an auxiliary breathing system like the Jackson–Rees modification of the Ayre's T-piece (Mapleson F) or the use of supplemental oxygen. Connecting the patient to the incorrect breathing circuit or choosing the wrong gas outlet will result in no fresh gas flow being delivered to the patient, leading to hypoxia. In electronically controlled machines, errors can occur when the correct circuit is not confirmed, or the wrong breathing circuit is selected on the user interface.

Circle Breathing System and Ventilator

Modern anaesthetic machines utilise a closed circle breathing system, which consists of a fresh gas supply, two unidirectional one-way valves (inspiratory and expiratory), a reservoir bag, a carbon dioxide absorber, an adjustable pressure-limiting (APL) valve, and a Y-piece for connection to the patient [16]. Removal of carbon dioxide allows the inhalational agents and anaesthetic gases to be recycled. Soda lime is the substance used to absorb the patients exhaled carbon dioxide, and this is stored in a canister and mounted vertically to the anaesthetic machine. Soda lime contains approximately 80% calcium hydroxide, 4% sodium hydroxide, 1% potassium hydroxide, and the remainder is water. Ventilators are an integral part of the modern anaesthetic machine and provide the means for an extended period of ventilation of the anaesthetised patient. They can be mechanically, pneumatically, or electronically controlled, with newer ventilators comparable to those used in intensive care. Many of the newer ventilators incorporate technology that facilitates more precise delivery of smaller tidal volumes required for neonatal and infants. Breathing systems are discussed in detail in Chapter 20.

Emergency Oxygen Flush

Because of the high pressures produced by the emergency oxygen flush it has been designed only to be activated by a non-locking button, which incorporates a self-closing valve to avoid accidental operation [11]. High-flow oxygen upward of 35 L/min is generated at pressures of up to 400 kPa. As the emergency oxygen flush bypasses the flowmeter and vaporiser, the gas flow only contains oxygen. It is sometimes used to inflate the breathing-circuit reservoir bag after a leak and must always be used cautiously; incorrect use could cause barotrauma. Similarly, because the oxygen flush bypasses the vaporiser, there is an inherent risk that using it will dilute the inhalational agents and may increase the risk of patient awareness [17].

Oxygen-Failure Warning Device

An early oxygen-failure warning system was the Ritchie whistle, which was introduced in the mid-1960s and was powered by the falling oxygen pressures in the system. Modern anaesthetic machines must have a built-in oxygen-failure device, which is situated upstream of the rotameter block. It is activated when the oxygen pressure falls below 200 kPa, which instigates an audible alarm above 60 decibels at a distance of 1 metre, which will only stop when sufficient oxygen pressure has been restored [18]. When the oxygen supply pressure falls below 137 kPa, the delivery of any other gases will be halted so that only oxygen can be delivered. The oxygen-failure alarm is designed to remain operational even in the absence of battery or mains power supplies.

Prevention of Hypoxic Gas Delivery

In order to prevent hypoxic gas delivery, several safety features have been developed:

- a pin-index system, non-interchangeable screw-thread connections, colour-coded and labelled cylinders, and colour-coded pipelines;
- colour-coded Schrader valves, which are size specific for each gas;
- colour-coded and non-kinkable pipeline hoses with gas-specific Schrader probes;
- an oxygen-failure alarm that is activated when the oxygen supply pressure falls below 200 kPa (some older machines may still feature the pneumatic Ritchie whistle);
- two means of supplying oxygen: pipelines and cylinders (a manual means of oxygen delivery such as a bag–valve mask should also be available on every machine);

- an oxygen analyser usually placed at the common gas outlet;
- a hypoxic guard or a Link-25 system that does not allow the user to deliver oxygen less than 25% of the total gas mix – for every 2.07 revolutions of the nitrous oxide flow-control spindle, the oxygen at the lowest oxygen flow rotates once;
- oxygen is always the last gas added to the fresh gas flow;
- use pressure gauges; and
- colour-coded flowmeters, and uniquely sized oxygen control spindle, which is always situated on the left in the UK.

Adjustable Pressure-Limiting Valve

The purpose of the APL valve is to enable the escape of exhaled or excess gases from the breathing system when a pre-set pressure has been exceeded (see Figure 19.5). This helps reduce the risk of causing barotrauma to the patient. It is also used to adjust the circuit pressure during spontaneous ventilation or manual ventilation with the reservoir bag [2]. The APL valve is a one-way spring-loaded valve, which can adjust the pressure required to open the valve. During spontaneous ventilation, the patient will generate positive pressure during expiration and therefore resistance to expiration should be minimal. When the dial is fully open, positive pressure from expiration causes the valve to open under a pressure of less than 1 cmH_2O (0.1 kPa). Screwing down the dial on the APL valve increases tension in the spring and the pressure required to open the valve during manual ventilation. In some modern machines, the APL valve is electronically adjustable and calibrated. When the dial is

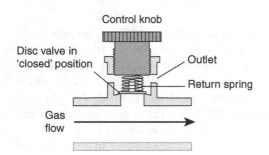

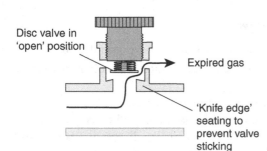

Figure 19.5 An APL expiratory valve (reprinted from T. Smith, C. Pinnock, and T. Lin (eds.). *Fundamentals of Anaesthesia*, 3rd ed. Cambridge: Cambridge University Press, 2009, p. 843)

fully closed it will release excess pressure at 60 cmH$_2$O (6 kPa) – this pressure occurs at a gas flow rate of 30 L/min [1].

Scavenging Systems

Scavenging describes the removal of expired waste anaesthetic gases and ensures that they do not vent into the operating theatre environment. Exposure to nitrous oxide and inhalational agents can have adverse effects on staff and these are therefore considered hazardous substances, which must be safely and effectively disposed of. Exposure to hazardous waste gases most commonly occurs from leaks around an ill-fitting face mask or supraglottic airway device, spillage during the refilling of a vaporiser, expired gas exhaled from the patient following emergence from anaesthesia, and from open-ended breathing circuits [19]. The volume of waste gases can be minimised by using low-flow anaesthesia and taking additional care when refilling vaporisers. An unscavenged operating theatre can show nitrous oxide levels up to 3,000 particles per million (ppm) compared with the recommended maximum accepted concentration of a 100 ppm (in the UK) time-weighted average over an 8-hour period [11].

Waste gases are commonly removed through two types of system: passive or active. Passive systems remove waste gases by relying on the expiratory effort of the patient to force it through additional tubing out into the atmosphere. The risks of this system are that the outflow of waste gases can become obstructed, which can generate a negative pressure or high positive pressures in the tubing. These effects can be mitigated by using pressure relief valves within the system. Passive systems offer less protection to theatre staff and are considerably less efficient than active systems.

The anaesthetic gas scavenging system (AGSS) is either connected to the outlet for the APL valve or directly to the circle system. The AGSS generates negative-pressure suction to remove waste anaesthetic gases towards a reservoir, which is then propelled into the outside atmosphere. However the system is powered, it must be able to accommodate 75 L/min of constant flow and be able to function at a peak rate of 135 L/min. The use of a pressure-limiting device within the system ensures that an excess negative pressure is not generated, which could interfere with patient ventilation [16]. Scavenging systems utilise a conical 30-mm connector to minimise the risk of it being incorrectly connected to a breathing circuit. Some systems will have a visual indicator situated on the back or to the side of the anaesthetic machine to check that the scavenging is functioning optimally. Irrespective of the system used, it is vital that the tubing is never occluded when attached to the patient as this could produce increased resistance to patient expiration.

Waste anaesthetic gases – especially desflurane and nitrous oxide – are also potent greenhouse gases, and new technology is being developed to reduce their impact on the environment. New scavenging devices aim to limit their release into the atmosphere by capturing, reusing, or destroying the gases, although there are still several unanswered questions regarding the feasibility of such technologies [20].

Suction Apparatus

Effective high-pressure suction should be available in some capacity – commonly it is attached to the anaesthetic machine. Suction is used to clear mucus, blood, and debris from the pharynx and trachea and should be able to maintain a negative pressure of at least

−400 mmHg at the outlet. The negative-pressure vacuum can be manually adjusted depending on the needs of the patient and incorrect use can cause trauma. Safely functioning suction should always be available and tested before anaesthetising any patient. Suction apparatus consists of a vacuum source, suction unit, suction tubing, and a Yankauer suction tip or catheter. The suction unit consists of a reservoir container, vacuum control regulator, and a vacuum gauge. The suction unit utilises a hydrophobic bacterial filter that removes 99.999% of bacteria and prevents fluid and smoke from contaminating the medical vacuum system.

Why It Is Important to Know How to Check an Anaesthetic Machine

Failure to perform an appropriate anaesthetic machine check can lead to serious patient harm. An inappropriate check or unfamiliarity with the anaesthetic machine, ventilator, vaporisers, or breathing circuit can compromise patient safety; in some cases, leading to hypoxic brain injury, awareness under general anaesthesia, cardiac arrest, and death. Causes of harm are multifactorial and commonly arise from human error, lack of knowledge, and a technical fault [21]. In most cases, adverse outcomes can be prevented by performing an appropriate check of the anaesthetic machine [22].

Checking the Anaesthetic Machine

It is essential that users ensure that all the mandatory manual and automated checks (where required) are performed prior to use. Checks should be in accordance with the most recent Association of Anaesthetists guidance [23]. In the case of ventilator failure, an alternative means of ventilating a patient should always be readily available, such as a self-inflating bag. Although an operating department practitioner or nurse often performs the routine checks, it remains the final responsibility of the end user (e.g., the anaesthetist or anaesthesia associate) to ensure that the anaesthetic machine is safe.

References

1. C. Sinclair, M. Thadsad, and I. Barker. Modern anaesthetic machines. *Continuing Education in Anaesthesia Critical Care and Pain* 2006; **6**: 75–78.

2. G. Briggs and J. Maycock. The anaesthetic machine. *Anaesthesia and Intensive Care Medicine* 2013; **14**: 94–98.

3. F. Rosewarne. The anaesthetic machine. In I. Harley and P. Hore (eds.), *Anaesthesia: An Introduction*, 5th ed. East Hawthorn: IP Communications, 2012, pp. 329–336.

4. S. J. Snow. *Blessed Days of Anaesthesia: How Anaesthetics Changed the World*. Oxford: Oxford University Press, 2008.

5. O. M. Watt. The evolution of the Boyle apparatus, 1917–67. *Anaesthesia* 1968; **23**: 103–118.

6. V. P Patil, M. G. Shetmahajan, and J. V. Divatia. The modern integrated anaesthesia workstation. *Indian Journal of Anaesthesia* 2013; **57**: 446–454.

7. C. L. Gurudatt. The basic anaesthesia machine. *Indian Journal of Anaesthesia* 2013; **57**: 438–445.

8. J. M. Feldman. The anesthesia ventilator. Available from: www.draeger.com/Library/Content/9049447_the_anesthesia_ventilator_8seitig_en_101209_fin.pdf.

9. P. J. Simpson and M. Popat. *Understanding Anaesthesia*, 4th ed. London: Elsevier, 2006.

10. B. Al-Shaikh and S. G. Stacey. *Essentials of Equipment in Anaesthesia, Critical Care and Perioperative Medicine*, 5th ed. London: Elsevier, 2018.

11. N. Robinson, G. Hall, and W. Fawcett. *How to Survive in Anaesthesia*, 5th ed. Cambridge: Cambridge University Press, 2017.

12. P. Greig and N. Crabtree. *Introducing Anaesthesia: A Curriculum-Based Guide*. Oxford: Oxford University Press, 2014.

13. A. Diba. The anaesthetic workstation. In A. J. Davey and A. Diba (eds.), *Ward's Anaesthetic Equipment*, 6th ed. London: Saunders, 2012, pp. 65–105.

14. A. P. J. Lake. Basal oxygen flow. *Anaesthesia* 2001; **56**: 1120–1121.

15. M. C. Kapoor and M. Vakamudi. Desflurane: revisited. *Journal of Anaesthesiology Clinical Pharmacology* 2012; **28**: 92–100.

16. J. Roberts and L. Darwin. Anaesthetic breathing systems. In D. Cottle and S. Laha (eds.), *Anaesthetics for Junior Doctors and Allied Professionals: The Essential Guide*. London: Radcliffe Publishing, 2013, pp. 39–45.

17. A. Crosby and S. Laha. The anaesthetic machine. In D. Cottle and S. Laha (eds.), *Anaesthetics for Junior Doctors and Allied Professionals: The Essential Guide*. London: Radcliffe Publishing, 2013, pp. 32–38.

18. E. S. Lin. Anaesthetic equipment. In T. Smith, C Pinnock, and T. Lin (eds.), *Fundamentals of Anaesthesia*, 3rd ed. Cambridge: Cambridge University Press, 2009, pp. 828–863.

19. M. C. Mushambi and S. Francis. Anaesthetic apparatus. In A. R. Aitkenhead, I. K. Moppett, and J. P. Thompson (eds.), *Smith and Aitkenhead's Textbook of Anaesthesia*, 6th ed. London: Elsevier, 2013, pp. 262–311.

20. M. Charlesworth and F. Swinton. Anaesthetic gases, climate change, and sustainable practice. *Lancet Planet Health* 2017; **1**: e216–e217.

21. J. L. Bourgain, Y. Coisel, D. Kern, et al. What are the main 'machine dysfunctions' to know? *Annales Françaises d'Anesthésie et de Réanimation* 2014; **33**: 466–471.

22. S. P. Mehta, J. B. Eisenkraft, K. L. Posner, et al. Patient injuries from anesthesia gas delivery equipment: a closed claims update. *Anesthesiology* 2013; **119**: 788–795.

23. Association of Anaesthetists. Checking anaesthetic equipment. Available from: www.aagbi.org/sites/default/files/checking_anaesthetic_equipment_2012.pdf.

Anaesthetic Breathing Systems

Cheryl Wayne-Kevan and Daniel Rodger

Introduction

Anaesthetic breathing systems are used to deliver oxygen and anaesthetic gases to patients and remove carbon dioxide. A breathing system is most commonly attached to an anaesthetic machine, which is designed to deliver the fresh gas flow to the patient via a face mask, a supraglottic device, or an endotracheal tube. The breathing system used can affect the composition of the gas and volatile anaesthetic mixture inhaled by the patient, and so it is important to understand the different breathing systems used in anaesthesia.

Anaesthetic breathing systems can be broadly categorised into two groups – non-rebreathing and rebreathing systems [1].

The essential components of a breathing system are:

- the reservoir bag (commonly available in 0.5-, 1- and 2-L sizes) (not Mapleson E);
- tubing (22-mm diameter for adult and 18-mm diameter for paediatric circuits);
- a fresh gas flow inlet;
- an adjustable pressure-limiting (APL) expiratory valve (not Mapleson E or F);
- connections (22-mm or 15-mm male to female fittings); and
- a carbon dioxide absorber (if a rebreathing system is being used).

The Ideal Breathing System

The ideal breathing system should be simple and safe to use; delivers the intended inspired gas mixture; permits different means of ventilation – spontaneous, manual, and controlled [2]; is sturdy and lightweight; is efficient and permits low gas flow without rebreathing of expired gas; and is suitable for spontaneous and controlled ventilation in all ages and sizes [3].

Useful Definitions

The following definitions are useful when considering breathing systems.

- The fresh gas flow (FGF) describes the mixture of anaesthetic gases and inhalational agents that leave the anaesthetic machine via the common gas outlet.
- The minute volume (MV) is the total gas breathed in one minute.
- Rebreathing describes when a patient inhales previously exhaled air or gases.
- Spontaneous breathing describes a patient breathing normally during anaesthesia without the need for mechanical ventilation.

- Controlled ventilation describes a mode of ventilation in which a set of bellows or mechanical ventilator delivers a pre-set volume or pressure to the patient's lungs; this is in contrast to a patient spontaneously breathing for themselves.
- Dead space at its most basic level is a volume where gases do not interact with the body. It can be thought of as ventilation without perfusion. This can be mechanical dead space (in the breathing system) or anatomical dead space (in the patient).
- The APL valve opens when the pressure in the breathing system reaches the level set to permit gases to leave. The valve is open for spontaneous ventilation and partially closed to deliver positive pressure during controlled ventilation.
- A coaxial arrangement of tubing locates one tube within another.
- The efficiency of a breathing system describes the flow rate of fresh gas required in comparison to the patient's minute volume in order to avoid the patient rebreathing their own expired gas.

Mapleson Breathing System Classification

In 1954, William Mapleson published an article in the *British Journal of Anaesthesia* in which he described a classification for anaesthetic breathing systems [4]. Each breathing system was assigned a letter from A to E (see Figure 20.1 and Table 20.1) [1]. The classification has proven flexible over the years and many modifications have entered practice, including the F, which is itself a modification of the E. This chapter discusses each of these breathing systems individually, outlining their use and efficiency and explaining a brief rationale for the choice of a circuit. Some systems are very efficient for spontaneously breathing patients, with little waste of gas, whereas others are efficient for ventilated patients; but none are efficient for both.

Mapleson A

The Mapleson A system is also known as the Magill's attachment. In this system, the APL valve is located at the patient end of the apparatus to reduce anaesthetic dead space. There are several limitations of this system. These include poor efficiency for controlled ventilation and not being appropriate for children less than 30 kg due to the increased dead space [2]. Despite being a very efficient breathing system for spontaneous breathing, it is rarely used in its original form today due to the bulkiness of having two tubes.

Lack Modification

There is also a coaxial modification of the Mapleson A system known as the Lack system. This was generally chosen by anaesthetists who wanted the versatility and compactness of the Magill circuit for spontaneous ventilation but with the APL valve at the 'proximal' anaesthetic machine end of the circuit, close to the reservoir bag [5], to facilitate ease of use when ventilating the patient manually. This also made connecting to the waste-gas scavenging more convenient. The fresh gas flow is delivered to the patient via the external tubing and expired gas is taken away from

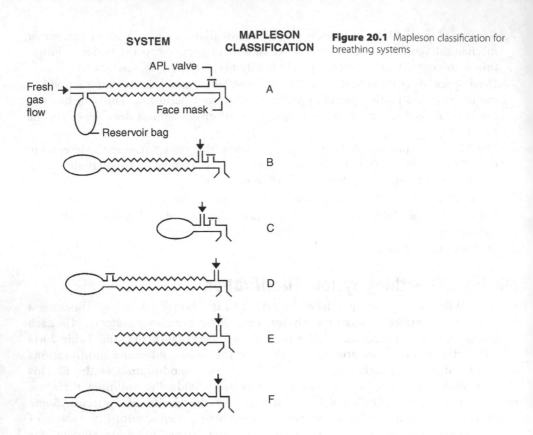

SYSTEM

MAPLESON CLASSIFICATION

Figure 20.1 Mapleson classification for breathing systems

the patient along the central tubing. It is also not suitable for prolonged controlled ventilation due to poor efficiency.

Mapleson B

The Mapleson B circuit is considered obsolete. It is very similar to the Mapleson C other than having additional tubing that acts as a reservoir between the reservoir bag and where the fresh gas flow enters.

Mapleson C

The Mapleson C circuit is lightweight and compact and was originally used for short transports before self-inflating resuscitation bags became available. It is ideal during resuscitation, in critical care, and the post-anaesthetic care unit as it assists ventilation and can apply continuous positive airway pressure when the APL valve is partially closed. Compared with a self-inflating bag it offers a much better assessment of the patient's lung compliance. It is seldom used for the induction of anaesthesia due to its inefficiency during spontaneous ventilation.

Table 20.1 Characteristics of Mapleson systems and comparing the FGF relative to the MV necessary to prevent rebreathing

Mapleson system	Modifications	Efficiency	
		Spontaneous breathing	Controlled ventilation
A (Magill)	Lack	High FGF > 1MV	Very Low FGF > 2–3MV
B		Moderate FGF > 2MV	Moderate FGF > 2MV
C		Moderate FGF > 2MV	Moderate FGF > 2MV
D	Bain	Very low FGF > 2–3MV	High FGF > 1MV
E	A modification of Ayre's T piece	Low FGF > 2–3MV Minimum flow 4 L/min	NA
F (Jackson–Rees)	A modification of E	Low FGF > 2.5–3MV	Low FGF > 1.5–2MV

Mapleson D

The Mapleson D circuit is most commonly seen in the form of the Bain system, which is a coaxial version of the system. In the Bain coaxial system the fresh gas flows through a narrower inner tube set within the outer tube where exhaled gas flows. The APL valve and reservoir bag are situated at the anaesthetic machine end, away from the patient. This system is most efficient when used for controlled ventilation. Because the fresh gas flow required to prevent rebreathing is so high, it is a very inefficient and uneconomical system for spontaneously breathing patients [2]. A Pethick test is performed with a Bain circuit to check the integrity of the inner tube within the coaxial system. This test should always be carried out before use as is it is possible for the inner fresh gas delivery hose to become twisted or for an occult disconnection that would result in increased dead space.

To perform the Pethick test, use the following steps:

- Occlude the patient end of the circuit (at the elbow).
- Close the APL valve. Fill the circuit, using the oxygen flush valve.
- Release the occlusion at the elbow and flush.
- The Venturi effect flattens the reservoir bag if the inner tube is patent.

Mapleson E and F

The Mapleson E or Ayre's T-piece was introduced in 1937. It is predominantly used for neonates, infants, and children weighing no more than 25–30 kg. The Ayre's T-piece is useful in spontaneously breathing children as there are no valves to increase the work of breathing. However, controlled ventilation can only be achieved by occluding the expiratory tubing and the lack of a bag means that there is no visual indication of the patient's breathing and using the fresh gas flow to inflate the chest.

The Mapleson F is a modification from the 1950s, which was created by adding an open-ended 500-mL reservoir bag that is connected to the expiratory limb of the T-piece and is known as the Jackson–Rees modification. The lack of a valve means that there is little additional work of breathing, but controlled ventilation requires occlusion of the open end of the bag and can be assisted by simultaneously squeezing the bag. This requires some degree of technical skill and manual dexterity.

The Circle System

The circle system is a rebreathing circuit that passes the patient's expired gases through a carbon dioxide absorber (usually soda lime) before returning them to the fresh gas flow to be breathed by the patient (see Figure 20.2). The circle system can therefore be extremely efficient as the expired gas can be reused after carbon dioxide removal, permitting lower fresh gas flows and thus reducing atmospheric pollution. This has the additional benefit of conserving heat and moisture and reducing the volume of waste anaesthetic gases that are released into the operating theatre environment. Efficient scavenging is also possible in the circle system as scavenging can be connected to the APL valve where excess gas can be vented into the active gas scavenging system.

The circle breathing system consists of:

- a reservoir bag;
- an APL valve;
- two one-way valves (inspiratory and expiratory);
- a carbon dioxide absorber;
- a Y-piece patient connector; and
- a fresh gas flow source.

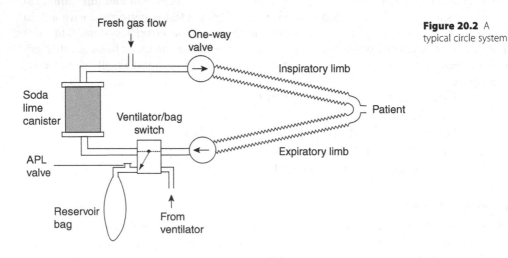

Figure 20.2 A typical circle system

Despite its benefits, there are some disadvantages to the circle system:

- the one-way valves required to ensure unidirectional flow can stick or fail due to condensation;
- inspired oxygen, end-tidal carbon dioxide, and inhalational agent concentrations must be carefully monitored throughout; and
- there is increased breathing resistance during spontaneous breathing.

Heat and Moisture Exchange Filter

An integral component for all types of breathing systems is the heat and moisture exchange (HME) filter. During normal breathing, inspired air is humidified and filtered by the upper airway. The delivery of dry gases via an endotracheal tube or supraglottic airway device bypasses this normal physiological process and can dry the respiratory mucosa. A disposable HME filter is attached to a catheter mount between the breathing system and the endotracheal tube or supraglottic airway device. The HME filter picks up water droplets from the expired gas, which retain some of the heat from the gas which has carried them. During inspiration, the incoming air collects the warm water droplets, and carries them as vapour into the patient's lungs – humidifying the inspired gas. Additionally, the HME filter also has an antibacterial capability, which can protect the patient and the breathing circuit from bacterial contamination [2].

In summary, it is essential that perioperative practitioners familiarise themselves with the features of each of the breathing circuits in common use. Very occasionally, circuits can develop faults, becoming disconnected or blocked. Perioperative practitioners should check the breathing circuits before use and change circuits in accordance with manufacturer's guidance and in line with the local policy, to ensure optimum patient care. It is also important to remember when using a breathing circuit in conjunction with an anaesthetic machine that all connections are secured by a 'push and twist'. The misuse of breathing circuits can compromise a patient's respiratory and cardiac function, which can lead to serious harm or death.

References

1. A. Donnelly and S. Dolling. Anaesthetic breathing systems. *Anaesthesia and Intensive Care Medicine* 2019; **20**: 90–94.

2. B. Al-Shaikh and S. G. Stacey. *Essentials of Equipment in Anaesthesia, Critical Care and Perioperative Medicine*, 5th ed. London: Elsevier, 2018.

3. T. K. Kaul and G. Mittal. Mapleson's breathing systems. *Indian Journal of Anaesthesia* 2013; **57**: 507–515.

4. W. W. Mapleson. The elimination of rebreathing in various semi-closed anaesthetic systems. *British Journal of Anaesthesia* 1954; **26**: 323–332.

5. C. L. Gwinnutt and M. Gwinnutt. *Clinical Anaesthesia (Lecture Notes)*, 5th ed. Oxford: Wiley-Blackwell, 2017.

Chapter 21

Pharmacological Agents in Anaesthetic Practice

Kathryn Newton, Peter Turton, and Brian Corrin

Introduction

Due to the wide range of drugs available, it is important for practitioners providing anaesthetic assistance to understand them. Clinical pharmacology can be divided into two broad categories. Pharmacokinetics describes the absorption, distribution, metabolism, and elimination of a drug whereas pharmacodynamics describes its effect and mechanism of action.

Pharmacokinetics

Pharmacokinetics describes four phases [1]: absorption, distribution, metabolism, and elimination, described below.

Absorption

A drug may be administered by many routes such as orally, intravenously, intramuscularly, subcutaneously, sublingually, rectally, or by inhalation. By each of these routes, drugs will be absorbed at a different rate, which may be very quickly (e.g., intravenously) or very slowly (e.g., subcutaneously). Furthermore, not all of a drug may be absorbed. Bioavailability describes the fraction (%) of an active drug that reaches the systemic circulation following administration. So, a drug that is administered intravenously will have a bioavailability of 100% because it is delivered directly into the systemic circulation. Conversely, a drug that is administered orally will have a much lower bioavailability because it must first travel through the gastrointestinal tract where it is subject to absorption before it gets to the systemic circulation. Some drugs may have very high bioavailability (because of high absorption) whereas some may have very low bioavailability (because of poor absorption, which will result in a higher dose being required orally relative to an equivalent intravenous dose).

Distribution

Once absorbed, the drug is required to reach the effect site such as the brain or heart in order to produce its therapeutic effect. Some drugs are distributed widely within the body whereas others tend to remain bound to certain molecules such as blood proteins. Drugs can only access certain parts of the body if they have suitable chemical properties. For example, the blood–brain barrier favours the entry of drugs with high lipid solubility or small size.

Metabolism

Most drugs in clinical use are transformed or metabolised in the liver by the enzymes of the cytochrome P450 superfamily. Drug administration can cause an increase in the activity (induction) or decrease (inhibition) of these enzymes. The administration of one drug can therefore alter the metabolism of another.

Elimination

Elimination is the removal of the drug or its by-products from the body, mostly by the kidneys but also by the liver and gut via bile. This is often described in terms of the half-life of the drug, which is the time taken for the amount of a drug in the body to be reduced by 50%. A drug with a short half-life will therefore only remain in the body for a brief period, whereas a long half-life will result in a longer duration of action.

It should be noted that the pharmacokinetics of any drug can be affected by many factors such as age or health. This means that a drug that has a rapid onset and elimination in a healthy young patient may have a slow onset and a prolonged action in an elderly patient.

Pharmacodynamics

The pharmacodynamics of a drug describe its interactions with the biology of the patient to produce its therapeutic and other effects. These interactions can take many forms such as binding to the active site of an enzyme, interacting with signalling proteins, or binding other molecules within the body.

Not all interactions with the body are beneficial, and pharmacodynamics also describes the mechanism of side effects such as toxicity. Whereas some drugs are relatively safe even in significant overdose, others may require very careful dosing or even regular monitoring of their plasma concentration to avoid serious complications. The therapeutic window represents the range between the lowest effective concentration of the drug and the highest acceptable concentration before the onset of toxicity. The therapeutic index (TI) is an expression of the ratio of the latter concentration to the former, so TI = toxic dose/effective dose.

Studies examining drugs demonstrate the effective dose, which is often described as ED_{50}, the dose which would be effective in 50% of the population, or ED_{95}, which would be effective in 95% of the population. Similarly, LD_{50} and LD_{95} refer to the lethal dose for 50% and 95% of the population.

Commonly Used Agents and When to Use Them

There are many different types of drugs used during an anaesthetic, and their usage may vary based on factors such as the type of operation being performed, the requirements of the patient, and even the individual preferences of the practising anaesthetist. One way to think about the different drugs used is to place them in the order in which they may be used during a general anaesthetic; Table 21.1 describes which commonly used agents are used at which point during a general anaesthetic. This list is by no means exhaustive and will contain agents that are beyond the scope of this chapter, such as premedications and intravenous fluids.

Routes of Administration

The route of administration describes the method by which the drug is delivered to the patient. Apart from the use of premedication, the oral route is not available to the

Table 21.1 Examples of commonly used drugs during general anaesthesia

Stage of anaesthetic	Example of drugs used for that stage	Aim of using each drug
Induction (opiate)	Fentanyl Alfentanil	Analgesia Obtund cardiovascular responses to laryngoscopy
Induction (intravenous induction agent)	Propofol Sodium thiopentone Ketamine Etomidate	Induce loss of consciousness May also be used for sedation
Induction (paralysing agent)	Suxamethonium Atracurium Rocuronium Vecuronium	Muscle relaxation for intubation and optimum surgical conditions
Maintenance of anaesthesia	Inhaled agents: • sevoflurane • isoflurane • desflurane • enflurane • nitrous oxide	Provide ongoing anaesthesia during an operation Gaseous induction
Antibiotics	Dependent on operation	Reduce risk of postoperative infections
Analgesia	Simple analgesics: • paracetamol Non-steroidal anti-inflammatories (NSAIDs): • diclofenac • parecoxib Opiates: • alfentanil • fentanyl • morphine • oxycontin	Opiates provide pain relief intraoperatively; this reduces heart rate and blood pressure, and thus reduces myocardial oxygen demand. Postoperative pain relief
Antiemetics	Ondansetron Cyclizine Dexamethasone	Prevent nausea and vomiting Treat postoperative nausea and vomiting
Vasopressor and inotropic agents	Many, but examples include: • metaraminol • phenylephrine • ephedrine • noradrenaline • adrenaline	Aim to raise blood pressure, either by constriction of blood vessels, or increasing cardiac force of contraction, or both Adrenaline has a role in anaphylaxis

Table 21.1 (cont.)

Stage of anaesthetic	Example of drugs used for that stage	Aim of using each drug
Anticholinergic agents	Atropine Glycopyrrolate	Treatment of bradycardia Treatment of excess secretions
Local anaesthetics (these may be used before or after induction or at the end of an operation)	Examples include: • lidocaine • bupivacaine • ropivacaine	Topical anaesthesia to skin Anaesthesia of subcutaneous tissues Nerve blockade for postoperative analgesia Intrathecal/epidural administration for pain relief and regional anaesthesia
Reversal of neuromuscular blockade	Neostigmine (with glycopyrrolate)	Reverse the effects of muscle relaxation

anaesthetist during a general anaesthetic. The commonest routes of administration are listed below (see also Figure 21.1):

- Intravenous: these are by far the most common, used for induction of anaesthesia.
- Inhalational: agents are delivered to the patient's respiratory system, either through spontaneous breathing of volatile agents, or delivered via mechanical ventilation.
- Regional: local anaesthetic is deposited around a nerve to provide analgesia to the region supplied by the nerve, preoperatively, intraoperatively, or postoperatively.
- Intrathecal: local anaesthetic and opiate agents are injected into the sub-arachnoid space to provide sensory and motor block to facilitate regional anaesthesia, for example during a Caesarean section or limb surgery. They may also be used prior to a general anaesthetic to provide analgesia [2].
- Epidural: local anaesthetic and opiate agents are injected into the epidural space to provide continuous analgesia via an indwelling catheter. Often used in obstetrics to provide analgesia in labour. Epidurals may also be used to provide analgesia during complex gastrointestinal surgery.
- Intramuscular: rarely used, but may be the chosen route of administration for specialist agents in obstetrics, such as ergometrine.
- Subcutaneous: used for infiltration of tissues with local anaesthetic agents.

The remaining sections in this chapter provide details of commonly used agents in anaesthetic practice.

Intravenous Induction Agents

The ideal intravenous induction agent is one that has a rapid onset/offset, does not cause disturbance on other organ systems, and offers both analgesic and antiemetic properties. It should induce unconsciousness within one arm–brain circulation time, that is, the time

Enteral	Oral
	Buccal
	Rectal
Parenteral	Intravenous
	Intramuscular
	Subcutaneous
	Intradermal
	Transdermal
	Inhalational
	Transtracheal
Topical	Skin
	Eyes
	Ears
	Intranasal
	Vaginal
	Urethral

Figure 21.1 Routes of drug administration (reprinted from T. Smith, C. Pinnock, and T. Lin (eds.), *Fundamentals of Anaesthesia*, 3rd ed. Cambridge: Cambridge University Press, 2009, p. 527)

taken to travel from the cannula where it is injected (usually the arm) to the brain, which usually equates to less than 30 seconds [3].

Propofol

Propofol is the most widely used intravenous induction agent. It comes in 1% and 2% (10 mg/mL and 20 mg/mL, respectively) preparations as an opaque white lipid–water emulsion. It produces general anaesthesia within one arm–brain circulation time. The induction dose is 1–2 mg/kg but this ought to be reduced in haemodynamically unstable patients due to producing a fall in systemic vascular resistance and, subsequently, blood pressure. Propofol causes respiratory depression and reduces airway and pharyngeal reflexes, making it an ideal agent for the insertion of a supraglottic airway device [4]. Propofol can also be used as an infusion for total intravenous anaesthesia (TIVA) (e.g., in patients with significant postoperative nausea and vomiting or for those undergoing surgery for cancer) as well as for sedation, both in theatre and also for patients who are intubated and ventilated [5, 6].

Sodium Thiopentone

Sodium thiopentone is stored as a pale-yellow powder in a glass vial containing nitrogen; 500 mg is reconstituted with 20 mL of water to create a solution of 25 mg/mL. The induction dose is 3–7 mg/kg and, in the UK, sodium thiopentone is predominantly used in obstetric anaesthesia [7]. It has a slightly quicker onset of action than propofol.

Ketamine

Ketamine has become an extremely versatile drug with uses in sedation, analgesia, induction of anaesthesia, and as a bronchodilator in severe asthma. It is different from propofol and sodium thiopentone in that it increases cardiac output, due to a rise in heart rate and blood pressure, making it an ideal choice in patients who are cardiovascularly unstable. Induction of anaesthesia can be produced intravenously (1–2 mg/kg) or intramuscularly (5–10 mg/kg); the onset of action is slower than other agents, with a state of hypnosis being reached in approximately 90 seconds. It will not cause respiratory depression but can lead to increased salivation and suppression of airway reflexes. It causes dissociative anaesthesia so the patient may experience hallucinations, exhibit nystagmus (eyes make repetitive and uncontrolled movements), and maintain their corneal reflex [8].

Etomidate

Etomidate is rarely used in the UK and has been withdrawn from use in other countries including the USA and Australia. The induction dose is 0.3 mg/kg and offers the advantage of minimal interference with the cardiovascular system; however, this is at the expense of suppression of the adrenal gland, and therefore a reduction in the hormones in cortisol and aldosterone, which play a key role in the stress response and are of particular importance in an unwell patient [9].

Inhalational Anaesthetic Agents

Every inhaled anaesthetic agent can be compared to a hypothetical perfect agent. Some properties of this perfect agent are as follows

- It should be non-flammable and non-explosive at room temperature.
- It should be stable in light.
- It should be either liquid and vaporisable at room temperature or a gas under these conditions.
- It should be stable at room temperature, with a long shelf life.
- It should be unreactive with the anaesthetic equipment, especially carbon dioxide absorbers.
- It should be environmentally friendly with no effect on ozone or global warming.
- It should be cheap and easy to manufacture.
- It should be pleasant to breathe and non-irritant to airways.
- It should have a fast onset and offset due to a low solubility in blood (low blood:gas solubility). This may seem counterintuitive, but an insoluble agent does not readily remain in solution in blood and therefore readily escapes solution and exhibits a high partial pressure.
- It should have high potency due to high oil:water solubility. An agent which is readily lipid soluble will exhibit high affinity for fatty tissues such as the brain.
- It should have minimal systemic effects such as on heart or kidneys.
- It should not react chemically with the body and should therefore not exhibit biotransformation. It should be excreted completely by the lungs.
- It should be safe for patients of all ages and levels of fitness. There should be no idiosyncratic reactions such as triggering malignant hyperpyrexia.

No agent in use can be considered perfect and therefore the choice of agent inevitably involves some degree of compromise. Volatile agents (sevoflurane, isoflurane, or desflurane) are introduced into the breathing circuit via a device called a vaporiser, which evaporates the anaesthetic agent in a predictable and controlled manner adjusted by dial on the top of the device [10]. Nitrous oxide is supplied as a gas and therefore requires no vaporiser, being added directly into the patient breathing circuit from the back bar on the anaesthetic machine.

Analogous to the ED_{50} described above, the potency of volatile anaesthetics is described by their minimum alveolar concentration (MAC). This describes the concentration of vapour in the alveoli of the lungs which prevents movement in 50% of subjects in response to surgical stimulus at an atmospheric pressure of 1 bar. A lower MAC indicates a more potent anaesthetic agent, but it should be noted that this number relates to healthy young volunteers and that the concentration of anaesthetic agent required by an individual patient may be much lower (such as in the elderly) or higher (in children). It should also be noted that administering an inhalational anaesthetic agent at a concentration equalling the MAC does not guarantee a lack of patient awareness and therefore vigilance is still required.

The volatile anaesthetic agents (isoflurane, sevoflurane, and desflurane) and the anaesthetic gas nitrous oxide enter the body via the lungs. Although the mechanism whereby anaesthesia is produced is not known precisely, the main site of action is in the brain. These agents must therefore be distributed from their source in the anaesthetic apparatus into alveoli within the lungs. They dissolve in the fluid lining the alveoli, pass into the pulmonary venous blood, which then leaves the pulmonary circulation and returns to the left atrium and from there blood flows into the left ventricle. This ventricle pumps arterial blood via the aorta into the cerebral circulation and thus the anaesthetic agent passes into its site of action in the brain.

During the induction of anaesthesia, anaesthetic agents move from areas of high concentration to areas of lower concentration. This phenomenon is called movement down a concentration gradient and is like the process whereby water flows down pipes from areas of high water pressure to areas of lower pressure. In biological systems, the concentration of a substance in these circumstances is referred to as its partial pressure. During induction, the partial pressure of the anaesthetic agent in the alveolus is higher than the partial pressure in blood and the agent, therefore, passes into the blood. Similarly, the partial pressure of the agent in the blood is higher than that in the brain and the agent passes into the brain where it exerts its effect. It is obvious that the partial pressures in the blood and brain will be very low at the beginning of induction, and absorption of anaesthetic agent is rapid because of the high partial-pressure gradients. As the process proceeds, however, the partial pressures of the agent in the blood and brain increase until they are equal to that in the alveolus. This is called the state of equilibrium and no further absorption of agent occurs because there are no remaining pressure gradients. In practice, a state of equilibrium is rarely produced. Agents that rapidly produce a high partial pressure in the alveolus tend to induce anaesthesia most quickly since the alveolar partial pressure is effectively the 'driving force' leading to the absorption of the agent.

When the supply of anaesthetic agents from the anaesthetic machine is stopped, the process reverses. Respiration reduces the partial pressure of the agent in the alveolus so that its passage is from the blood into the alveolus. The partial pressure of the agent in the blood is thus reduced below that in the brain, so that the anaesthetic agent passes from the brain into the blood and the system of pressure gradients is thus reversed, the anaesthetic agent being gradually eliminated via the lungs, as illustrated in Figure 21.2. Although respiratory elimination is the main mechanism for ridding the body of volatile anaesthetic agents and gases, some agents also undergo limited metabolism in the liver.

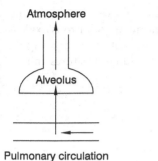

Atmosphere

Alveolus

Pulmonary circulation

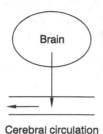

Brain

Cerebral circulation

Figure 21.2 The elimination of volatile anaesthetic agents and gases (reprinted from A. Davey and C. S. Ince (eds.), *Fundamentals of Operating Department Practice*. Cambridge: Cambridge University Press, 2000, p. 145)

Sevoflurane

Sevoflurane is frequently used in both induction and maintenance of anaesthesia. It is well suited for inhalational induction due to its pleasant odour and does not cause irritation of the airway and respiratory tract like other agents; it does, however, cause respiratory depression and hypotension in the absence of a reflex tachycardia.

Isoflurane

Isoflurane is commonly used in the maintenance of anaesthesia. It has a pungent smell and leads to coughing, airway irritability, and breath holding so it is not used for inhalational induction. It may cause respiratory depression, hypotension, and subsequent reflex tachycardia as the autonomic nervous system attempts to minimise a reduction in cardiac output.

Desflurane

Like isoflurane, desflurane has a pungent smell and can result in coughing, airway irritability, and breath holding and therefore is not selected for induction of anaesthesia. As the boiling point of desflurane is 23.5 °C it requires the use of an electronic vaporiser such as the Ohmeda Tec 6, which heats desflurane to 39 °C to avoid the output fluctuating. It has the most rapid onset/offset profile followed by sevoflurane and then isoflurane; this makes it a popular choice for operations of long duration.

Nitrous Oxide

The MAC of nitrous oxide is 104%, meaning that it is not suitable as a sole agent for maintaining general anaesthesia at standard atmospheric pressure as it would not be possible to achieve a concentration of 104%. However, as the effect of anaesthetic agents is cumulative and synergistic, nitrous oxide at a concentration of approximately 50% is often used in combination with the volatile anaesthetic agents mentioned above for both induction and maintenance of anaesthesia. Nitrous oxide provides an increase in the speed of onset of anaesthesia at induction (second gas effect) while reducing the concentration of volatile agent required to achieve an adequate level of anaesthesia intraoperatively. This can be especially useful as nitrous oxide causes less haemodynamic disturbance than the volatile agents. Furthermore, it is extremely insoluble in blood, resulting in a very fast onset and offset of action, and is not unpleasant to inhale. The other significant use of nitrous oxide is as Entonox™, which is a 50:50 mixture of nitrous oxide and oxygen – it provides analgesic effects, making it suitable for painful procedures such as manipulation of fractures and for women in labour [11].

Xenon

The inert gas xenon shows considerable promise as an anaesthetic agent with a MAC of 71%. It is extremely insoluble and gives rapid induction and emergence. It is produced by fractional distillation of air at extremely low temperatures. As a naturally occurring and chemically unreactive gas, it is non-polluting. It has minimal cardiovascular effects and is not a trigger for malignant hyperthermia. However, due to cost and equipment issues, it is not yet used clinically.

Environmental Effects of Inhalational Agents

The inhalational agents are mostly eliminated by simple exhalation and are not significantly altered by the body. They are vented into the active gas scavenging system or into the room, and eventually pass into the atmosphere. There is a growing awareness of the contribution of inhaled anaesthetic agents to the greenhouse effect and climate change, especially desflurane and nitrous oxide. It is therefore possible that, in the future, their use may be limited to a clinical necessity rather than clinician preference, and alternative techniques such as TIVA will be more actively encouraged (see Chapter 15).

Muscle Relaxants

Overview of Muscular Contraction

Each muscle fibre is supplied by a single axon terminal that terminates close to the muscle fibre. This connection between nerve and muscle is termed the neuromuscular junction and is the area in which muscle contraction originates. As an action potential arrives at the nerve terminal, calcium ions enter the unmyelinated portion of the nerve. This rise in calcium concentration within the nerve causes the release the acetylcholine (ACh) from vesicles within the nerve terminal (see Figure 21.3). ACh diffuses across the synapse (the space between the pre- and post-synaptic membranes) and binds to nicotinic acetylcholine receptors (nAChRs) on the post-synaptic membrane. On binding, nAChRs allow sodium, potassium, and calcium ions across the membrane, until a threshold potential is reached. This leads to the opening of sodium channels, causing depolarisation of the muscle membrane. Muscle cells then release calcium from the sarcoplasmic reticulum, and muscle contraction is initiated [12].

It is through the blocking of nAChRs that muscle relaxation is achieved. This is done through two classes of agent: depolarising neuromuscular blocking drugs (NMBDs) and non-depolarising NMBDs.

Depolarising NMBDs

Suxamethonium is the commonly used depolarising NMBD. It acts by mimicking the ACh molecule, binding to nAChRs, and causing the inflow of ions that leads to contraction.

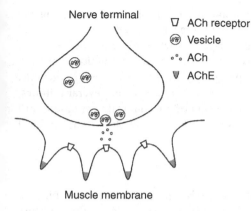

Nerve terminal

∇ ACh receptor

Vesicle

ACh

∇ AChE

Muscle membrane

Figure 21.3 Neuromuscular junction (reprinted from M. E. Cross, and E. V. E. Plunkett (eds.), *Physics, Pharmacology and Physiology for Anaesthetists: Key Concepts for the FRCA*. Cambridge, Cambridge University Press, p. 305)

However, suxamethonium has a longer duration of action than ACh, and stops ACh from binding to the receptor, and preventing any further transmission of electrical activity. Once suxamethonium is broken down, the nAChR can be bound by ACh again, and muscular contraction resumes.

Suxamethonium is administered intravenously (at a dose of 1–2 mg/kg) after induction of anaesthesia. Shortly after administration, characteristic muscle fasciculation can often be seen, and endotracheal intubation can be performed [13].

Reported side effects include bradycardia, hyperkalaemia, anaphylaxis, muscle pain due to fasciculation, and a rise in intraocular pressure. Suxamethonium should not be used in patients with burns (more than 10% of their body surface area) for 24 hours from the initial burns injury and should be avoided in the first 6 months of a spinal injury; in both situations, extra-junctional nAChRs form, which release potassium into the circulation [14].

More serious complications of suxamethonium use are malignant hyperthermia and a prolonged neuromuscular block, sometimes referred to as 'suxamethonium apnoea'.

Malignant hyperthermia is a rare condition in which calcium ions in the muscle cell continue to be released from its calcium store, the sarcoplasmic reticulum, leading to muscle rigidity. Energy in the form of adenine triphosphate is required to push calcium back into the sarcoplasmic reticulum, and this energy expenditure leads to the generation of heat and carbon dioxide. Eventually, potassium is released into the circulation, and lactate accumulates through cell death.

Malignant hyperthermia occurs after the administration of either suxamethonium or on commencing inhalation of a volatile agent. Signs include a raised end-tidal carbon dioxide on, with a characteristic step-wise increase in the plateau phase of the graph with subsequent breaths, increased temperature, tachycardia, sweating and muscle rigidity. The treatment includes stopping the offending agent (in the case of volatiles, switching from the volatile agent to an intravenous infusion of propofol), aggressive cooling of the patient and correction of electrolyte abnormalities. A specific antidote, dantrolene, is available and should be administered on suspicion of malignant hyperthermia. It works by binding to a receptor on the surface of the sarcoplasmic reticulum (the ryanodine receptor), and preventing the release of calcium from the sarcoplasmic reticulum [15] (see Chapter 28).

A prolonged block at the neuromuscular junction occurs when there is a deficiency of the enzyme responsible for the breakdown of suxamethonium. Such a reduction in plasma cholinesterase may be acquired (e.g., during pregnancy or liver disease) or genetic. Depending on the genetic abnormality, the block may be prolonged for several minutes, or up to several hours. Treatment is to continue sedation and mechanical ventilation until the effects wear off, though fresh frozen plasma is a source of plasma cholinesterase and will reverse the effects of suxamethonium.

Non-depolarising NMDBs

Non-depolarising agents act by binding to the nAChR and blocking ACh itself from binding to the receptor, but unlike suxamethonium, they do not lead to changes in ion flow or cause muscle fasciculation. This process is called competitive inhibition.

There are two types of non-depolarising agents, based on their chemical structures. Common *aminosteroid* agents include rocuronium and vecuronium, while *benzylisoquinolinium* agents include atracurium and mivacurium. Unlike suxamethonium, these agents are not dependent on plasma cholinesterase for their breakdown; aminosteroids tend to be metabolised by the liver, while benzylisoquinolinium agents spontaneously break down within the plasma by the process of Hoffmann degradation. This is a non-enzymatic, temperature-dependant process resulting in the spontaneous degradation and deactivation of the atracurium molecule. This means that a prolonged block on administration does not occur in patients with plasma cholinesterase deficiency; however, other commonly used agents, such as the antibiotic gentamicin, can prolong the effects of a neuromuscular block.

Rocuronium and vecuronium have minimal effects on the cardiovascular system. Rocuronium is used for its rapid onset, and intubation can be achieved within 60 seconds when high doses (0.9 mg/kg) are administered. It is for this reason that rocuronium is often used in preference to suxamethonium for Rapid Sequence Induction (RSI). In normal doses (0.6 mg/kg), intubating conditions can be achieved in under 2 minutes.

Atracurium is given at a dose of 0.5 mg/kg and can achieve intubating conditions within 2–3 minutes. Its main side effect is the release of histamine, which can cause either a localised or systemic rash, but may cause hypotension in bronchospasm [14].

Monitoring and Reversal of Neuromuscular Blockade

As previously discussed, muscular contraction is dependent on ACh binding to its receptor. Acetylcholinesterases (AChE) are enzymes that break down ACh. Therefore, an agent which can block the action of AChE will prevent the breakdown of ACh, so that more ACh is available to bind to its receptor. Non-depolarising agents can be reversed by using anti-cholinesterases, such as neostigmine. Neostigmine has effects away from the neuromuscular junction and can cause severe bradycardia. For this reason, neostigmine is usually given in combination with glycopyrrolate. Other side effects include increased salivation and abdominal pain.

Neostigmine can be used to prevent both types of non-depolarising agent; however, sugammadex can be used specifically to reverse the effects of rocuronium. Sugammadex works by encapsulating rocuronium, removing it from circulation, and reversing its effects.

It can be given in high doses to quickly reverse neuromuscular blockade, for example in a difficult intubation in which the procedure is abandoned [16].

Monitoring of neuromuscular blockade is achieved using a peripheral nerve stimulator. Peripheral nerve stimulators deliver an electrical stimulus to nerve fibres, with resulting muscular contraction. The devices have a variety of modes, but the commonest is the train-of-four (ToF) mode. In ToF mode, the device delivers four electrical stimuli, 0.5 seconds apart. These electrical stimuli cause the muscle to visibly twitch. The number of twitches seen corresponds approximately to the percentage of nAChRs that are currently occupied. Only one twitch is seen at 95% occupancy, and the fourth twitch starts to fade above 70% occupancy, disappearing completely above 90% occupancy. In general, the reversal of neuromuscular blockade by neostigmine can be performed when two or more twitches are observed [17].

Local Anaesthetics

General Principles

Local anaesthetic agents act by diffusing through the cell membranes of nerve cells and binding to the internal surface of the sodium channel. This prevents the sodium channel from opening, and stops the influx of sodium into the cell in response to changes in the resting membrane potential. This in turn prevents the formation of an action potential, and therefore prevents depolarisation along the nerve, preventing the transmission of pain signals from the site of tissue injury to the brain [18].

Local anaesthetics can be used in several different ways; subcutaneous infiltration of local anaesthetic can provide loss of sensation to skin when performing painful procedures such as suturing or performing venepuncture. They are used in nerve blocks to provide regional anaesthesia, providing analgesia during and after a procedure within the distribution of the nerve blocked. Local anaesthetics are also used in intrathecal and epidural anaesthesia to provide analgesia by blocking nerve roots across several spinal levels. Finally, some local anaesthetics (mostly lidocaine) are increasingly used intravenously as an infusion for pain relief postoperatively, although it should be noted that cardiotoxicity contraindicates bupivacaine and levobupivacaine for intravenous use.

Local anaesthetics are divided by their chemical structures, either *esters* or *amides*. Examples of esters in clinical practice are cocaine, used in nasal surgery for its vasoconstriction properties, and procaine. Examples of amides (and the more commonly used agent clinically) are lidocaine, bupivacaine, and ropivacaine. The decision about which local anaesthetic to use is guided by the individual characteristics of each agent [19]. In general terms, the duration of a local anaesthetic is determined by the level of protein binding; agents with limited protein binding have a short duration of action, while those that are heavily protein bound have a longer duration of action. The duration of action can also be extended by reducing the uptake and therefore removal of the local anaesthetic from the injection site. Hence, adrenaline is often used in conjunction with lidocaine to provide a longer duration.

It should be noted also that the efficacy of local anaesthetic infiltration may be reduced in inflamed tissue as the acidic conditions of these tissues prevents the dissociation of the local anaesthetic molecules necessary for their action [20].

Absorption and Toxicity

Absorption of local anaesthetic into the systemic circulation, and consequent systemic effects, is dependent on the site into which it is administered. Subcutaneous administration leads to low systemic absorption, whereas intercostal administration, for example, to provide pain relief for rib fractures, has the highest absorption, due to the close proximity of the target nerve to blood vessels. Raised plasma concentrations of local anaesthetics can lead to local anaesthetic toxicity. For this reason, bupivacaine is limited to a dose of 2 mg/kg, and lidocaine, 3 mg/kg (or 7 mg/kg if administered with adrenaline) [21].

Cardiovascular Drugs

The cardiovascular system can be manipulated by different pharmacological pathways, with a wide variety of agents available to the anaesthetist depending on the clinical situation. This section focuses on the commonly used vasopressors and antihypertensives used in the perioperative period and in critical care but is by no means exhaustive; it also presumes prior understanding of the physiology of the cardiovascular system.

Vasopressors by Bolus

The commonly used vasopressors that are typically administered in the form of a bolus include metaraminol, phenylephrine, and ephedrine (the former two can also be administered as an infusion). These are crucial in maintaining blood pressure following anaesthesia – whether that is regional (e.g., spinal) or general; this is particularly important for those patients with underlying cardiac disease, in order to ensure their coronary arteries are perfused.

Metaraminol is sympathomimetic agent, acting at the alpha receptors, which causes an increase in systemic vascular resistance (SVR) resulting in a blood pressure rise, and is usually associated with a fall in heart rate. SVR describes the resistance used in the circulatory system to create blood pressure. Metaraminol is a clear colourless solution, presented as 10 mg in a 1-mL ampoule and is reconstituted in 20 mL to form a solution of 0.5 mg/mL. Dosing of 0.5–2 mg is titrated to effect.

Phenylephrine is also a sympathomimetic agent acting at the receptor specifically. It leads to a rise in SVR and blood pressure with a reflex bradycardia. It is a clear colourless solution presented as 10 mg in a 1-mL ampoule and is reconstituted in 100 mL to form a solution of 100 micrograms/mL. It is administered as 50–100-microgram boluses, titrated to effect.

Ephedrine is a sympathomimetic acting at both alpha and beta receptors. Its greater affect at beta receptors than metaraminol and phenylephrine leads to an increase in cardiac output and heart rate as well as blood pressure. It is presented as a clear colourless solution as 30 mg in 1 mL and is reconstituted to 10 mL to form a solution of 3 mg/mL. Dosing is titrated to effect in 3-mg boluses [22].

Adrenaline (see following section) is administered in the cardiac arrest situation as 1 mg (10 mL minijet of 1:10,000).

Vasopressors by Infusion

Patients who are unstable (e.g., septic, ruptured abdominal aortic aneurysm) may require continuous vasopressor support – as mentioned above, metaraminol and phenylephrine can be used but this is usually temporary until central venous access is established and then alternative agents discussed below can be commenced.

Noradrenaline acts at alpha and beta receptors (alpha $\gg$ beta). It is administered to increase SVR and blood pressure. Dosing is 0.05–0.5 micrograms/kg per minute.

Adrenaline acts at alpha and beta receptors. It is dosed at 0.01–0.5 micrograms/kg per minute. It increases both SVR and heart rate – care needs to be taken at increasing doses due to the risk of arrhythmias [23].

Anticholinergics

These agents act as antagonists at muscarinic ACh receptors and therefore are useful in treating isolated bradycardia.

Atropine (600 micrograms in 1-mL ampoule or 500 micrograms in a 10-mL minijet) leads to a significant increase in heart rate although an initial bradycardia may be seen following a first small dose.

Glycopyrrolate also causes an increase in heart rate (200 micrograms/mL in 1-mL and 3-mL ampoules) [24].

Antihypertensives

In some situations, a reduction in blood pressure may be required, for example, an acute intracranial event, response to laryngoscopy, or poorly controlled hypertension in a patient requiring urgent surgery. Labetalol has actions at both alpha and beta receptors; therefore, its use leads to a reduction in blood pressure and heart rate. It is dosed at 5–20 mg and titrated to effect. This also can be used as an infusion [25].

Antiemetics

Management of nausea and vomiting in the perioperative period is an important task for the anaesthetist. Risk factors for postoperative nausea and vomiting (PONV) include patient factors (female sex, non-smoker), surgical factors (middle ear and ophthalmic surgery), and anaesthetic factors (use of opioids, volatile anaesthetics, and nitrous oxide).

The physiology underpinning nausea and vomiting is complex. At a basic level, there is an area in the brain called the vomiting centre which receives input from various sources such as the gut, middle ear, sensory organs, and, most importantly, the chemoreceptor trigger zone, which is rich in dopamine (D_2) and serotonin (5-HT) receptors. ACh is also key in neural transmission from the ear [26]. Antiemetics have been designed to act at these receptors in order to reduce the incidence of PONV; however, if a patient is at high risk from PONV then the anaesthetist should consider alternative techniques rather than rely on antiemetics, for example, multimodal anaesthesia including the use of regional techniques where possible, including TIVA [27].

Dopamine Antagonists

Examples include metoclopramide (also a prokinetic and has action at 5-HT$_3$ receptors) and prochlorperazine (also used in treatment of psychiatric conditions).

Side effects include extrapyramidal effects such as dystonias and akathisia.

Anithistamines

Examples include cyclizine and promethazine. Side effects include tachycardia.

5-HT$_3$ Antagonists

Ondansetron is the most commonly used antiemetic and acts at 5-HT$_3$. It also has a role in managing nausea and vomiting in patients undergoing chemo- and/or radiotherapy.

Side effects include headache, flushing, and bradycardia following intravenous administration.

Miscellaneous

Other agents used include steroids (e.g., dexamethasone) which have an unclear mechanism of action. They are also used to reduce inflammation and are thought to have an analgesic effect [28].

Analgesia

General Principles

The management of pain is an important aspect of the anaesthetist's role and there is a wide variety of approaches to do this. The decision of what type of, and how much, analgesia to administer depends on both the patient (who may have a history of chronic pain and therefore already be taking regular analgesia at home) and the procedure to be performed (major procedures will obviously require more pain relief than a minor one).

Non-opioid Analgesia

Paracetamol is a simple analgesic which is used regularly in the perioperative period to manage mild to moderate pain. It can be given orally, intravenously, or rectally. It also exhibits antipyretic action. An adult dose is 4 g/day in divided doses and 15 mg/kg in children. If a dose is exceeded, such as in paracetamol overdose, there is risk of acute liver failure due to a build-up of toxic metabolites, which are usually cleared by the liver when given at a therapeutic dose. Its mechanism of action is not fully understood but possibly acts at the COX-3 enzyme (see below) [29].

Non-steroidal anti-inflammatory drugs (NSAIDs) are also commonly used to treat mild to moderate pain. They can be given orally, intravenously, or rectally. They help to reduce the dose of opioid required. They work by inhibiting the enzyme cyclo-oxygenase (COX), of which there are subtypes (COX-1, COX-2, and COX-3) [30]. Non-specific COX inhibitors include ibuprofen, diclofenac, and ketorolac. A specific COX-2 inhibitor is parecoxib which is given intravenously. Side effects of NSAIDs include gastric irritation and bronchospasm (contraindicated in asthmatics whose attacks were precipitated by aspirin or other NSAIDs); they should be avoided in patients with renal impairment as they can reduce blood flow to the kidneys and make their kidney function worse.

Other adjuncts for analgesia include opiate-sparing techniques such as magnesium sulphate, lignocaine, ketamine, clonidine, antidepressants, antiepileptics, and regional anaesthesia but these are beyond the scope of this chapter [31].

Opioids

Opioid is a term for both naturally occurring and synthetic substances that act at opioid receptors whereas opiates refer only to naturally occurring substances with that action. Opioids are used to treat moderate to severe pain. They also have an important role during the induction of anaesthesia by both reducing the cardiovascular response to laryngoscopy (tachycardia and hypertension) and reducing the dose of induction agent required to result in unconsciousness (important in the unstable patient) [32]. Their side-effect profile is extensive and includes respiratory depression, nausea and vomiting, constipation, sedation, bradycardia/hypotension, histamine release, pruritus, and muscle rigidity [33]. It is important to know if a patient takes any opioid medications at home as they are likely to need a higher dose than normal, intra- and postoperatively. This section discusses the commonly used opioids but there are many others such as oxycodone, methadone, pethidine, and buprenorphine, which are not considered here.

Morphine is a naturally occurring opioid, which comes in a variety of presentations for oral, rectal, intramuscular, and intravenous administration. The dose of intravenous morphine is 0.1–0.2 mg/kg. It provides longer-term analgesia compared with the other opioids discussed below and is particularly useful in managing visceral pain.

Fentanyl is a short-acting synthetic opioid with a rapid onset of action. It is stored as a clear colourless solution for injection as 50 micrograms/mL. The dose typically used is 1–2 micrograms/mL but higher doses are used when wanting to blunt the laryngoscopy response/reduce the dose of induction agent. It can also be added to spinal and epidural anaesthesia.

Alfentanil is another short-acting synthetic opioid with a slightly faster onset of action than fentanyl. A typical dose used is 10 micrograms/kg as a co-induction agent and as short-acting analgesia intraoperatively.

Remifentanil is a synthetic opioid with an ultra-short duration of action. It is presented as a white powder in a glass ampoule. It is usually reconstituted with 0.9% sodium chloride to form a solution of intravenous infusion. It can be used in conjunction with a propofol infusion (TIVA) or alongside a volatile agent, often desflurane, for longer surgeries, to allow for rapid wake up at the end of the procedure [34].

Antibiotics

Antibiotics are frequently given preoperatively for preventative (prophylactic) reasons for certain surgical procedures. The goal is to ensure that the concentration is highest at the time of incision. Antibiotics work by either killing bacteria (bactericidal drugs) or by limiting bacterial growth (bacteriostatic drugs) and therefore allowing the body's own defences to combat the organism. In principle, there are five main ways antibiotic drugs are toxic to bacteria while being minimally toxic to animal cells:

(1) inhibition of bacterial cell wall synthesis (e.g., cephalosporins and penicillins;

(2) inhibition of bacterial protein synthesis (e.g., tetracyclines and clindamycin);

(3) alteration of bacterial cell membranes (e.g., polymixins and bacitracin);

(4) inhibition of bacterial nucleic acid synthesis (e.g., quinolones and metronidazole); and

(5) antimetabolite activity (e.g., sulphonamides and trimethoprim).

It is clinically significant to note that along with neuromuscular blocking agents, antibiotics are a major cause of life-threatening anaphylaxis during the perioperative period [35].

References

1. F. Roberts and D. Freshwater-Turner. Pharmacokinetics and anaesthesia. *Continuing Education in Anaesthesia Critical Care and Pain* 2007; **7**: 25–29.

2. G. Hocking and J. A. W. Wildsmith. Intrathecal drug spread. *British Journal of Anaesthesia* 2004; **93**: 568–578.

3. E. I. Eger. Characteristics of anaesthetic agents used for induction and maintenance of general anaesthesia. *American Journal of Health System Pharmacy* 2004; **61**: S3–S10.

4. K. S. Khan, I. Hayes, and D. J. Buggy. Pharmacology of anaesthetic agents I: intravenous anaesthetic agents. *Continuing Education in Anaesthesia Critical Care and Pain* 2014; **14**: 100–105.

5. Z. Al-Rifai and D. Mulvey. Principles of total intravenous anaesthesia: practical aspects of using total intra-venous anaesthesia. *BJA Education* 2016; **16**: 276–280.

6. J. Jacobi, G. L. Fraser, D. B. Coursin, et al. Clinical practice guidelines for the sustained use of sedatives and analgesics in the critically ill adult. *Critical Care Medicine* 2002; **30**: 119–141.

7. R. J. Hamer-Hodges, J. R. Bennett, M. E. Tunstall, and R. F. Knight. General anaesthesia for operative obstetrics with special reference to the use of thiopentone and suxamethonium. *British Journal of Anaesthesia* 1959; **31**: 152–163.

8. M. S. Kurdi, K. A. Theerth, and R. S. Deva. Ketamine: current applications in anaesthesia, pain and critical care. *Anaesthesia Essays and Researches* 2014; **8**: 283–290.

9. H. C. Hemmings. The pharmacology of intravenous anaesthetic agents: a primer. *Anaesthesiology News* 2010; October: 9–16.

10. K. S. Khan, I. Hayes, and D. J. Buggy. Pharmacology of anaesthetic agents II: inhalation anaesthetic agents. *Continuing Education in Anaesthesia Critical Care and Pain* 2014; **14**: 106–111.

11. N. El-Wahab and N. Robinson. Analgesia and anaesthesia in labour. *Obstetrics Gynaecology and Reproductive Medicine* 2011; **21**: 137–141.

12. J. C. Calderon, P. Bolanos, and C. Caputo. The excitation–contraction coupling mechanism in skeletal muscle. *Biophysical Reviews* 2014; **6**: 133–160.

13. J. Appiah-Ankam and J. M. Hunter. Pharmacology of neuromuscular blocking drugs. *Continuing Education in Anaesthesia Critical Care and Pain* 2004; **4**: 2–7.

14. S. S. Tripathi and J. M. Hunter. Neuromuscular blocking drugs in the critically ill. *BJA Education* 2006; **6**: 119–123.

15. P. K. Gupta and P. M. Hopkins. Diagnosis and management of malignant hyperpyrexia. *BJA Education* 2017; **17**: 249–254.

16. J. M. Hunter. Reversal of neuromuscular block. *BJA Education* 2020; **20**: 259–265.

17. C. D. McGrath and J. M. Hunter. Monitoring of neuromuscular block. *Continuing Education in Anaesthesia Critical Care and Pain* 2006; **6**: 7–12.

18. J. F. Butterworth and G. R. Strichartz. Clinical use of local anaesthetics in anaesthesia. *Anaesthesiology* 1990; **72**: 711.

19. D. E. Becker and K. L. Read. Essentials of local anaesthetic pharmacology. *Anaesthesia Progress* 2006; **53**: 98–109.

20. D. E. Becker and K. L. Read. Local anaesthetics: review of pharmacological considerations. *Anaesthesia Progress* 2012; **59**: 90–102.

21. L. E. Christie, J. Picard, and G. L. Weinberg. Local anaesthetic systemic toxicity. *BJA Education* 2015; **15**: 136–142.

22. M. N. Bangash, M. Kong, and R. M. Pearse. Use of inotropes and vasopressor agents in critically ill patients. *British Journal of Pharmacology* 2012; **165**: 2015–2033.

23. L. Stratton, D. A. Berlin and J. E. Arbo. Vasopressors and inotropes in sepsis.

Emergency Medicine Clinics of North America 2017; **35**: 75–91.

24. V. P. Nair and J. M. Hunter. Anticholinesterases and anticholinergic drugs. *Continuing Education in Anaesthesia Critical Care and Pain* 2004; **4**: 164–168.

25. D. B. Scott. The use of labetalol in anaesthesia. *British Journal of Clinical Pharmacology* 1982; **13**: S133–S135.

26. S. Chatterjee, A. Rudra, and S. Sengupta. Current concepts in the management of postoperative nausea and vomiting. *Anaesthesiology Research and Practice* 2011; **2011**: 748031.

27. X. Cao, P. F. White, and H. Ma. An update on the management of postoperative nausea and vomiting. *Journal of Anaesthesia* 2017; **31**: 617–626.

28. S. Pierre and R. Whelan. Nausea and vomiting after surgery. *Continuing Education in Anaesthesia Critical Care and Pain* 2013; **13**: 28–32.

29. C. V. Sharma and V. Mehta. Paracetamol: mechanisms and updates. *Continuing Education in Anaesthesia Critical Care and Pain* 2014; **14**: 153–158.

30. B. Doleman, J. Loenardi-Bee, T. P. Heinink, J. Lund, and J. P. Williams. Pre-emptive and preventive NSAIDs for postoperative pain in adults undergoing all types of surgery. *Cochrane Database of Systematic Reviews* 2018; **3**: CD012978.

31. K. Kumar, M. Kirksey, S. Duong, and C. Wu. A review of opioid-sparing modalities in perioperative pain management: methods to decrease opioid use postoperatively. *Anaesthesia and Analgesia* 2017; **125**: 1749–1760.

32. C. C. Hug Jr. Opioids: clinical use as anaesthetic agents. *Journal of Pain Symptom Management* 1992; **7**: 350–355.

33. P. Lavand'homme and A. Steyaert. Opioid-free anaesthesia opioid side effects: tolerance and hyperalgesia. *Best Practice and Research Clinical Anaesthesiology.* 2017; **31**: 487–498.

34. A. F. Nimmo, A. R. Absalom, O. Bagshaw, et al. Guidelines for the safe practice of total intravenous anaesthesia (TIVA). *Anaesthesia* 2019; **72**: 211–224.

35. T. Cook and N. Harper. Anaesthesia, surgery and life-threatening allergic reactions: report and findings of the Royal College of Anaesthetists' 6th National Audit Project: perioperative anaphylaxis. Available from: www .nationalauditprojects.org.uk/downloads/ NAP6%20Report%202018.pdf.

Chapter 22

Fundamentals of Emergency Obstetric Care

Victoria Cadman and Rebecca Helen Lowes

Introduction

Working in the obstetric theatre can be challenging and demanding, especially in an emergency context. Caring for the obstetric patient requires a high level of technical skill, knowledge, and experience. Roughly one in four pregnant women in the UK give birth in the operating theatre and more than one in ten births are by an emergency lower-segment Caesarean section (LSCS) [1]. Moreover, it is now more common to operate on women during pregnancy for non-obstetric reasons, though where possible this is delayed until after delivery. This chapter explores some of the foundational knowledge required to provide safe and effective obstetric care with a focus on the emergency context.

Emergencies

What Is an 'Emergency' Procedure?

Perceptions of what defines an emergency can differ. To provide clarity and enable equity in decision making, the UK's National Confidential Enquiry into Patient Outcome and Death (NCEPOD) determined a classification system. This system enables the optimum utilisation of theatre services and ensures that patients are operated on within an appropriate time frame.

The NCEPOD classification of intervention is as follows [2]:

- **Immediate**: Immediate life, limb, or organ-saving intervention, resuscitation simultaneous with intervention. Normally within minutes of the decision to operate.
- **Urgent**: Intervention for acute onset or clinical deterioration of potentially life-threatening conditions that may threaten the survival of limb or organ, for fixation of many fractures and for the relief of pain or other distressing symptoms. Normally within hours of the decision to operate.
- **Expedited**: Patient requiring early treatment where the condition is not an immediate threat to life, limb, or organ survival. Normally within days of the decision to operate.
- **Elective**: Intervention planned or booked in advance of routine admission to hospital. Timing to suit patient, hospital, and staff.

Emergency Anaesthesia

There are many patient factors which are assessed to prepare for elective surgery. These may include age, physical and mental health of the patient, and the American Society of Anaesthesiologists' physical status classification [3]. These factors are often considered at length during preoperative assessment, to assess a patient's co-morbidities and predict the perioperative risk. However, in an emergency the opportunity to acquire this information is diminished, or non-existent, owing to an increased risk to the patient. Emergency anaesthetic techniques, and cognitive aids – posters, flowcharts, checklists, or mnemonics – are used to minimise the risk and improve patient outcomes.

Rapid Sequence Induction during Pregnancy

Preoperative fasting is unlikely or unknown in emergency situations and therefore rapid sequence induction (RSI) is commonplace, with cricoid pressure (Sellick's manoeuvre) in the UK. The technique is performed to minimise the likelihood of aspiration of stomach contents, particularly due to pregnancy and labour-related anatomical and physiological changes, and to secure and protect the airway [4]. Despite a lack of good-quality evidence to support its efficacy during RSI [5, 6], cricoid pressure continues to be routinely used for pregnant women undergoing a general anaesthetic and is used by nearly all anaesthetists for women having a RSI for an LSCS [7].

The gold standard of airway management in obstetric anaesthesia remains RSI with tracheal intubation because of the increased risk of regurgitation and aspiration. However, there is emerging evidence emerging that supraglottic devices may be as effective at reducing the risk of aspiration, even in pregnancy [8]. Following a failed intubation, the most common rescue supraglottic airway device used for an LSCS is the i-gel® [7]. Performing a RSI in an emergency context is often highly pressurised and patient anxiety will likely be very high, so communication with the patient is key to reassure them, should this technique be employed.

Anatomical and Physiological Changes during Pregnancy

Before we consider anaesthesia in obstetric patients, it is first important to identify the altered anatomy and physiology in pregnancy and understand the points at which it impacts on and differs to routine anaesthesia. Please refer to Table 22.1.

The development of the fetus, known as gestation, lasts approximately 40 weeks (280 days), with 'full term' being defined as being at 37–42 weeks [11]. During this time, the woman's body undergoes significant anatomical and physiological adaptation as identified in Figure 22.1. The location of the placenta and presentation of the fetus (such as transverse or breech position) also pose a significant risk to life during labour and birth, and these require careful consideration and clinical management. These changes impact on the surgical and anaesthetic management of the patient and can exacerbate the management of a difficult airway.

Other variations in anatomy and physiology may also significantly impact the safe delivery of the fetus and these may include placenta praevia, pre-eclampsia, Haemolysis, Elevated Liver enzyme levels, and Low Platelet levels (HELLP) syndrome, gestational diabetes, female genital mutilation, and obesity.

Obstetric Anaesthesia

A variety of surgeries are performed in obstetric theatres and the care provided is unique in the multidisciplinary team care for both the mother and fetus ('dual life'), and the birth partner. Most obstetric procedures are performed under regional anaesthesia as this is safer

Table 22.1 Pregnancy-related changes in anatomy and physiology, the clinical implications, and clinical management (adapted from [9])

System	Changes	Clinical implications	Clinical management
Cardiovascular	↑ in blood volume, ↑ in size of heart, ↑ heart rate, ↓ systemic vascular resistance, ↑ stroke volume (approx 30%), blood pressure can vary, ↓ in diastolic pressure to term, may be ECG changes, ↓ peripheral resistance	Hypotension	For Caesarean section: volume preloading, intravenous ephedrine or phenylephrine infusion [10] Left lateral tilt of 15°
Haematology	↑ in blood plasma (up to 50%), red blood cells can ↑ by 20%, ↑ risk of anaemia, ↑ in coagulability	↑ risk of venous thromboembolism	Manage blood loss effectively and efficiently – mass haemorrhage protocols
Respiratory	Capillary engorgement of nasal, pharyngeal mucosa and larynx, ↓ in residual and reserve volumes, minute ventilation ↑ and oxygen consumption ↑, tidal volume ↑ (approximately 45%), PaCO$_2$ levels ↓	↑ secretions, oedema around the neck and airway	More likely to become hypoxic Use of a McCoy laryngoscope blade
Digestive	Gums can swell and bleed easily, ↑ intragastric pressure	↑ risk of reflux and aspiration during intubation	RSI with cricoid pressure Antacids such as sodium citrate and ranitidine to ↓ acidity
Reproductive	↑ breast volume, enlarged uterus, development of the placenta and fetus.	Implications on positioning and intubation, pressure of the inferior vena cava thus ↓ venous return, pushes heart upwards and rotated forwards	Oxford HELP® pillow Left lateral tilt when patient is on back Selection of a short 'stubby' handle/ selection of laryngoscopes for laryngoscopy Awareness of the site of the placenta and transfusion protocols
Endocrine	Human chorionic gonadotrophin (bHCG) produced, progesterone, oxytocin produced, oestrogen, levels of cortisol ↑, thyroid gland is enlarged	Oestrogen and progesterone cause hypertrophy of pancreatic beta cells and ↑ insulin secretion and insulin resistance	Management tools for diabetes such as checking blood glucose levels

↑ = increase and ↓ = decrease.

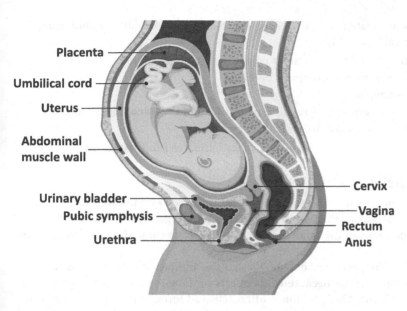

Figure 22.1 Normal third-trimester pregnancy anatomy

Placenta

Umbilical cord

Uterus

Abdominal muscle wall

Urinary bladder

Pubic symphysis

Urethra

Cervix

Vagina

Rectum

Anus

and results in less maternal and neonatal morbidity than general anaesthesia. Procedures requiring a general anaesthetic often require extreme urgency when assessed as having the potential for morbid outcomes or a risk to life. A general anaesthetic may also be due to patient choice, owing to the emotive nature of the procedure (e.g., the management of intrauterine fetal death).

While most anaesthetics undertaken in pregnant women occur within an obstetric or maternity department, all practitioners must be aware of the impact of pregnancy on anaesthesia. While surgery during pregnancy is generally avoided, or performed under regional anaesthesia, advancements in safety and technology mean it is increasingly likely that pregnant women may undergo surgery as part of treatment related to emergencies, trauma, and maternal malignancy. Pregnancy results in a variety of changes in both the anatomy and physiology of a woman, and many of these require a change or adaptation in anaesthetic provision.

Spinal and Epidural Anaesthesia

Epidurals are often used during labour, for an emergency LSCS, or procedures following delivery. In preparation for instrumental or LSCS delivery, it is possible to increase the effect of analgesia by 'topping-up' an epidural, and this is often with 0.5% bupivacaine, though some variations and 'rapid top-up' techniques using lidocaine–bicarbonate–adrenaline have been suggested, which halve the onset time [12]. It is, however, important to note that approximately 12% of epidurals fail, therefore a 'top-up' block may not be effective and, depending on the urgency, general anaesthesia or rapid sequence spinal anaesthesia may be performed [13]. A general anaesthetic is the quickest approach to anaesthetise a patient requiring a category 1 LSCS (see

Table 22.3) but is associated with increased morbidity and mortality. Rapid sequence spinal anaesthesia includes [14]:

- no-touch spinal technique (i.e., without palpating anatomic landmarks);
- consideration of omission of the spinal opioid;
- limiting spinal attempts;
- allowing the start of surgery before full establishment of the spinal block; and
- being prepared for conversion to general anaesthesia.

For more information on spinal and epidural anaesthesia, refer to Chapter 18.

General Anaesthesia

There will remain some circumstances where general anaesthesia is indicated such as severe fetal distress, maternal haemorrhage, and other extreme emergencies. While many aspects of general anaesthesia remain the same in obstetrics, there are some slight differences and factors to consider.

In terms of intubation, evidence has shown that the 'ramped' position is beneficial for intubation in obstetric patients because of its effects on functional residual capacity and laryngoscopy view [15, 16]. This position is often achieved through use of a head-elevated laryngoscopy pillow (HELP) and may form part of a modified checklist for RSI in obstetric patients, as shown in Figure 22.2.

General anaesthesia patients will not have the residual benefits of having had a spinal and may be given a transverse abdominis plane block for postoperative analgesia. This peripheral block is usually guided by ultrasound and put in place using a sterile technique, immediately post surgery. It provides effective analgesia after an LSCS by blocking several abdominal wall nerves [18].

Accidental awareness during general anaesthesia (AAGA) is another important consideration within obstetrics. The NAP5 report into AAGA confirmed obstetrics as being a high-risk area for occurrence of AAGA [19]. This identified that Caesarean sections provided a point of the accumulation of several risk factors for AAGA identified elsewhere in the report, resulting in much higher reporting (incidence 1:670 compared to 1:19,000). Such risk factors included RSI, use of thiopental, use of neuromuscular blocking drugs, omission of opioids at induction, difficult airway management, obesity, inadequate time for the volatile agent to take effect before the start of surgery, and the high incidence of emergency out-of-hours surgery resulting in reduced rates of consultant care.

Drugs Used in Obstetrics

Drugs that are used specifically within the obstetric context are listed in Table 22.2. As some drugs can transfer across the placenta, there are drugs that need to be avoided as these can be harmful to the developing fetus at any stage of pregnancy. Because of this, a pregnancy test is of key importance prior to any form of anaesthesia, as a woman may not know she is pregnant yet. In earlier stages of pregnancy, such drugs can lead to malformations due to their effects on the rapidly dividing tissues. During the later stages of pregnancy, the effects are more on the functional development of the fetus, and those given nearer delivery or during labour can affect the neonate. Drugs that should particularly be avoided are non-steroidal anti-inflammatory drugs and benzodiazepines. It is also essential for the

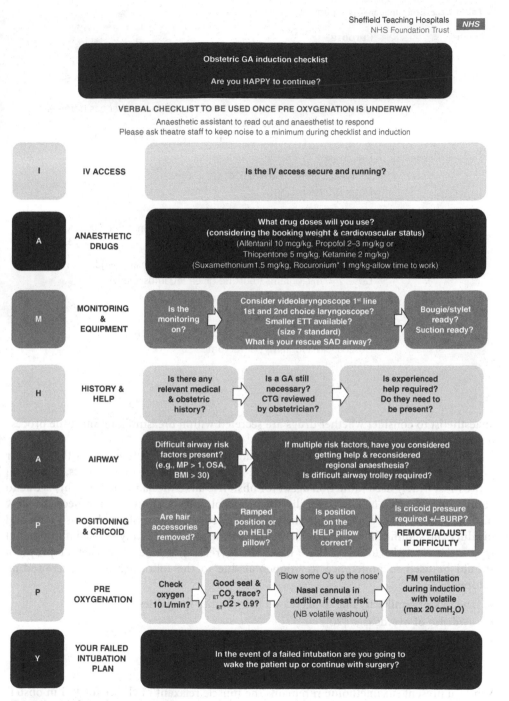

Sheffield Teaching Hospitals
NHS Foundation Trust   NHS

Obstetric GA induction checklist

Are you HAPPY to continue?

VERBAL CHECKLIST TO BE USED ONCE PRE OXYGENATION IS UNDERWAY
Anaesthetic assistant to read out and anaesthetist to respond
Please ask theatre staff to keep noise to a minimum during checklist and induction

I — **IV ACCESS** — Is the IV access secure and running?

A — **ANAESTHETIC DRUGS** — What drug doses will you use?
(considering the booking weight & cardiovascular status)
(Alfentanil 10 mcg/kg, Propofol 2–3 mg/kg or
Thiopentone 5 mg/kg, Ketamine 2 mg/kg)
(Suxamethonium1.5 mg/kg, Rocuronium* 1 mg/kg-allow time to work)

M — **MONITORING & EQUIPMENT** — Is the monitoring on? → Consider videolaryngoscope 1st line 1st and 2nd choice laryngoscope? Smaller ETT available? (size 7 standard) What is your rescue SAD airway? → Bougie/stylet ready? Suction ready?

H — **HISTORY & HELP** — Is there any relevant medical & obstetric history? → Is a GA still necessary? CTG reviewed by obstetrician? → Is experienced help required? Do they need to be present?

A — **AIRWAY** — Difficult airway risk factors present? (e.g., MP > 1, OSA, BMI > 30) → If multiple risk factors, have you considered getting help & reconsidered regional anaesthesia? Is difficult airway trolley required?

P — **POSITIONING & CRICOID** — Are hair accessories removed? → Ramped position or on HELP pillow? → Is position on the HELP pillow correct? → Is cricoid pressure required +/–BURP? REMOVE/ADJUST IF DIFFICULTY

P — **PRE OXYGENATION** — Check oxygen 10 L/min? → Good seal & $_{ET}CO_2$ trace? $_{ET}O2 > 0.9$? → 'Blow some O's up the nose' Nasal cannula in addition if desat risk (NB volatile washout) → FM ventilation during induction with volatile (max 20 cmH_2O)

Y — **YOUR FAILED INTUBATION PLAN** — In the event of a failed intubation are you going to wake the patient up or continue with surgery?

*Rocuronium 1 mg/kg needs reversal with Sugammadex-only use if prolonged surgery > 2 hrs anticipated
Remember max 2 intubation attempts (3rd by experienced colleague)
REMOVE CRICOID and/or lateral tilt if difficulty encountered   RB/FR/MW update 09/2019

Figure 22.2 An example of an obstetric RSI checklist (taken from Sheffield Teaching Hospitals NHS Foundation Trust [17]); CTG, cardiotocography; ETT, endotracheal tube; GA, general anaesthetic; MP, Mallampati score; OSA, obstructive sleep apnea; SAD, supraglottic airway device;

Table 22.2 Drugs that are used specifically within the obstetric context

Drug	Purpose
Syntocinon	Uterotonic Synthetic analogue of oxytocin, responsible for uterine contraction Maintains myometrial contraction and reduces bleeding Used routinely for elective LSCS delivery as the mother has not released any during the process of labour Dose: initial 5 IU at delivery, then infusion of 40 IU over 4 h
Ergometrine	Uterotonic Stimulates uterine contraction Dose: 500 micrograms
Syntometrine	Uterotonic Dose: combination of syntocinon 5 IU and ergometrine 500 micrograms
Carboprost	Prostaglandin Used in severe atony unresponsive to sytocinon and ergometrine Dose: 250 micrograms (must be given intramuscularly)
Misoprostol	Prostaglandin Can be used to induce labour Can be given as treatment for post-partum haemorrhage Dose: 600 micrograms per rectum

anaesthetist to consider whether drugs are secreted within breastmilk or affect the process of lactation.

Should a general anaesthesic be required, one of the key differences in the care for pregnant women is the induction agent used. Rarely used outside of obstetrics, thiopental is the most widely used induction agent for obstetric anaesthesia in the UK. This is due to conflicting evidence on the suitability of propofol and its effects on the neonate. Low induction doses of propofol result in significant neonatal depression whereas thiopental produces no significant neonatal effects, and so propofol should only be used if thiopental is contraindicated. However, there has been increasing debate over whether propofol should be used in preference to thiopental due to the following issues surrounding thiopental:

- the lack of familiarity due to decreased use in other specialties;
- evidence of overdosage [20];
- evidence of underdosage contributing to AAGA [21];
- the risk of an accidental swap with an antibiotic; and
- the supply and cost.

While at present suxamethonium remains the muscle relaxant of choice for RSI in obstetrics, there is increasing discussion for a move to rocuronium [16]. Rocuronium when given at high dose has a similar onset to suxamethonium and can be reversed with sugammadex to return to spontaneous ventilation. In terms of the effect of rocuronium on the neonate in comparison to suxamethonium, no significant differences between 5-min and 10-min Apgar scores and umbilical cord arterial blood gases have been found [22].

Obstetric Procedures

Obstetric procedures are unique as the birthing partner (e.g., father, friend, family member, or doula) often routinely accompanies the mother during labour and birth. It is important to include the birthing partner in the birthing experience as much as is appropriate and, should a general anaesthetic be required, birthing partners should be reassured and escorted from theatre as quickly as possible with regular communication from the team, as this will be an anxious time for them.

Modern births are centred around patient preference and choice, and this should continue in the operating theatre environment where possible. These may include the use of music, hypnosis, hypnobirthing techniques, and skin-to-skin contact. An array of health professionals will be present in theatre during obstetric procedures and their roles can vary depending on local policy.

Patients may often need to be positioned several times during obstetric procedures and the requirement to change position can be exhausting and painful for the mother, so consideration should be given for the use of Entonox® during contractions if safe to do so. Common positions include sitting, supine (with lateral tilt), lithotomy, and Lloyd–Davies. The operating table should be placed in a convenient position for all potential positions.

Caesarean Section

The most associated procedure with obstetric patients is an LSCS and this is the most common major surgical intervention in some countries [23]. LSCSs now account for over 25% of births in the UK and are indicated for several reasons, either as an elective or emergency procedure. The classification of the urgency of an LSCS currently in use is provided in Table 22.3.

Indications for an elective LSCS are regularly reviewed based on perinatal outcomes to inform planning for future pregnant women and their deliveries. In the UK, current National Institute for Health and Care Excellence guidelines consider the following indications for which an LSCS should routinely be offered to women [10]:

- a singleton, breech presentation at term, when external cephalic version is either unsuccessful or contraindicated;
- placenta praevia;

Table 22.3 Classification of the urgency of Caesarean section currently used in the UK [24]

Category	Definition
1: Emergency	Immediate threat to life of woman or fetus (perform as soon as possible)
2: Urgent	Maternal or fetal compromise which is not immediately life-threatening (perform as soon as possible)
3: Scheduled	Needing early delivery but no maternal or fetal compromise
4: Elective	At a time to suit the woman and maternity team

- a morbidly adherent placenta;
- women with HIV who are not receiving anti-retroviral therapy, or who are receiving anti-retroviral therapy with a viral load of 400 copies per mL or more; and
- women with primary genital herpes simplex virus infection occurring in the third trimester.

A LSCS is not routinely offered for reasons of multiple pregnancy, predicting failure to progress from cephalopelvic disproportion, reducing mother-to-child transmission of maternal infections, body mass index (BMI), preterm birth, and small for gestational age, as there is insufficient evidence that an LSCS improves these outcomes. Women can request to have an LSCS when there is no other indication. This can be for a variety of reasons and health professionals need to be sympathetic to these, promoting autonomy and advocating discretion while being mindful of the impact of birth on physical and psychological health. A common reason for a maternal request for an LSCS includes anxiety due to a previous traumatic birth.

During an LSCS the patient is positioned in a supine position with a left lateral tilt of 15° to reduce compression of the inferior vena cava. Despite the limited evidence to support or disprove the clinical value of a lateral tilt it remains standard obstetric practice [25]. Cell salvage is being increasingly used, particularly for women at risk from postpartum haemorrhage [26].

Other Obstetric Procedures

While LSCS accounts for most of the workload within obstetric theatres, there are several other procedures that are also undertaken. These are summarised below.

- **Assisted delivery** – this may be termed 'trial of forceps' and may either use forceps (Keillands or Neville–Barnes) or suction (Ventouse or Kiwi). Depending on each individual hospital's policy and/or the position of the baby, these may be attempted in the delivery room, or the mother may be taken to theatre. A failed assisted delivery needs to convert to an LSCS quickly.
- **Repair of tear** – tears are graded 1–4. The higher degree the tear, the more clinically significant. The repair of lower-degree tears is routinely carried out in the delivery room. More severe tears require regional anaesthesia and so are undertaken in theatre. Tears which are significant or mismanaged can have a lasting impact on physical, sexual, and mental well-being.
- **Removal of placenta** – when the placenta fails to deliver it needs to be removed in theatre promptly to avoid haemorrhage and infection.
- **Cervical cerclage** (Shirodkar suture) – also known as a cervical stitch – is a treatment for a weak cervix when the cervix opens too early in a pregnancy, resulting in late miscarriage or preterm birth. The procedure is carried out around week 12–14 and removed towards the end of pregnancy.

Unanticipated Events in Emergency and Obstetric Theatres

Though emergency and obstetric theatres teams are prepared for unplanned surgery, unanticipated events such as a major haemorrhage, cardiac arrest, anaphylaxis, and failed intubation pose an additional risk. Most emergencies are managed using protocols such as a mass haemorrhage or 'can't intubate can't ventilate' protocol and these should be accessible and rehearsed often by the team. Unanticipated obstetric emergencies such as fetal morbidities or neonatal or maternal death can be highly distressing for all parties [27].

Maternal death is the death of a woman while pregnant or within 42 days of the termination of pregnancy, irrespective of the duration and site of the pregnancy [28]. According to the World Health Organization, maternal mortality is unacceptably high with 75% of these attributed to one of the following [29]:

- severe bleeding (mostly bleeding after childbirth);
- infections (usually after childbirth);
- high blood pressure during pregnancy (pre-eclampsia and eclampsia);
- complications from delivery; and
- unsafe abortion.

There is a higher incidence in women who have pre-existing physical or mental health problems or from a minority ethnic background [30]. In the UK, all maternal deaths must be reported and, between 2016 and 2018, 217 women died during or up to 6 weeks after pregnancy. The causes were the following: cardiac disease, 23%; blood clots, 15%; mental health conditions, 13%; epilepsy and stroke, 13%; sepsis, 11%; bleeding, 9%; other physical conditions, 7%; cancer, 3%; pre-eclampsia, 2%; and other causes, 4% [31].

The death of a fetus or neonate requires sensitive management. Death can occur *in utero*, which is referred to as intrauterine fetal death, or as a stillbirth where the baby is delivered but there are no signs of life. As the former still requires a mode of birth, labour may be induced with a subsequent vaginal delivery, LSCS, or prolonged expected management. This is dependent on factors such as maternal choice, stage of pregnancy, and the physical and mental well-being of the mother [32].

Legal and Ethical Considerations in Obstetrics

In the UK, the fetus has no legal status until birth so while the fetus remains *in utero*, care of the mother remains the absolute priority [33]. This can pose ethical dilemmas, such as to deliver the preterm fetus to save the mother's life during a cardiac arrest or the right of the mother to refuse treatment against the advice of clinicians. Practitioners must respect the mother's right to autonomy, often ignoring their own moral convictions while remaining vigilant to coercion from third parties and advocating consent based on a woman's mental capacity to act.

Legal cases linked to obstetrics are often guided by case law, which also sets a precedent for future decisions. It will be interesting to see how the social, moral, and legal status of the fetus develops as technology continues to advance, particularly in the field of *in utero* imaging, fetal surgery, and ectogestation.

Surgery in Pregnancy

Although elective surgery is ideally avoided during pregnancy, urgent or emergency surgery may be necessary due to trauma, maternal malignancy, or acute conditions such as appendicitis. The complications of surgery during pregnancy include fetal loss or damage in early pregnancy, and early delivery in later pregnancy. Regional anaesthesia is preferred during pregnancy where feasible in order to minimise the exposure of the fetus to drugs and to minimise the physiological impact of anaesthesia. However, general anaesthesia may be inevitable. If general anaesthesia is necessary during pregnancy, the effects of pregnancy on the mother must be borne in mind as well as the effects of anaesthesia on the fetus. As gastric emptying is delayed in pregnancy antacid premedication and RSI with full pre-oxygenation should be considered. Drugs are chosen carefully, aiming to use well-established agents that are known to be safe in pregnancy.

In later pregnancy, the gravid uterus needs to be considered. A wedge or left lateral tilt should be used to improve venous return and maintain haemodynamic stability. From 24 weeks, the fetal heart should be monitored by cardiotocography, and the obstetric team must be informed and available in case of fetal distress or early delivery. Prior to this stage, the fetal heartbeat may be confirmed before and after surgery by auscultation or Doppler probe to confirm fetal survival.

Fetal Surgery

Advances in diagnostic techniques have led to innovation and advances in surgery. One such area that is evolving because of this is that of fetal surgery. Detection of congenital abnormalities has enabled the development of surgical techniques to correct these to optimise the outcome for the fetus. These can be performed as minimally invasive endoscopic procedures, open procedures, or as ex utero intrapartum therapy. This is indicated when there is an abnormality that has significant morbidity but can be corrected *in utero*. Examples include congenital diaphragmatic hernia, some forms of spina bifida, and congenital heart defects. Such surgeries provide additional considerations for the anaesthetist as *in utero* fetal anaesthesia and analgesia is also required.

References

1. Royal College of Obstetricians and Gynaecologists. RCOG statement on emergency Caesarean section rates, 2013. Available from:www.rcog.org.uk/en/news/ rcog-statement-on-emergency-caesarean-section-rates/.

2. National Confidential Enquiry into Patient Outcome and Death. The NCEPOD classification of intervention, 2004. Available from: www.ncepod.org.uk.

3. American Society of Anaesthesiologists. ASA Physical Status Classification System. Available from: www.asahq.org/standards-and-guidelines/asa-physical-status-classification-system (accessed August 2020).

4. A. Birenbaum, D. Hajage, S. Roche, et al. Effects of cricoid pressure compared with a sham procedure in the rapid sequence induction of anaesthesia. The IRIS randomized clinical trial. *Journal of the American Medical Association, Surgery* 2019; **154**: 9–17.

5. C. M. Algie, R. K. Mahar, H. B. Tan, et al. Effectiveness and risks of cricoid pressure during rapid sequence induction for endotracheal intubation. *Cochrane Database of Systematic Reviews* 2015; **11**: CD011656.

6. J. Butler and A. Sen. Cricoid pressure in emergency rapid sequence induction. *Emergency Medicine Journal* 2005; **22**: 815–816.

7. N. Desai, J. Wicker, A. Sajayan, and C. Mendonca. A survey of practice of rapid sequence induction for Caesarean section in England. *International Journal of Obstetric Anesthesia* 2018; **36**: 3–10.

8. Y. Metodiev and M. Mushambi. Supraglottic airway devices for Caesarean delivery under general anaesthesia: for all, for none, or for some? *British Journal of Anaesthesia* 2020; **125**: E7–E11.

9. N. Yanamandra and E. Chandraharan. Anatomical and physiological changes in pregnancy and their implications in clinical

practice. In E. Chandraharan and S. Arulkumaran (eds.), *Obstetric and Intrapartum Emergencies: A Practical Guide to Management*. Cambridge: Cambridge University Press, 2013, pp. 1–8.

10. National Institute for Health and Care Excellence. Caesarean section clinical guideline [CG132]. Available from: www .nice.org.uk/guidance/cg132.

11. Royal College of Obstetricians and Gynaecologists. A to Z of medical terms. Available from: https://www.rcog.org.uk/ for-the-public/a-z-of-medical-terms/.

12. J. Allam, S. Malhotra, C. Hemingway, et al. Epidural lidocaine–bicarbonate–adrenaline vs levobupivacaine for emergency Caesarean section: a randomised controlled trial. *Anaesthesia* 2008; **63**: 243–249.

13. P. H. Pan, T. D. Bogard, and M. D. Owen. Incidence and characteristics of failures in obstetric neuraxial analgesia and anesthesia: a retrospective analysis of 19,259 deliveries. *International Journal of Obstetric Anesthesia* 2004; **13**: 227–233.

14. S. M. Kinsella, K. Girgirah, and M. J. L. Scrutton. Rapid sequence spinal anaesthesia for category-1 urgency Caesarean section: a case series. *Anaesthesia* 2010; **65**: 664–669.

15. R. Hignett, R Fernando, A. McGlennan, et al. A randomized crossover study to determine the effect of a 30° head-up versus a supine position on the functional residual capacity of term parturients. *Anaesthesia and Analgesia* 2011; **113**: 1098–1102.

16. M. C. Mushambi, S. M. Kinsella, M. Popat, et al. Obstetric Anaesthetists' Association and Difficult Airway Society guidelines for the management of difficult and failed tracheal intubation in obstetrics. *Anaesthesia* 2015; **70**: 1286–1306.

17. Sheffield Teaching Hospitals NHS Foundation Trust. Obstetric GA induction checklist: are you HAPPY to continue? Available from: https://sheffieldteachin ghospitals.github.io/SODA-course/ documents/2018/I%20AM%20HAPPY% 202017%20(5).pdf.

18. R. Champaneria, L. Shah, M. J. Wilson, et al. Clinical effectiveness of transversus abdominus plane (TAP) blocks for pain relief after Caesarean section: a meta-analysis. *International Journal Obstetric Anesthesia* 2016; **28**: 45–60.

19. J. J. Pandit, J. Andrade, D. G. Bogod, et al. The 5th National Audit Project (NAP5) on accidental awareness during general anaesthesia: summary of main findings and risk factors. *Anaesthesia* 2014; **69**: 1089–1101.

20. S. Yentis and P. Clyburn, and M. Knight, on behalf of the MBRRACE-UK anaesthetic chapter writing group. Lessons for anaesthesia. In M. Knight, S. Kenyon, P. Brocklehurst, et al. (eds.) on behalf of MBRRACE-UK, *Saving Lives, Improving Mothers' Care: Lessons Learned to Inform Future Maternity Care from the UK and Ireland Confidential Enquiries into Maternal Deaths and Morbidity 2009–12*. Oxford: National Perinatal Epidemiology Unit, University of Oxford, 2014, pp. 65–71.

21. F. Plaat, N. Lucas, and D. G. Bogod. AAGA in obstetric anaesthesia. In J. J. Pandit and T. M. Cook (eds.), *NAP5. 5th National Audit Project of the Royal College of Anaesthetists and the Association of Anaesthetists of Great Britain and Ireland. Accidental Awareness during General Anaesthesia in the United Kingdom and Ireland. Report and Findings*. London: The Royal College of Anaesthetists, 2014, pp. 133–143.

22. M. Kosinova, P. Stourac, M. Adamus, et al. Rocuronium versus suxamethonium for rapid sequence induction of general anaesthesia for Caesarean section: influence on neonatal outcomes. *International Journal of Obstetric Anesthesia* 2017; **32**: 4–10.

23. T. Boerma, C. Ronsmans, D. Y Melesse, et al. Optimising Caesarean section use 1. Global epidemiology of use and disparities in Caesarean sections. *Lancet* 2018; **392**: 1341–1348.

24. D. N. Lucas, S. M. Yentis, and S. M. Kinsella. Urgency of Caesarean section: a new classification. *Journal of the*

Royal Society of Medicine 2000; **93**: 346–350.

25. C. Cluver, N. Novikova, G. Justus Hofmeyr, and D. R. Hall. Maternal position during Caesarean section for preventing maternal and neonatal complications. *Cochrane Database of Systematic Reviews* 2013; **3**: CD007623.

26. UK Cell Salvage Action Group. Intraoperative cell salvage in obstetrics: ICS Technical Factsheet 8. Available from: www .transfusionguidelines.org/transfusion- practice/uk-cell-salvage-action-group/ technical-factsheets-and-frequently-asked- questions-faq.

27. Å. Wahlberg, M. Andreen Sachs, K. Johannesson, et al. Post-traumatic stress symptoms in Swedish obstetricians and midwives after severe obstetric event: a cross-sectional retrospective survey. *BJOG* 2017; **124**: 1264–1271.

28. Organisation for Economic Co-operation and Development. Glossary of statistical terms: maternal death: Available from: https://stats.oecd.org/glossary/detail.asp? ID=6332.

29. World Health Organization. Maternal mortality. Available from: www.who.int/ news-room/fact-sheets/detail/maternal- mortality (accessed August 2020).

30. M. Knight, K. Bunch, D. Tuffnell, et al. (eds.) on behalf of MBRRACE-UK. *Saving Lives, Improving Mothers' Care: Lessons Learned to Inform Maternity Care from the UK and Ireland Confidential Enquiries into Maternal Deaths and Morbidity 2014–16*. Oxford: National Perinatal Epidemiology Unit, University of Oxford, 2018.

31. MBRRACE-UK. Saving lives, improving mother' care: lessons learned to inform maternity care from the UK and Ireland Confidential Enquiries into maternal deaths and morbidity 2016–18. Available from: www .npeu.ox.ac.uk/assets/downloads/ mbrrace-uk/reports/maternal-report- 2020/MBRRACE-UK_Maternal_ Report_Dec_2020_v10_ONLINE_ VERSION_1404.pdf.

32. Royal College of Obstetricians and Gynaecologists. Late intrauterine fetal death and stillbirth (Green-top Guideline No. 55). Available from: www.rcog.org.uk/ en/guidelines-research-services/guidelines/ gtg55/.

33. K. X. Cao, A. Booth, S. Ourselin, et al. The legal frameworks that govern fetal surgery in the United Kingdom, European Union, and the United States. *Prenatal Diagnosis* 2018; **38**: 475–481.

Chapter

23

Care of the Bariatric Patient

Hannah Abbott

Introduction

The word 'bariatric' is from the Greek word *barros*, which means large or heavy and is used to refer to the treatment of patients who are overweight or obese [1]. More recently, however, the term bariatric has also become associated with weight-loss surgery. While both terms may be used in clinical practice, obesity has more specific definitions while bariatric is a broader term. Fundamentally, however, the terms 'overweight and obesity' refer to the abnormal or excessive accumulation of fat which can impact health [2].

The global population is becoming heavier with obesity rates having almost tripled since 1975; and in 2016 over 1.9 billion adults were overweight or obese [2]. This is consistent with the trend in England where the majority (63%) of adults in 2018 were overweight or obese [3]. As a consequence, increased numbers of patients presenting for surgery and anaesthesia will be overweight/obese and thus experience the associated co-morbidities and specific perioperative challenges. This chapter explores the specific areas for consideration when caring for bariatric patients undergoing any surgical procedure.

Defining Obesity

Patients presenting for surgery will have their height and weight recorded. This is typically carried out in pre-assessment; however, it may also be on admission, particularly if the pre-assessment was completed by telephone. In order to determine whether a patient is overweight or obese, these measurements are used to calculate the body mass index (BMI), which is patient's weight in kilograms divided by the square of the height in meters (kg/m^2) [4] – the computer system does the calculation and will give a numerical value of the BMI. These numerical values correspond to different classifications of obesity/nutritional status as shown in Table 23.1. While the BMI is widely used, it is important to remember that this does not differentiate between fat and lean muscle and therefore has limited reliability in those with an athletic build. It also does not reflect fat distribution, which may impact some care considerations and the likelihood of some co-morbidities.

It is therefore suggested that the BMI is used in conjunction with waist circumference as a measure of abdominal obesity and associated metabolic risk factors. The desirable waist circumference is less than 94 cm for men and 80 cm for women [3]. The relationship between waist and height can be helpful in indicating the type of obesity and the associated perioperative challenges. Patients whose waist measurement is greater than half their height are considered to have central obesity, which increases the risk of a difficult airway, cardiovascular disease, thrombosis, and metabolic syndrome. In contrast, patients who

Table 23.1 Classification by BMI (from [4])

Classification/nutritional status	BMI
Underweight	Below 18.5
Normal range	18.5–24.9
Overweight/ pre-obese	25.0–29.9
Obesity class I	30.0–34.9
Obesity class II	35.0–39.9
Obesity class III	Over 40

have peripheral obesity accumulate fat outside the abdominal capacity and are lower risk [5].

Waist measurement is therefore particularly relevant in perioperative care as it allows practitioners to consider both the risk level and any specific equipment, for example, table width extenders or appropriate surgical instruments, such as retractors.

Physiological Changes in the Bariatric Patient

Obesity is a complex physiological condition with multi-factorial causation and affects many physiological systems, resulting in a number of co-morbidities [6]. All of these can have an impact on the perioperative care of the patient. This chapter, however, focuses on the most common and their impact on clinical practice.

Respiratory Function

The most significant impact on respiratory function occurs in patients with a BMI over 45, when significant impairment is likely. Obese patients have a decreased functional residual capacity, which, when combined with their increased minute oxygen demand and increased work of breathing, results in rapid oxygen desaturation following apnoea [6, 7]. Obesity also increases the likelihood that the individual will have asthma, due to a number of predisposing factors including reduced lung volume and narrowing of airways, changes to the smooth muscle, and an inflammatory state associated with obesity [6, 7]. It has been suggested that the observed wheezing in the obese patient may be due to airway closure rather than asthma as weight loss can result in the subsidence of symptoms [7]. Patients may also have developed pulmonary hypertension due to their obesity and this increases the morbidity and mortality risk of surgery and anaesthesia [6].

Obstructive Sleep Apnoea

Obstructive sleep apnoea (OSA) is a breathing disorder where there are periods of reduced or ceased breathing during sleep, and it occurs in 10–20% of patients with a BMI over 35; however, this is often undiagnosed. OSA has significant implications for perioperative care as it significantly increases the risks of postoperative desaturation, respiratory failure, postoperative cardiac events, and admission into intensive care; it is also associated with difficult airway and laryngoscopy [7].

It is essential that OSA is considered in the preoperative assessment of obese patients and the STOP-Bang questionnaire is a common tool which was developed specifically for surgical patients and has been validated for patients with a BMI over 30 [8]. The STOP-Bang tool asks the patient about:

Snoring – whether the patient knows they snore;

Tiredness – whether the patient experiences tiredness or falling asleep during the day;

Observation – whether anyone has seen the patient gasping or stop breathing during sleep; and

Pressure – whether the patient has high blood pressure.

It also includes some additional data: BMI, Age, Neck measurement, and Gender. Based on the information, a score is provided which indicates the risk of OSA [9].

Cardiovascular System

In obesity, the cardiovascular system has to adapt to the increased physical mass and meet the associated increased metabolic demands. Obesity will therefore result in increased blood pressure and increased cardiac output and workload. Patients with untreated OSA may also present with pulmonary hypertension and heart failure, of which heart failure is the greatest risk factor for perioperative complications. Obesity is associated with arrhythmias, particularly increasing the risk of atrial fibrillation [6, 7].

Thrombosis

All perioperative patients must be assessed for their risk of thrombosis. However, obesity is a known factor and must be considered in line with the other procedural and patient-specific risk factors [10]. Obesity is associated with a higher incidence of venous thromboembolism (VTE), stroke, and myocardial infarction. Appropriate methods of intraoperative VTE prophylaxis need to be selected, which may include intermittent pneumatic calf compression devices and/or thromboembolic device (TED) stockings. There is limited evidence supporting the use of TED stockings in obesity; however, they are commonly provided to all patients on admission; it is essential that there are sufficient size combinations available, particularly to cater for shorter leg length with a large diameter, as incorrectly sized TED can cause vascular occlusion [7, 11, 12]. In addition to this mechanical prophylaxis, heparin (low-molecular-weight or low-dose unfractionated) is recommended [13]; however, this must be balanced against the risk of blood loss. Patients should be encouraged to mobilise as soon as possible and it is particularly important to remind them to continue this throughout their recovery at home, as thrombosis most frequently occurs after discharge. However, it is suggested that this risk can be reduced by the continuation of thromboprophylaxis medication [14].

Diabetes

There is a clear association between obesity and insulin resistance and hence bariatric patients are more likely to have diabetes than those within the normal weight range. The patient's history of glycaemic control should be explored at pre-assessment as poor control increases the risk of wound infections and acute renal failure. Good glycaemic control is also essential during the perioperative period as failure to achieve this is associated with increased morbidity [6, 7].

Gastrointestinal System

Bariatric patients are at a higher risk of reflux due to mechanical and hormonal changes [6]. It is therefore considered good practice to administer preoperative metoclopramide and oral ranitidine as a prophylactic measure for all bariatric patients, even if reflux is not reported [15]. For patients with a history of reflux, a rapid sequence induction technique will typically be employed.

Psychological Considerations for the Bariatric Patient

In order to deliver holistic care to the patient, it is essential that the patient's psychological needs are also considered. Obesity has been associated with mood and anxiety disorders; this relationship is linked to both hormonal and social factors [6]. Bariatric patients are likely, therefore, to have encountered negative societal attitudes and so it is important that effective care planning does not reinforce these attitudes or add to existing feelings of discrimination or shame. For example, by ensuring that there is appropriately sized equipment at every stage is important to avoid patient embarrassment.

Preoperative Assessment and Preparation

Bariatric patients will undergo a full preoperative assessment in the same way as all patients. While there are several physiological changes associated with obesity, it is important to remember that many bariatric patients are relatively healthy, with a comparable perioperative risk to those of normal weight. The specific assessments for the bariatric patient therefore focus on OSA, thrombosis, and respiratory assessment. As with all preoperative diagnostic testing, this is based on the assessment of clinical need to impact the management of the patient; obesity alone is not a sole indicator for preoperative testing [7].

The chance of a difficult intubation is 30% higher in obese patients [16] and therefore it is important to complete a full airway assessment. Additionally, in bariatric patients, it is useful to record the neck circumference as difficult intubation has been associated with a circumference of over 60 cm [17]; the ratio of neck circumference to thyromental distance is also considered an indicator of difficult intubation [18]. A further qualitative assessment has been suggested as a submental sign assessment; a positive submental sign, where the submental space consists of a non-complaint tissue mass preventing palpation of the hyoid bone, is considered indicative of difficult intubation [19].

When preparing the patient for surgery, it is essential that there are suitably sized gowns, disposable underwear (if appropriate), and name bands available, to ensure patient dignity is not compromised. Patients with beards may be asked to trim or shave these as they can impair bag–mask ventilation, which is more challenging in obesity [7]; such requests must be handled sensitively.

Preparation of the Theatre

The team brief prior to the start of the list is a fundamental process to enable sharing of key patient information, thus ensuring safe, individualised care [12]; this is therefore an essential opportunity to plan the care for bariatric patients. Considerations at this meeting may

Table 23.2 Specific equipment considerations for the bariatric patient (from [5])

Patient positioning/handling	Operating table with appropriate weight limit Hover mattress, slide sheet, and transfer equipment Gel padding to reduce risk of pressure sores Wide strapping to secure the patient Table extenders and/or arm boards to accommodate the patient on the operating table Equipment for ramping; due to raising the patient's head and upper body in this position, the anaesthetist may benefit from a step when the patient is in this position
Patient monitoring	Large blood pressure cuff or forearm cuff of sufficient size (a range of sizes is suggested) Neuromuscular monitoring (typical monitoring for all patients when muscle relaxants are used) Depth of anaesthesia monitoring
Intravenous access	Long-length cannulas Ultrasound machine to enable location of veins
Airway and ventilation	Tracheal tubes – size should be based on ideal weight and a smaller size should be available Difficult airway equipment as intubation may be difficult Video laryngoscope Ventilator which has pressure modes and positive end expiratory pressure
Other	Long needles for regional anaesthesia Calf compressors of sufficient size

include any specific risk factors related to the patient, the manual handling plan, and whether there are sufficient team members to safely move and position the patient. This therefore allows any issues to be addressed prior to the arrival of the patient.

The theatre will be checked and prepared as usual. However, some additional/specific equipment may be required for bariatric patients as shown in Table 23.2.

There may also be a preference to anaesthetise in the operating theatre as this avoids transporting the anaesthetised patient and the risk of desaturation associated with disconnection of the breathing system. If this is the plan, the anaesthetic practitioner needs to ensure all their equipment is available in theatre and the rest of the team need to be aware of this, in order to limit preparation noise at induction.

Anaesthetic Care

Where appropriate, regional anaesthetic techniques offer several advantages for bariatric patients; however, there must still be a plan for conversion to general anaesthesia. Even where regional techniques alone are not appropriate for surgery, they may still be employed for the purposes of postoperative pain relief, to limit the use of opioids. It is suggested that the sitting position is preferable for spinal and epidural techniques as this optimises patient comfort and success rate [20]; however, patients with central obesity may find this position difficult.

Where general anaesthesia is required, pre-oxygenation is essential prior to induction as this increases the tolerance to apnoea and so is crucial where there is an increased risk of difficult intubation. It is suggested that the patient is placed in the 'ramping' position for induction – in this position the tragus of the ear is level with the sternum and the arms are away from the chest. This ramping position is beneficial for oxygenation and ventilation, in addition to improving laryngoscopy view. The goal at induction is to minimise the risk of desaturation and hence there should be minimal time from induction to commencement of ventilation, following successful intubation [5, 7].

Tracheal intubation and ventilation is the preferred airway management option due to the increased work of spontaneous breathing in bariatric patients. Supraglottic airways may occasionally be used for selected patients undergoing short surgical procedures where the patient can remain head up throughout; however, there must be a plan for conversion to intubation if required; for example, due to an inability to maintain sufficient oxygen saturations [7].

Research into the pharmacology of anaesthetic drugs has shown that there are changes to the apparent volume of drug distribution in obese patients. This is because obese patients have an increased fat mass per kilogram of total body weight, resulting in an overall decrease in lean body mass per kilogram [21]. This is a consideration when selecting anaesthetic drugs; for example, propofol is lipophilic and so the suggested dosing for propofol infusion is the 'adjusted body weight' (ideal plus 40% excess) [5]. In contrast, atracurium is hydrophilic with a similar distribution in obese and non-obese patients and hence the dosage is calculated using the lean body mass. It is believed that the high proportion of body fat in obese patients acts as a reservoir for volatile anaesthetic agents, which may increase emergence time and the risk of residual airway obstruction. While it has been suggested that the low blood:gas partition coefficient in desflurane could be beneficial, a randomised control trial has not shown any significant difference between sevoflurane and desflurane in the recovery of obese patients [15, 22].

Extubation must be carefully planned and the reversal of neuromuscular blockade monitored with a nerve stimulator. Prior to extubation there must be a full reversal with the return of airway reflexes, and the patient should be breathing with acceptable tidal volumes. The patient should be extubated awake and in the sitting position. It is suggested that a nasopharyngeal airway may be beneficial for patients with OSA to minimise the risk of partial airway obstruction in emergence [5, 7].

Patient Positioning and Manual Handling

All patients are risk assessed prior to manual handling; however, this is of particular importance when planning care for bariatric patients. The planning process should ensure that there is appropriate equipment and sufficient staff available to ensure efficient care delivery. This is also to prevent embarrassment for the patient if it becomes obvious that there are delays while additional staff are sought to move them.

Where possible, the patient can be encouraged to self-transfer to the operating table. However, some bariatric patients may have limited mobility, and hence this may not be possible. Due to the design of theatres and the ceiling-mounted equipment, it is not usually possible to have a ceiling-mounted hoist/track and hence lateral transfer is performed using sliding boards [23]. A hover mattress is advised for transferring the bariatric patient as this creates a cushion of air that reduces friction and allows the team to 'glide' the patient between the bed and table.

It is essential to check the safe operating load of the equipment to ensure this is suitable for the weight of the patient. Sufficient table attachments are also required in order to position the patient and ensure they are secure on the table; when completing this, it is important to consider how moving the patient to position them and moving the patient during surgery may change the weight distribution due to the movement of the excess tissue [23].

When positioning the bariatric patient, particular care must be taken in relation to pressure-area care as obese patients have an increased risk of pressure ulcers due to greater skin–weight ratio, reduced vascularity, and reduced perfusion in adipose tissue [1]. When positioning bariatric patients, it is therefore important to ensure that table attachments are not causing pressure and that suitable pressure-relieving material, such as gel which redistributes pressure, is used.

Postoperative Care

The bariatric patient will be monitored in the post-anaesthetic care unit (PACU), with particular attention to respiratory function to observe for hypoventilation. Postoperative oxygen therapy should continue until the patient is mobile; it has been suggested that postoperative incentive spirometry and continuous positive airway pressure (CPAP) in the PACU improves the return of pulmonary function [15]. This is not, however, part of the UK guidance, which advocates the use of inhaled oxygen in the PACU unless this is not sufficient to maintain adequate oxygen saturation [7]. For patients with known OSA, they will also be cared for in the seated position and their own CPAP will recommence in the PACU; postoperative opioids are avoided where possible for these patients as they cause respiratory depression [5].

The patient should be positioned in a seated or semi-seated, 45° head-up tilt position. It is beneficial if the bed/trolley is electronically controlled as this minimises manual handling for the team. When moving the patient in the PACU it is essential that there are sufficient staff and that sliding sheets are used to prevent skin damage from friction and sheer. PACU practitioners should also check the location of any catheters and wound drains, to ensure that the tubing has not become buried in soft tissue which can cause pressure damage in the skin folds [1].

Bariatric patients can be discharged from the PACU when they meet the normal discharge criteria and, in addition, they have a normal respiratory rate with no hypopnea/apnoea for a minimum of an hour, and oxygen saturation has returned to preoperative values with/without oxygen [7].

The postoperative recovery continues on the ward where the patient will be encouraged to mobilise as soon as possible. Oxygen therapy is continued until oxygen saturations return to the patient's baseline levels and monitoring continues until the baseline can be maintained without supplementary oxygen [7].

Specific Surgery: Bariatric Surgery

The chapter has considered the care of bariatric patients undergoing any perioperative procedure. However, there are some surgical procedures specific to this patient group. Bariatric surgery is an effective way of achieving and maintaining weight loss for obese patients who have typically exhausted all other methods. It is an overarching term for a range of surgical procedures including gastric banding, Rouex-en-Y gastric bypass, and sleeve gastrectomy. The aim of bariatric surgery is to reduce the stomach volume, thus achieving satiety after small volumes of food, and hence reducing calorie intake [11].

Patients undergoing bariatric surgery are required to follow a specific preoperative diet for 2 weeks prior to surgery. This is a low-fat, low-calorie, and low-carbohydrate diet that is designed to reduce glycogen stores, in particular those in the liver, which will reduce the size of the liver overall, thus improving the surgical access to the stomach [11].

The Obesity Surgery Mortality Risk Stratification (OS-MRS) score is used to assess the risk factors associated with mortality. This considers BMI, gender, age, hypertension, and risk factors for pulmonary embolism, resulting in a numerical score which corresponds to the risk of mortality. While this may be considered a useful tool for all bariatric patients, it has only been validated for use in those undergoing gastric bypass surgery [7].

It is also essential to know if a patient presenting for any surgical procedure has had previous bariatric surgery. This is because patients with a gastric band are at increased risk of aspiration and hence intubation is recommended [7].

References

1. A. Rush. Bariatric care: pressure ulcer prevention. *Wound Essentials* 2009; **4**: 68–74.

2. Wold Health Organization. Obesity and overweight. Available from: www.who.int/news-room/fact-sheets/detail/obesity-and-overweight (accessed June 2020).

3. NHS Digital. Statistics on obesity, physical activity and diet, England, 2020. Available from: https://digital.nhs.uk/data-and-information/publications/statistical/statistics-on-obesity-physical-activity-and-diet/england-2020.

4. World Health Organization Regional Office for Europe. Body mass index: BMI. Available from: www.euro.who.int/en/health-topics/disease-prevention/nutrition/a-healthy-lifestyle/body-mass-index-bmi (accessed June 2020).

5. Society for Obesity and Bariatric Anaesthesia. Anaesthesia for the obese patient (SOBA single-sheet guideline). Available from: www.sobauk.co.uk/guidelines-1.

6. V. E. Ortiz and J. Kwo. Obesity: physiologic changes and implications for preoperative management. *BMC Anesthesiology* 2015; **15**: 97–109.

7. Association of Anaesthetists of Great Britain and Ireland. Peri-operative management of the obese surgical patient 2015. *Anaesthesia* 2015; **70**: 859–879.

8. F. Chung, Y. Yang, and P. Liao. Predictive performance of the STOP-Bang score for identifying obstructive sleep apnea in obese patients. *Obesity Surgery* 2013; **23**: 2050–2057.

9. Toronto Western Hospital. STOP-Bang questionnaire. Available from: www.stopbang.ca (accessed June 2020).

10. National Institute for Health and Care Excellence. Venous thromboembolism in over 16s: reducing the risk of hospital-acquired deep vein thrombosis or pulmonary embolism. Available from: www.nice.org.uk/guidance/ng89/chapter/recommendations.

11. H. Abbott. Laparaoscopic adjustable gastric band; the care of Chloe Brown. In H. Abbott and S. Wordsworth (eds.), *Perioperative Practice Case Book*. London: Open University Press, 2016, pp. 167–176.

12. H. Abbott. Perioperative assessment. In H. Abbott and M. Ranson (eds.), *Clinical Examination Skills for Healthcare Professionals*, 2nd ed. Keswick: M&K Publishing, 2017, pp. 171–192.

13. M. K. Gould, D. A. Garcia, S. M. Wren, et al. Prevention of VTE in nonorthopedic surgical patients: Antithrombotic Therapy and Prevention of Thrombosis, 9th ed. American College of Chest Physicians Evidence-Based Clinical Practice Guidelines. *Chest* 2012; **141**: e227S.

14. I. Raftopoulos, C. Martindale, A. Cronin, et al. The effect of extended post-discharge chemical thromboprophylaxis on venous thromboembolism rates after bariatric surgery: a prospective comparison trial. *Surgical Endoscopy* 2008; **22**: 2384–2391.

15. A. Subharwal and N. Christelis. Anaesthesia for bariatric surgery. *Continuing Education in Anaesthesia* 2010; **10**: 99–103.

16. L. H. Lundstrfm, A. M. Mfller, C. Rosenstock, et al. High body mass index is a weak predictor for difficult and failed tracheal intubation: a cohort study of 91,332 consecutive patients scheduled for direct laryngoscopy registered in the Danish Anesthesia Database. *Anesthesiology* 2009; **110**: 266–274.

17. J. B. Brodsky, H. J. M. Lemmens, J. G. Brock-Utne, et al. Morbid obesity and tracheal intubation. *Anesthesia and Analgesia* 2002; **94**: 732–736.

18. S. M. Crawley and A. J. Dalton. Predicting the difficult airway. *BJA Education* 2015; **15**: 253–257.

19. M. J. Javid. Examination of submental space as an alternative method of airway assessment (submental sign). *BMC Research Notes* 2011; **4**: 221.

20. J. Hamza, M. Smida, D. Benhamou, et al. Parturient's posture during epidural puncture affects the distance from the skin to the epidural space. *Journal of Clinical Anesthesia* 1995; **7**: 1–4

21. J. Ingrande, J. B. Brodsky, and H. J. M. Lemmens. Lean body weight scalar for the anesthetic induction dose of propofol in morbidly obese subjects. *Anesthesia and Analgesia* 2011; **113**: 57–62.

22. M. C. Vallejo, N. Sah, A. L. Phelps, et al. Desflurane versus sevoflurane for laparoscopic gastroplasty in morbidly obese patients. *Journal of Clinical Anaesthesia* 2007; **19**: 3–8.

23. Health and Safety Executive. Risk assessment and process planning for bariatric patient handling pathways. Available from: www.hse.gov.uk/research/rrpdf/rr573.pdf.

Fundamentals of Decontamination and Sterilisation

Chapter

24

Martin Kiernan and Roger King

Introduction

Infection prevention is one of the key features of perioperative care and a working knowledge of the principles of sterilisation, disinfection, and infection control are essential for effective and safe perioperative practice. The modern operating department is often perceived and expected to be the pinnacle of cleanliness and sterility in a healthcare setting. This is vital for preventing cross-contamination and to reduce the incidence of surgical site infections.

Decontamination is defined as the combination of methods including cleaning, disinfection, and sterilisation used to make a reusable item safe for further use on patients and for handling by staff. The term refers to the whole cycle. Aseptic technique is fundamental to ensure patient and staff safety with regard to infection and its associated risks. All staff and visitors should understand the infection prevention and control principles (see Chapter 7) related to their role and responsibility. Perioperative practitioners must adhere to national and local protocols and understand how the transmission of pathogens can lead to infection and how the decontamination cycle can mitigate the risk of infection.

Why Do We Need to Decontaminate?

Decontamination is critically important due to concerns about preventing healthcare-associated infection, made more challenging by the increase in prevalence of microorganisms that are resistant to antimicrobials and an ever-increasing scrutiny of healthcare standards. Failure to decontaminate even non-invasive reusable equipment has been implicated in cross-infection with associated mortality. For example, a coroner's report described a patient death that was caused by a failure to effectively decontaminate a non-disposable laryngoscope handle appropriately between each patient use [1].

Regardless of the degree of pathogenicity, if one patient's microorganisms are transmitted to another through inadequate decontamination, this is an avoidable complication of healthcare and should not be tolerated in a modern healthcare setting.

Legislation Relating to Decontamination in Healthcare Settings in the UK

UK legislation falls under the remit of the Department of Health and Social Care and the executive agency the Medicines and Healthcare products Regulatory Agency (MHRA). As of 2021, the Department of Health and Social Care guidance includes the relevant documents listed in Table 24.1.

Table 24.1 Department of Health and Social Care documents

Title	Agency	Publication date	Scope of the document
Decontamination of Surgical Instruments (HTM 01-01)	Department of Health	July 2016	Health Technical Memorandum 01-01 explains the management of decontamination and the various ways to sterilise reusable medical devices. There are five parts to the document: • Part a: management and provision • Part b: common elements • Part c: steam sterilisation • Part d: washer-disinfectors • Part e: alternatives to steam for the sterilisation of medical devices
Management and decontamination of flexible endoscopes (HTM 01-06)	Department of Health	June 2016	Health Technical Memorandum 01-06 describes the processes involved in safe reprocessing of endoscopes. The document consists of five parts: • Part a: policy and management • Part b: design and installation • Part c: operational management • Part d: validation and verification (including storage/drying cabinets) • Part e: testing methods
Decontamination in primary care dental practices (HTM 01-05)	Department of Health	March 2013	Health Technical Memorandum 01-05 advice on patient safety when decontaminating reusable instruments in primary care dental practices
Top 10 tips on benchtop steam sterilisers	MHRA	January 2013	This guidance covers: • processing • loading items • checking performance • washing • record keeping
Top 10 tips on endoscope decontamination	MHRA	August 2013	This guidance covers: • quality • staff training • compatibility • identification • channel connection • manual cleaning • chemical compatibility • process validation • preventative maintenance • incident reporting

Decontamination also comes under the remit of the Health and Social Care Act 2008: code of practice on the prevention and control of infections. This legislation describes the core requirements providing the National Framework for decontamination regulation. It specifies that a healthcare provider must designate a lead for decontamination and that there must be an organisational decontamination policy. Other requirements include:

- decontamination of reusable medical devices takes place in appropriate facilities;
- appropriate procedures are followed for the purchase or acquisition, maintenance, and validation of decontamination equipment;
- staff are trained in decontamination processes and hold appropriate competences for their role; and
- a record-keeping regime is in place to ensure that decontamination processes are fit for purpose and use the required quality systems.

The Decontamination Life Cycle

The decontamination life cycle describes all the stages that an instrument passes through when in use. Before entering the cycle, the instrument first must be acquired (through purchase or loan) and a key part of the procurement process is the consideration of the methods of decontamination available in the organisation and whether the device is able to be managed in the existing system or an alternative is needed.

Once acquired, an instrument or device then enters the circle. As an example, for a sterile instrument, it begins with cleaning, then disinfection to render the item safe for the next step, which is an inspection to determine whether the device is still functioning as it is and that no damage has occurred. If the item is damaged it may leave the circle temporarily for repair or leave permanently to go for scrap. After passing inspection, the item is then packaged, sterilised, and transported to a storage facility, ready for use. Following use, the item is safely transported back to the decontamination facility for cleaning and the cycle begins again (see Figure 24.1). At all stages of the process the item should be tracked, enabling both inventories to be maintained and to enable traceability.

Cleaning, Disinfection, and Sterilisation

Three distinct processes make up any decontamination procedure and all may be adequate depending on the subsequent use following the process. In practice, these processes may be applied sequentially, with the final goal of producing a sterile instrument. In some instances, however, the first two stages alone (cleaning and disinfection) may be sufficient. The decision as to which of these processes is the final one is often made based on the long-established Spaulding classification (see Table 24.2) [2]. The decision also rests on the compatibility of the item with a chosen decontamination procedure; for example, many may not survive a heat/pressure form of decontamination. The system is based on the patient's risk of infection from the degree of invasiveness and exposure that various types of intervention can create.

There has been some recent discussion exploring whether these criteria should be revisited. Some critics argue that 'low' risk devices that are only cleaned can be a transmission risk. This is because the cleaning process can leave viable pathogens for transfer and colonisation, which can act as a reservoir for future transmission [3–5]. It must be noted that many items in use in the perioperative setting are according to the criteria

Table 24.2 Spaulding classification

Risk level	Application	Recommended process
High (critical)	Introduced into sterile body areas or in contact with a break in the skin or mucous membrane	Sterilisation
Intermediate (semi-critical)	In contact with intact mucous membranes	Disinfection
Low (non-critical)	In contact with intact skin only	Cleaning

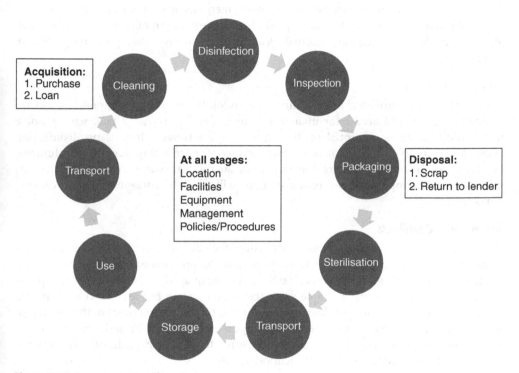

Figure 24.1 Decontamination life cycle

considered to be 'low risk' (e.g., blood pressure cuffs and patient support surfaces) and these items have been implicated in infection outbreaks when not adequately decontaminated [6].

Cleaning

Any surfaces that have residues, dried blood, or tissue remaining on them will reduce the efficacy of the sterilisation/disinfection process. Cleaning is an initial process that results in the removal of these contaminants (often referred to as 'soil' or 'contamination') from a surface to the extent necessary for further processing or use. The term contaminants includes microorganisms as well as other extraneous materials that may be organic (e.g., blood and tissues) or inorganic (e.g., dust).

Four modes of washing procedures are used to clean surgical instruments and flexible endoscopes. These range from basic manual cleaning methods, ultrasonic baths, thermal washer–disinfectors, and automated endoscope reprocessing devices. The Department of Health and Social Care recommends automated methods over manual ones as it is difficult to validate the consistency of a manual process. Due to their design or component materials, some instruments such as flexible endoscopes cannot always be processed in an automated washer–disinfector and so must be manually pre-cleaned before being placed in an automated reprocessor.

Manual Cleaning

Manual cleaning may be undertaken by one of two methods: immersion or non-immersion.

To minimise the risk to personnel, splashing and the creation of spray must be avoided at all times. Staff carrying out manual cleaning must always wear personal protective equipment.

Ultrasonic Cleaners

Ultrasonic cleaners are ideal for instruments with joints or multiple components that are difficult to clean and access for manual cleaning. They comprise a tank with a single ultrasonic transducer mounted on the bottom and a timer. There is no disinfection stage. More complex models may include facilities for irrigating devices with lumens. Caution must be taken to ensure that an item cleaned in this way is compatible with this method; for example, rubber products that will absorb ultrasonic waves, causing damage.

Determining Cleanliness

From a practical perspective, a surface that is described as 'clean' is visually free of soil and quantified as below specified levels of analytes (such as proteins or other specific components of contamination). If required, cleanliness can be quantified using adenosine triphosphate measurement, where a simple swab test may indicate the level of contamination present [7]. Following effective cleaning and moving on to the next process, the method of disinfection or sterilisation will be dependent upon the materials the device is made from. This is because some equipment may be sensitive to high temperatures and therefore incompatible with some disinfecting chemical agents.

Disinfection

The effectiveness of any disinfection process is dependent on the number of microorganisms present on the item. It is worth noting that any disinfection process begins with effective cleaning. The principal purpose of disinfection is to reduce the presence of microorganisms to a level that will minimise the risk of infection occurring. There are, however, some microorganisms, particularly spore-forming bacteria and some non-enveloped viruses, that are more challenging to destroy by conventional chemical disinfection. For example, bacterial spores (formed when the vegetative form of some organisms such as *Clostridioides* spp. and *Bacillus* spp. dies off) are the most resilient life form on Earth and can tolerate chemicals and extremely high temperatures, making them difficult to denature and kill. A spore is an organism in a dormant phase that can be reactivated when the right conditions are present.

Disinfection methods commonly involve contact with a chemical such as chlorine, peracetic acid, or hydrogen peroxide. The effectiveness of the disinfectant is dependent on a range of factors, primarily the concentration of the chemical and the time exposed to the surface in question, and to some extent the temperature and the acidity or alkalinity of the chemical.

The Importance of Contact Time

The contact time is how long a surface needs to have wet contact with a disinfectant to result in a meaningful reduction in microorganisms. A 99.9% reduction in microorganisms (also known as a 3 log reduction) means that 1,000,000 bacteria are reduced to 1,000, and for some (but not all) organisms this is a low enough amount to reduce the risk of transmission. The higher the log reduction, the more effective the product is at reducing microorganisms, so a 6 log reduction reduces microorganisms by 99.9999%. Often, the log reduction is dependent on how long the disinfectant remains in contact with the target surface and the organisms on it. This means that by observing the contact time or the 'wet time' you are efficiently and effectively disinfecting the surface you are applying your disinfectant product to. Contact times to achieve a meaningful kill for disinfectants differ significantly from 10 seconds to 10 minutes. Disinfectant products should include instructions that direct you to ensure that the surface is visibly wet for the recommended contact time. Disinfectant manufacturers report the results of their product against microbiological testing using an accredited laboratory-standard testing method.

However, not all organisms are killed at the same rate as they may have different physical characteristics; for example, enveloped viruses have a lipid layer that makes them easier to kill than the viruses without this coating. Different contact times are dependent on the microorganisms that the product has demonstrated efficacy against, and the length of time required to kill these microorganisms at the concentration. For example, a disinfectant may have a contact time for norovirus of 30 seconds, but the contact time for the hepatitis B virus might be 60 seconds. Unless you know which microorganism you are trying to kill, the longest contact time is the one that should be followed since there could be many different microorganisms present on surfaces. A high-quality disinfectant will kill a wide range of microorganisms with a short contact time. This is important as it may be difficult to maintain a wet surface for the contact time that a manufacturer may recommend.

Several factors may affect contact time, including temperature and humidity. Under some conditions such as high temperatures, low humidity, and airflow it can be difficult even for disinfectants with contact times as short as 3 minutes to stay wet. It is particularly challenging for disinfectants with a high alcohol content, which evaporate quickly. If the disinfectant does dry on the surface before the contact time is reached, label instructions usually require reapplication to ensure that the contact or wet time is met. A clean surface is also a critical component of disinfection as prior cleaning is necessary to remove material and biofilms, to allow the disinfectant to work as intended. Some products clean and disinfect in one, and these are a practical and time-saving choice.

Thermal Washer–Disinfectors

A thermal washer–disinfector is a purpose-designed washing machine for processing surgical instruments and other medical devices, which both cleans and thermally disinfects (without removing spores) in a single process. Versions are available for instrumentation, hollowware, anaesthetic accessories, and non-invasive medical devices. They utilise a mechanical cleaning action in combination with a detergent. A pass-through double-door option is preferable to prevent contamination.

Washer–disinfectors should be purchased against an appropriate specification and be capable of being validated in accordance with HTM 01-01, part d. There are several different models of washer–disinfector that meet current standards. The size, model, and type should be measured against throughput requirements, together with the availability of space. Logbooks and records should be kept by a designated 'user' and include a description of all loads, cycle details, monitoring records, and details of routine testing and maintenance.

Automatic Endoscope Reprocessor Devices

Automatic endoscope reprocessor (AER) devices are used specifically for processing the flexible endoscopes. They have a lower operating temperature than thermal washer–disinfectors and their disinfection action is achieved by chemicals and not heat. They incorporate additional connectors and tubing to enable water, detergents, and disinfectants to flow through endoscope lumens. Channel patency testing ensures that lumens are decontaminated, and leak testing is also undertaken.

Purchase of these devices is more complicated than standard thermal washer–disinfectors as the compatibility with the endoscope (via manufacturer-specific channel connectors) and disinfectant choice also need to be considered. As with any other form of decontamination, pre-cleaning to remove soil that could reduce the effectiveness of the decontamination procedure should be undertaken.

Sterilisation

Sterilisation is a process that results in a surface or product that is free from all viable microorganisms. This can be achieved in several different ways, including physical or chemical methods.

Physical Methods

Heat sterilisation is the most common method used to sterilise surgical instruments and can be divided into either dry or moist heat sterilisation. Dry sterilisation requires both a longer exposure time and a higher temperature than the moist heat method and is usually carried out in hot air ovens at temperatures from 150 °C to 180 °C in order to achieve the destruction of microorganisms by the oxidation of cell constituents. In contrast, the principal method of destruction via moist heat sterilisation are the denaturing of the structural proteins and enzymes of the microorganisms. This is achieved by exposing the microorganisms to hot or boiling water or steam under pressure. Steam under pressure is probably the most popular method for moist heat sterilisation and rapidly inactivates most types of microorganisms on contact, but the immediate release of energy on condensation is believed to be particularly effective at inactivating more resistant forms of microorganisms, such as bacterial spores. It is carried out in autoclaves where steam under pressure can achieve temperatures in excess of 100 °C, where time and pressure are used to titrate the rate of destruction of spore-bearing organisms. Raising the temperature greatly reduces the pressure and the time needed to achieve sterilisation but this may not be suitable for certain fragile instruments or devices.

Table 24.3 Sterilisation time (from [8])

Temperature (°C)	Pressure (kPa)	Sterilisation time (minutes)
121–124	200	15
126–129	250	10
134–138	300	5

For the sterilisation process to effectively access all the items in the autoclave, displacement of air in the autoclave chamber creates a negative pressure and this allows steam to distribute and access all materials in the chamber.

The sterilisation time is measured from the moment that all materials in the sterilisation chamber have reached the required temperature. The sterilisation time, pressure, and temperature are all relevant to each other. Examples of time temperature and pressure ranges are given in Table 24.3.

Modern autoclaves have automated monitoring systems that ensure that the required parameters for sterilisation are achieved and provide a log of detailed records of the process.

The process of moist heat sterilisation triggers the change in appearance of the 'autoclave tape', which is one indication to the practitioner that the package has undergone a sterilisation process; thus, along with other factors, it provides evidence that the contents are sterile. Stripes on the autoclave tape should be uniform and even. Any packaging which has incomplete or blurred stripes on the autoclave tape should be withdrawn from use, the batch number noted, and the failure reported through the appropriate channels.

Physicochemical systems may utilise both heat and a chemical. Gas sterilisation using ethylene oxide, for example, requires dilution of the toxic gas, thus reducing the risk of residual chemicals remaining on the items. There is a toxicity risk with these methods, and they may be used when no other sterilisation method is suitable; for example, electronic items that cannot be sterilised by heat. As with other methods of sterilisation, strict protocols and checks carried out by highly trained staff are required. The concentration of gas, humidity, temperature, and exposure time along with the type of items to be sterilised affect the efficiency of these systems but in practice these are all slow processes as elimination of any remaining toxic chemical must be ensured and confirmed by appropriate testing. In practice, ethylene oxide sterilisation is primarily carried out by manufacturers of items undertaking bulk sterilisation of items that may be single use and where time is not of the essence or specialist decontamination facilities. Some types of catheters and flexible fibre-optic endoscopes are other examples of equipment that may require these specialist sterilisation methods, or they may be subject to gas-plasma sterilisation techniques using hydrogen peroxide.

Gas plasma is considered as the fourth state of matter, which is effectively a cloud of ions and electrons. Plasma can be generated by strong electrical fields and these, together with chemicals such as hydrogen peroxide or acetic acid, generate free radicals, which interact with the cell membranes, enzymes, or nucleic acids to disrupt the life functions of these microorganisms. At the end of the process, excess gas is removed and the sterilisation chamber returned to atmospheric pressure by introducing filtered air. The by-products of the cycle – water vapour and oxygen – are not toxic, removing the requirement for aeration. Sterilised materials can be handled safely, either for immediate use or storage. The process operates in the range of 37–44 °C and has a cycle time of 75 minutes. However, if any moisture is present on the objects, the vacuum will not be achieved and the cycle immediately ceases [9].

It is worth acknowledging that once the instrument tray has been opened and thus exposed to the ambient air, in theory it is no longer sterile because it is not possible to work in an operating department with sterile air, regardless of the efficiency of the ventilation/air-conditioning system.

Facilities for Undertaking Decontamination

The great majority of the decontamination of invasive surgical instruments is undertaken within specialist designed centralised departments, often known as sterile service departments (SSDs) or even off-site regional centres. These areas process a mixture of standard theatre trays, supplementary instruments, and smaller, more general, packs for wards and other departments.

The Department of Health and Social Care published a design guide for SSDs called Health Building Note (HBN) 13 (Department of Health 2004). The document sets out the rooms required, suggests a typical floor layout, and offers advice as to the mechanical services (including ventilation) required. The critical features include:

- work and staff flow that prevents cross-contamination between segregated clean and dirty work zones;
- a controlled and monitored inspection, assembly, and packing (IAP) room that meets the standard of ISO Class 8 (BS EN ISO 14644; International Standards Organisation 1999);
- a dedicated wash room with pass-through washer–disinfectors that exit their load into the IAP area;
- either double-door pass-through sterilisers or single-door sterilisers with a loading area separated from the IAP room; and
- gowning rooms for both the wash and IAP rooms.

Packaging

Instruments that have been processed by an SSD will be supplied within sterilisation containers and wrapped, although in some instances instruments are not necessarily wrapped prior to sterilisation. If instruments are packaged, the materials used must comply with BS EN ISO 11607 (International Standards Organization 2006) standard. Packaging should be compatible with the chosen sterilisation process and may be flexible or rigid. Following AER processing, flexible endoscopes are unwrapped and must be used within 3 hours of reprocessing or stored in drying cabinets that extend the storage time and disinfected state for up to 30 days.

Commonly used types of packaging include:

- valved or filtered rigid sterilisation containers;
- dual-layered reusable barrier fabric wraps;
- paper/film peel pouch wraps;
- paper systems using two layers of disposable wraps;
- disposable paper two-layer bonded single paper wrap; and

- inner paper wrap with a reusable barrier fabric outer wrap.

Packaging systems normally feature a colour-change display as a label or printed on the package itself. This provides assurance that the item passed through an effective sterilisation process. If the display has not changed to the indicated colour, the tray or instrument should never be used, the batch number noted, and the failure reported through the appropriate channels.

Practical Aspects of Sterilisation and Disinfection

Practitioners should consider themselves, the environment, all equipment/items, and the patient in planning for care delivered in perioperative areas. Standard practices such as suitable attire for the environment, hand hygiene, the use of personal protective equipment, checking the integrity of packaging, the expiry date of medications, testing dates of equipment, and essential integrity checks of items such as sterilised instruments are daily considerations.

Understanding decontamination, sterilisation, and disinfection techniques enables the practitioner to undertake essential safety checks. These include ascertaining that all items have been processed appropriately and that relevant disposal or recycling procedures are followed while ensuring that all items required for each patient conform with local and national policies for every case.

References

1. Medicines and Healthcare products Regulatory Agency. MDA/2011/0096 reusable laryngoscope handles. Available from: https://mhra-gov.filecamp.com/s/yw DEZLgX0nEPtNCx/fo/3gd4DFg85VgXQo G9/fi/f22KmJZol3Qswky0.

2. E. H. Spaulding. Chemical disinfection of medical and surgical materials. In E. A. Lawrence and E. S. Block (eds.), *Disinfection, Sterilisation and Preservation*. Philadelphia, PA: Lea & Febiger, 1968, pp. 517–531.

3. G. McDonnell and P. Burke. Disinfection: is it time to reconsider Spaulding? *Journal of Hospital Infection* 2011; **78**: 163–170.

4. T. Lewis V. Patel, A. Ismail, and A. Fraise. Sterilisation, disinfection and cleaning of theatre equipment: do we need to extend the Spaulding classification? *Journal of Hospital Infection* 2009; **72**: 361–363.

5. E. T. Curran M. Wilkinson and C. Bradley. Chemical disinfectants: controversies regarding their use in low risk healthcare environments (part 1). *Journal of Infection Prevention* 2019; **20**: 76–82.

6. R. Branch and A. Amiri. Environmental surface hygiene in the OR: strategies for reducing the transmission of health care-associated infections. *AORN Journal* 2020; **112**: 327–342.

7. C. E. McCafferty, D. Abi-Hanna, M. J. Aghajani, et al. The validity of adenosine triphosphate measurement in detecting endoscope contamination. *Journal of Hospital Infection* 2018; **100**: e142–e145.

8. G. E. McDonnell. Antisepsis, disinfection, and sterilization: types, action and resistance, 2nd ed. Washington DC: ASM Press, 2017.

9. W. A. Rutala and D. J. Weber, Healthcare Infection Control Practices Advisory Committee. Guideline for disinfection and sterilization in healthcare facilities, 2008. Available from: www.cdc.gov/ infectioncontrol/pdf/guidelines/ disinfection-guidelines-H.pdf.

Chapter 25

Management and Use of Medical Equipment

Julie Quick and Laura Garbett

Introduction

Perioperative practitioners will use a range of medical equipment and devices to assist them in their role caring for patients and it is essential that they understand how to use and manage them safely. The World Health Organization [1] defines medical equipment as a piece of equipment that requires maintenance, repair, user training, and decommissioning. A medical device is defined as a piece of equipment used to prevent, diagnose, treat, monitor, or alleviate an illness or disease. It can also modify anatomy or control conception [2].

There are three main types of medical devices:

- general medical devices: for example, a heart valve, X-ray equipment, or a dressing;
- active implantable devices: for example, a cardiac pacemaker, nerve stimulator, or a cochlear implant;
- in vitro medical devices: for example, pregnancy test or blood group reagent.

Regulation 15 of the Health and Social Care Act 2008 [3] ensures that equipment used to deliver care and treatment is used only for its intended purpose and that it is maintained, stored, and cleaned appropriately. Failure to adhere to the legislation can result in substandard material that can lead to poor surgical outcomes. One example of this is the Poly Implant Prothèse (PIP) breast-implant scandal in 2009, when implants were manufactured using a cheaper, non-medical-approved silicone that was prone to rupturing, causing inflammation, scarring, and pain to millions of women around the world [4].

Since 2017, more stringent compliance requirements have been implemented, including the European Medical Devices Regulation [5]. After January 2021, following the UK leaving the European Union, devices are awarded a UK Conformity Assessed (UKCA) mark for goods sold within Great Britain. For goods sold in Northern Ireland, a European Conformity (CE) or UKNI mark will be required. Approved devices are registered with the Medicines and Healthcare products Regulatory Agency (MHRA) within the UK. The MHRA is responsible for ensuring that medical devices work effectively and are safe to use [2]. Each medical device sits in one of three classes, dependent upon the risk posed if used incorrectly or it malfunctions [2]:

- class I: low risk (e.g., surgical instruments, stethoscopes, and bandages);
- class II: moderate risk (e.g., an ECG monitor);
- class III: high risk (e.g., a defibrillator, pacemaker, or breast implant).

Procurement

Having access to good-quality, affordable, and appropriate medical equipment and devices is essential to promote health [1]. In England and Wales, the National Health Service (NHS) Supply Chain is responsible for managing the sourcing, delivery, and supply of healthcare products to the NHS as well as other healthcare organisations. To transform this process, the 'future operating model', launched in 2017, enhances efficiency and effectiveness of procurement [6]. This model is organised into 11 category towers covering different areas of procurement spend (see Figure 25.1). Consequently, this model offers a single national price and benefits all healthcare trusts, whatever their size [6].

Not all equipment is available through this process. Within the operating theatre it may be necessary to trial equipment or loan items such as specialist surgical instrumentation, and where these are required, booking is done in advance through the procurement department, following organisation policy and procedures for their supply and use.

Training

All perioperative practitioners have a professional obligation to take reasonable care for the safety of themselves, patients, and colleagues [7, 8]. Part of this responsibility is to ensure that any equipment required in the course of their job is used for the purpose it is designed for, in line with the manufacturer's instructions [9]. It is also a legal requirement that employers must ensure employees are trained and competent in the use of any equipment that they may use [10]. To support the training of employees, manufacturers often provide national and local training, as well as updates on their equipment and demonstration of new and loan equipment.

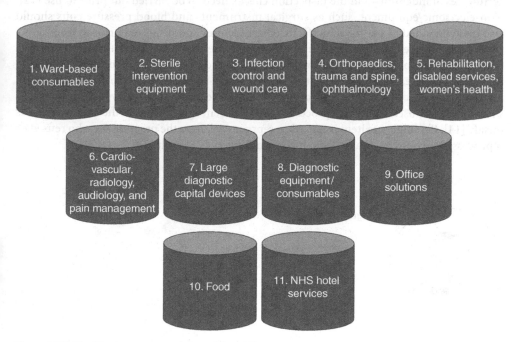

Figure 25.1 The 11 category towers (adapted from [6])

Instructions for Use

All practitioners rely on medical equipment to be in good working order to ensure a safe and effective service to the patient. Equipment should be checked for functionality and safety before and after use, following manufacturer guidance [11]. Local instructions for use may need to be provided, particularly when one piece of equipment is used in conjunction with another. Any equipment that is used by an employee falls under The Provision and Use of Work Equipment Regulations [12]. Practitioners should ensure that the equipment selected is:

- checked by authorised designated personnel on delivery and before use;
- used in accordance with the manufacturer's recommendations for its intended use only; and
- used only by employees who have been instructed in its use.

Maintenance, Repair, and Reporting

Electronic equipment should have a planned, regular maintenance contract, with each piece of equipment recorded on an asset register which documents service history and planned replacement dates. Within healthcare organisations, the electrical biomedical engineering department (EBME) is responsible for scheduling maintenance and servicing of all electronic equipment. Some of the more specialist or complex equipment requires manufacturers to service this type of equipment. The EBME will liaise with company engineers as well as the theatre manager and designated clinical staff to schedule maintenance at a time when the equipment is not in use. Some departments may have spare equipment to ensure that theatre utilisation is not disrupted during servicing. Loan or trial equipment should have certificates of indemnity and the inspection checks need to be carried out prior to use [12]. Non-electronic equipment, such as surgical instruments and blood pressure cuffs should also be maintained as per the manufacturer's guidelines and inspected prior to use.

Medical devices used within the operating theatre may have limitations to their use. Some devices are only licensed for single use and should be only used on one patient during a single procedure, and then discarded [13]. All single-use items have the symbol shown in Figure 25.2 on the device or the packaging. Single-use items such as hypodermic needles should never be used again or reprocessed. To use them again, even on the same patient, is unsafe [14]. If a single use item is reused or reprocessed, then the practitioner who reused or reprocessed it could be legally liable if harm occurred as a result [14].

Figure 25.2 Single-use symbol

Some devices such as pneumatic compression devices are intended for single patient use, which means they may, following manufacturer guidelines, be reused, or reprocessed for use on the same patient [14].

Despite legislation and local protocols, each year accidents involving medical equipment leave staff and patients seriously injured and, in rare cases, these accidents can be fatal [15]. In certain circumstances, accidents involving medical devices need to be reported to the MHRA via the 'yellow card' reporting system, ideally within 24 hours. This includes:

- when someone is injured (or almost injured) by a medical device, either because its labelling or instructions are not clear, it is broken; or has been misused; and
- when a patient's treatment is interrupted because of a faulty device.

In this situation, the equipment is retained and must not be discarded, repaired, or returned to the manufacturer until the MHRA has carried out its own investigation. The MHRA may recall or issue an alert regarding faulty medical devices to preserve patient safety. If the accident involves an employee, this will also need to be reported following the Reporting of Injuries, Diseases and Dangerous Occurrences Regulations [16]. In the UK, any risks from medical devices that need to be disseminated to other organisations is done so via the NHS England National Patient Safety Alerting System [17], which issues alerts to any potential risks to patient safety.

Decontamination and Sterilisation

Equipment must be cleaned and decontaminated prior to its service, repair, inspection, or transportation. This is essential to protect those individuals who are working with or have been in contact with that item of equipment. This is because under the Health and Safety at Work Act 1974 [18] workers have a legal right not to be exposed to any form of risk from contaminated equipment.

A safe system of working must be implemented so that individuals are able to provide such a service and a responsible person should be nominated to deal with issues, training, documentation, and any other legislative requirements. Further legislation is found in the Control of Substances Hazardous to Health (COSHH) regulations, which relate to both chemical and biological hazards.

There may be rare occasions where it is not prudent to decontaminate equipment, as may be the case in an investigation into equipment failure or any incident that has resulted in direct harm to either a patient or staff member. However, a few key steps may still be taken to ensure that the recipient is aware of the condition in which they will receive the equipment in question:

- a warning label to inform the user of the hazard prior to opening the package;
- the inner package should not be able to contaminate the outer package;
- the packaging should be strong enough to withstand handling during transport from sender to recipient; and
- a declaration of contamination status should travel with the item and this should contain relevant information to inform of contamination.

Decommissioning

At some point, all equipment will need to be replaced due to wear and tear and a decommissioning policy on removing the medical device from use is an essential element of the management of equipment [11]. Decommissioning aims to make equipment safe to remove from use, and the manufacturer should be contacted for advice on correct methods for disposal.

Use of Medical Equipment

The Electrosurgical Unit

The electrosurgical unit, often referred to as a diathermy machine, is an integral part of the modern operating theatre. It is used to produce a controllable source of heat over different waveforms, which can cut and coagulate tissue during surgery [19]. All perioperative practitioners involved in the use of electrosurgery should be trained and familiar with its working principles due to the risk of serious harm, which could cause a surgical fire and thermal injury to the patient and user [20].

Electrosurgery consists of an insulated active electrode in the form of a diathermy point, pencil, or forceps [9]. The active electrode is connected to an electrosurgical generator by a cable. A return electrode is also required to earth the current back to the generator and, in the two types of electrosurgical units detailed below, this is achieved differently:

Monopolar Diathermy

Monopolar diathermy is versatile and effective for many types of surgery and is the most frequently used modality (see Figure 25.3). The circuit consists of:

- the electrosurgical generator;
- an active electrode;
- the patient; and
- a patient return electrode.

It involves the passage of a high-frequency current directly through the patient from the active electrode to a return electrode attached to the patient. The electrosurgical generator produces a current of over 200 kHz compared with a standard household electrical current of 60 Hz. This does not result in electrocution of the patient because nerve and muscle

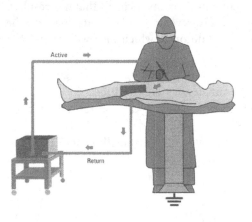

Figure 25.3 Monopolar circuit

stimulation cease above 100 kHz, and so the electrical current can safely pass through the patient. The return electrode can be in the form of an adhesive plate, often called a diathermy pad, or a specialist mattress that the patient lies on during surgery. Electrothermal injuries may result from incorrect return electrode application, active electrode insulation failure, and coupling [20]. Therefore, the following considerations are needed by practitioners when selecting and applying the correct return electrode:

- The size of the electrode needs to be proportionate to the patient to prevent the current concentrating on a small area.
- The site selected must be well vascularised, as close to the operative site as possible and free from hair and scars.
- Bony prominences such as the hip or knee joints, which could result in poor electrical conductivity, should be avoided.
- Ensure the electrode is dry after skin preparation. If wet, then reapply a new one.
- The electrode may become dislodged when the patient is moved – check the pad once the patient is positioned or repositioned during surgery.

The smoke plume generated from the use of electrosurgery units and lasers contains toxic vapours, which are invisible to the naked eye [21]. Inhalation of the surgical smoke can cause damage to the respiratory system and therefore exposure to the diathermy plume should be adequately controlled [22]. This can be achieved by effective local exhaust ventilation using on-tip extraction suction [23]. However, the use of surgical plume extraction equipment remains limited, despite growing evidence of the risks posed by surgical smoke to staff and patients.

Bipolar Diathermy

Bipolar diathermy is used for more minor procedures, and it does not have the versatility of different waveforms that monopolar diathermy has. However, the main advantage over monopolar diathermy is that it does not require a return electrode, which removes the risk of a return-electrode burn. The double-lumen lead carries the electrical current to one of the tips of the forceps and returns it via the other, with the tissue that is between the forceps forming part of the circuit (see Figure 25.4). Bipolar diathermy is primarily used on more

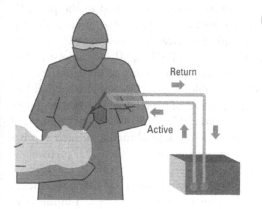

Figure 25.4 Bipolar circuit

sensitive areas such as the digits, extremities, and bowel as there is greater accuracy and less tissue damage due to the lower concentration of the current. The circuit consists of:

- an electrosurgical generator;
- a double-lumen lead; and
- the patient's tissue.

Waveforms

Electrosurgical generators can produce different waveforms by varying the duty cycle to achieve distinct tissue effects that are relevant to the type of surgery being performed. The duty cycle describes the ratio or percentage of the on-time [22]. A lower duty cycle produces less heat, and a higher duty cycle produces more heat. A constant waveform creates heat rapidly, vaporising tissue and producing a 'cutting' effect. An intermittent waveform produces less heat and a 'coagulating' effect because the modified waveform has a lower duty cycle. There are also blend waveforms; they are not a mixture of the cut and coagulation waveforms but are interruptions in the waveform cycle to produce different tissue effects. Moving from blend 1 to 3 leads to a progressively lower duty cycle and so blend 1 can vaporise tissue with minimal haemostasis while blend 3 offers minimal cutting but maximum haemostasis.

Avoiding Adverse Events

Most adverse events involving electrosurgical units can be prevented if attention is paid to common causes such as:

- checking all equipment prior to use, including the insulation of active electrodes;
- careful handling and storage of electrosurgery equipment while in use;
- ensuring the patient is not in contact with, or in close contact to, any metal when positioned on the operating table to avoid arcing of the current;
- use of surgical smoke extractors;
- correct application of the return electrode; and
- perioperative practitioner training prior to use of equipment.

Intermittent Pneumatic Compression Devices

Intermittent pneumatic compression (IPC) devices are garments applied to the patient's legs during and after surgery to prevent hospital acquired venous thromboembolism (VTE). This is a leading cause of perioperative mortality, and all surgical patients should be assessed as soon as possible after admission to identify their risk of VTE [24]. An assessment is performed by using an assessment tool based on national guidance such as that published by the Department of Health and Social Care [25] – see Table 25.1. VTE prophylaxis should be used as a prescribed plan of care for patients deemed at risk of developing hospital-acquired VTE as it reduces the incidence of deep vein thrombosis (DVT) and consequent pulmonary embolism [24]. VTE prophylaxis includes non-invasive mechanical methods, such as anti-embolism stockings and intermittent pneumatic compression devices, as well as pharmacological treatments such as low-molecular-weight heparin.

IPC devices consist of an electric pump that provides compression to a pair of garments wrapped around the lower limb, to intermittently apply pressure to the legs. It mimics the natural action of the leg muscles to increase blood flow through the veins, helping to prevent

Table 25.1 VTE risk assessment screening tool adapted from Department of Health [25]

Surgical VTE risk	Tick below	Contraindication to chemical or mechanical prophylaxis	Tick below	Pharmacological and mechanical prophylaxis guide
High		**Chemical contraindications**		**Pharmacological prophylaxis**
Hip and knee replacement		High risk of bleeding		Consideration of enoxaparin or other anticoagulant as per surgeon's preference
Intra-abdominal surgery		Adverse reaction to heparin		
Surgery lasting longer than 45 mins and age > 45		Severe hepatic disease		
Lower limb cast/ immobilisation		On current anticoagulation [date stopped]		
Severe respiratory disease		**Mechanical contraindications**		**Mechanical prophylaxis**
Pregnant or up to 6 weeks post-partum		Fragile skin		Consider applying intermittent pneumatic compression device or thrombo-embolus deterrent (TED) stocking as per surgeons preference
Hormone replacement therapy		Dermatitis/cellulitis		
Oestrogen-containing contraception		Severe lower limb oedema		
Obesity (BMI > 30)		Recent skin graft		
Known thrombophilia or increased blood clotting		Severe peripheral vascular disease		
Acute inflammatory bowel disease		Burns		
Low		**VTE education for staff**		**Complications of mechanical prophylaxis**
All other surgery		Signs and symptoms of VTE		Compartment syndrome
Family history of VTE		How to apply TED stockings		PE
				Muscle necrosis
				Peroneal nerve palsy

Table 25.1 (cont.)

Surgical VTE risk	Tick below	Contraindication to chemical or mechanical prophylaxis	Tick below	Pharmacological and mechanical prophylaxis guide
		How to apply automatic compression devices		
		Importance of mobilisation		
		Importance of hydration		
		Length of interventions		

a DVT by reducing venous stasis [24]. IPC devices are manufactured in thigh or calf length sizes, and selection is based upon the VTE risk to the patient and the procedure the patient is undergoing. There are few contraindications to the use of mechanical compression; they include patient allergy to the garment's material, severe cardiac insufficiency, and peripheral arterial occlusive disease [26]. Complications are rare if used correctly but there have been reports of discomfort, dry skin, and tissue necrosis [24]. IPC devices are therefore clinically effective in reducing the risk of hospital-acquired VTE and should therefore be continued until the patient's mobility is significantly improved [24].

Tourniquets

For centuries, tourniquets have been used to control the return of blood in a limb or digit as an attempt to reduce blood loss and save limb or life. Despite the introduction of modern medical devices such as diathermy to control blood loss, the use of tourniquets has continued not only to prevent bleeding during surgery to provide a bloodless operating field [27].

The application of a tourniquet involves the practitioner applying pressure to the extremity to be operated on in the form of a manual or pneumatic cuff, and subsequent exsanguination of the limb or digit through elevation. Single-cuffed tourniquets are commonly used in orthopaedic and plastic surgery, but a double-cuffed tourniquet is used when providing intravenous regional anaesthesia; for example, a Bier's block, to isolate the circulation in the limb.

While the use of tourniquets is common, harm to the patient, even when used correctly, is always a risk, particularly in the older patient [28]. To reduce the risk of tourniquet-acquired injuries, pre- and intraoperative considerations should include [29, 30]:

- identification of potential patient risk factors such as pre-existing skin damage and co-morbidities such as peripheral vascular disease and cardiac disease;
- selection of the correct size cuff for the patient;
- avoidance of bony prominences;
- application of the cuff at the greatest circumference on the limb where muscle bulk is greatest;
- application of padding under the cuff;

- prevention of antiseptic solution pooling under the tourniquet, which could cause chemical burns; and
- timing of antibiotics.

The occlusion pressure applied by the tourniquet depends upon several factors, including the patient's age and the application site, and should be kept to a minimum to prevent injury to the patient. Ideally, the pressure range for an adult should 200–300 mmHg but this should always be confirmed with the surgeon before inflation [29]. Some modern pneumatic tourniquets calculate the limb occlusion pressure automatically based on the patient's blood pressure [30]. When the duration of the tourniquet inflation extends beyond 2 hours, the surgeon may request deflation of the tourniquet for 10 to 15 minutes to allow reperfusion of the limb or digit [30].

Tourniquet use is not without risk and too little pressure can result in intraoperative bleeding [27]. The duration and pressure of the tourniquet should be monitored throughout use and documented, as physiological changes can occur shortly after inflation [28]. Complications associated with prolonged use and high tourniquet pressures range from minor tissue damage, including bruising and friction, to more serious conditions such as compartment syndrome and nerve damage [30]. Monitoring the patient during and after surgery is therefore essential to assess and manage potential tourniquet injury. Hypertension and tachycardia could indicate pain, and a rise in temperature to the affected limb may indicate tourniquet injury. Hypotension, metabolic acidosis, and hyperkalaemia can occur upon tourniquet deflation due to the release of anaerobic metabolites into the circulation [29]. Cardiac arrests and raised intracranial pressure have also been reported following tourniquet deflation [30].

Postoperatively, neurovascular and tissue viability assessments should be performed noting:

- vital signs;
- limb or digit temperature and colour;
- the skin condition under the cuff;
- distal pulses; and
- the surgical wound site, including blood loss.

The type of tourniquet used, cuff size, padding, and site applied as well as inflation time and pressure settings should all be documented, and any concerns should be reported to the surgeon or anaesthetist.

Intraoperative Cell Salvage

The use of intraoperative cell salvage devices has become increasingly common over the decade and they are now routinely used for some elective and emergency surgeries, and usually recommended where a blood loss of more than 500 mL is expected. These devices should only be used by practitioners who have received the appropriate training, run on the automatic mode (where available), and only used according to the manufacturers' instructions. To reduce to incidence of error, each hospital should use just one type of cell salvage device [31].

A cell salvage device facilitates the collection of blood from the surgical field and allows it to be collected, filtered, washed, and returned to the same patient. This is known as autologous blood transfusion (see Figure 25.5) and contrasts with an allogenic blood

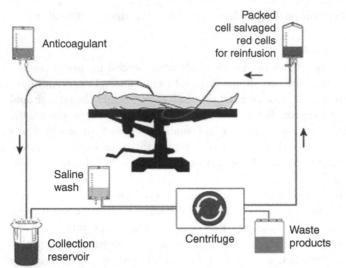

Anticoagulant

Packed
cell salvaged
red cells
for reinfusion

Saline
wash

Collection
reservoir

Centrifuge

Waste
products

Figure 25.5 Autologous red blood cell transfusion (autotransfusion)

transfusion, which describes a patient receiving donated blood. Cell salvage devices can differ in the method of collection and processing (continuous or semi-continuous), the fixed bowl size, available modes, and the anticoagulant used.

The patient's blood is mixed with an anticoagulant as it is aspirated using low-pressure suction to collect the blood in a reservoir and then passes through a filter. The red blood cells are separated using centrifugation and then washed using normal saline. This process results in the production of washed and packed red cells suspended in normal saline, which can then be reinfused to the patient; this is usually recommended within 4 hours of processing [32].

Cell salvage devices have both advantages and disadvantages [32]. The advantages are:

- reduced transmission of infection;
- no risk of ABO incompatibility;
- they are acceptable for some Jehovah's Witness patients (or others with concerns about receiving allogenic blood);
- a reduced demand for allogeneic blood; and
- a reduced risk of adverse transfusion reactions.

  Their disadvantages are:

- the initial cost of the device;
- the ongoing cost of disposables;
- they require staff training and competencies;
- the complex equipment; and
- a risk of air and fat embolism.

Summary

In conclusion, this chapter has identified the importance of the management of equipment in the operating department. This includes understanding its intended use and undertaking the required training to ensure patient and user safety. Perioperative practitioners must adhere to the relevant regulations and legislation to ensure the safe use and management of medical equipment.

References

1. World Health Organization. Medical devices. Available from: www.who.int/health-topics/medical-devices#tab=tab_1 (accessed March 2020).

2. Medicines and Healthcare products Regulatory Agency. Medical devices: how to comply with the legal requirements in Great Britain. Available from: www.gov.uk/guidance/medical-devices-how-to-comply-with-the-legal-requirements (accessed September 2021).

3. Health and Social Care Act 2008 (Regulated Activities) Regulations 2014. Available from: www.legislation.gov.uk/ukdsi/2014/9780111117613/contents.

4. National Health Service. PIP breast implants. Available from: www.nhs.uk/conditions/PIP-implants/ (accessed September 2021).

5. European Medical Devices Regulation on medical devices. Available from: https://eur-lex.europa.eu/legal-content/EN/TXT/HTML/?uri=CELEX:32017R0745&from=EN.

6. Department of Health. The future operating model for NHS procurement: transforming the landscape of NHS procurement, June 2017. Available from: www.nhsbsa.nhs.uk/sites/default/files/2017-06/FOM_general_guide_0.pdf.

7. Healthcare and Professions Council. *Standards of Proficiency for Operating Department Practitioners*. London: HCPC, 2014.

8. Nursing and Midwifery Council. The Code: professional standards of practice and behaviour for nurses, midwives and nursing associates. Available from: www.nmc.org.uk/globalassets/sitedocuments/nmc-publications/nmc-code.pdf.

9. Association for Perioperative Practice. *Standards and Recommendations for Safe Perioperative Practice*. Harrogate: AfPP, 2016.

10. Health and Safety Executive. Are you a user of work equipment? Available from: www.hse.gov.uk/work-equipment-machinery/user.htm (accessed September 2021).

11. Medicines and Healthcare products Regulatory Agency. Managing medical devices: guidance for health and social care organisations. Available from: https://assets.publishing.service.gov.uk/government/uploads/system/uploads/attachment_data/file/982127/Managing_medical_devices.pdf.

12. The Provision and Use of Work Equipment Regulations 1998. Available from: www.legislation.gov.uk/uksi/1998/2306/made.

13. E. Wilkinson. The implications of reusing single-use medical devices *Nursing Times* 2006; **102**: 23.

14. Medicines and Healthcare products Regulatory Agency. Single use medical devices. Available from: https://assets.publishing.service.gov.uk/government/uploads/system/uploads/attachment_data/file/743384/Single_use_medical_devices_leaflet_250918.pdf.

15. Health and Safety Executive. Equipment safety. Available from: www.hse.gov.uk/healthservices/equipment-safety.htm (accessed September 2021).

16. Reporting of Injuries, Diseases and Dangerous Occurrences Regulation. Available from: www.hse.gov.uk/riddor/ (accessed September 2021).

17. National Health Service. NHS England and NHS improvement national patient safety alerts. Available at: www.england.nhs.uk/

patient-safety/patient-safety-alerts/ (accessed September 2021).

18. Health and Safety at Work etc. Act 1974. Available from: www.legislation.gov.uk/uk pga/1974/37/contents.

19. Royal College of Obstetricians and Gynaecologists. Diathermy. Available from: https://elearning.rcog.org.uk/abdom inal-surgery/diathermy.

20. Medicines and Healthcare products Regulatory Agency. Electrosurgery – top tips. Available from: https://assets .publishing.service.gov.uk/government/up loads/system/uploads/attachment_data/fil e/477600/Electrosurgery_top_tips_ Nov_15__2_.pdf.

21. Health and Safety Executive. Diathermy and surgical smoke. Available from: www .hse.gov.uk/healthservices/diathermy-emissions.htm (accessed September 2021).

22. E-S. Mohsen, S. Mohamed, and E. Saridogan. Safe use of electrosurgery in gynaecological laparoscopic surgery. *The Obstetrician and Gynaecologist* 2020; **22**: 9–20.

23. I. Alkatout, T. Schollmeyer, N. A. Hawaldar, et al. Principles and safety measures of electrosurgery in laparoscopy. *Journal of the Society of Laparoscopic and Robotic Surgeons* 2012; **16**: 130–139.

24. National Institute for Health and Care Excellence. Venous thromboembolism in over 16s: reducing the risk of hospital-acquired deep vein thrombosis or pulmonary embolism. Available from: www.nice.org.uk/guidance/ng89/chapter/ Recommendations#risk-assessment.

25. Department of Health. *Risk assessment for Venous Thromboembolism (VTE)*. London: Department of Health, 2010.

26. E. Rabe, H. Partsch, N. Morrison, et al. Risks and contraindications of medical compression treatment: a critical reappraisal. An international consensus statement. *Phlebology: The Journal of Venous Disease* 2020; **35**: 447–460.

27. L. Barr, U. Shridhar Iyer, A. Sardesai, et al. Tourniquet failure during total knee replacement due to arterial calcification: case report and review of the literature. *Journal of Perioperative Practice* 2010; **20**: 55–58.

28. J. L. Deloughry and R. Griffiths. Arterial tourniquets. *Continuing Education in Anaesthesia, Critical Care and Pain* 2009; **9**: 56–60.

29. K. Kumar, C. Railton, and Q. Tawfic. Tourniquet application during anesthesia: 'What we need to know?' *Journal of Anaesthesiology Clinical Pharmacology* 2016; **32**: 424–430.

30. Association of periOperative Registered Nurses. Guideline quick view: pneumatic tourniquets. *AORN Journal* 2020; **111**: 720–723.

31. A. A. Klein, C. R. Bailey, A. J. Charlton, et al. Association of Anaesthetists guidelines: cell salvage for peri-operative blood conservation 2018. *Anaesthesia* 2018; **73**: 1141–1150.

32. L. Kuppurao and M. Wee. Perioperative cell salvage. *Continuing Education in Anaesthesia Critical Care and Pain* 2010; **10**: 104–108.

<table>
<tr><td>Chapter</td></tr>
<tr><td>26</td></tr>
</table>

Fundamentals of the Surgical Scrub Role

Lindsay Keeley

Introduction

This chapter identifies and explores the fundamental aspects of the perioperative practitioner essential to the surgical scrub role [1, 2]. All healthcare professionals involved in perioperative practice are responsible for providing a safe environment for patient care [3]. In addition, organisations undertaking surgical interventions must have standardised, structured, and safe practice in place [3]. The World Health Organization Surgical Safety Checklist 'Five Steps to Safer Surgery' [4] and the National Safety Standards for Invasive Procedures [5] standardise the critical elements of procedural care, ensuring it is evidence based.

There are three phases of perioperative care: preoperative, intraoperative, and postoperative [3]. The role of the perioperative practitioner within the operating theatre is multifaceted, providing practical clinical expertise and competence that incorporate a wide range of technical and non-technical skills [6]. The scrub practitioner is a recognised member of the perioperative team, performing a crucial role in preparing the operating theatre environment for surgical procedures [3, 7]. They ensure it is clean, ready, and safe to receive the surgical patient [3, 7].

The scrub practitioner must have acquired key competencies, technical skills, and theoretical underpinning knowledge of anatomy and physiology [6]. In addition, they should be capable of anticipating the requirements needed during a surgical procedure and respond effectively in an emergency when faced with a complex and challenging situation. This work is not done in isolation but as part of the larger perioperative team, requiring assistance from the circulating practitioner [6]. The circulator uses critical skills and core knowledge of the perioperative environment by providing expertise and support to meet the patient's needs.

Duties and Responsibilities

The scrub practitioner is responsible for providing a safe environment for the patient during the intraoperative phase of care and has a crucial role in preventing a surgical site infection (SSI) [3, 7], planning, anticipating, and responding to the needs of the surgeon and the surgical team throughout the procedure.

The scrub practitioner and the multidisciplinary team have a direct influence on a patient's surgical outcome, determined by their competence, knowledge, and underpinning skills regarding aseptic technique [3, 7, 8, 9]. Attention, therefore, is crucial in maintaining aseptic technique throughout the interoperative procedure by using standard and transmission-based precautions as an approach to preventing an SSI [3, 7, 8, 10].

Practitioners who participate in the surgical procedure are responsible and accountable for providing and reconciling sterile instrumentation, equipment, and all supplementary items [9, 11]. They are required to maintain the sterile field's integrity, safety, and efficiency, by implementing recognised practices to prevent wound contamination [7, 8, 9, 10]. This is explored in Chapter 24. The focus and management of holistic care should be concentrated around the patient on the operating table, where each surgical team member knows exactly what to do, when to do it, and how to do it. Scrub practitioners are frequently required to make intuitive decisions based on experiential knowledge, often referred to as the 'gate keeper' [9], allowing the surgeon to concentrate on the task in hand, free from distractions.

Surgical hand antisepsis, gowning, and gloving is a standard procedure performed by the scrub practitioner to prevent and reduce the risk of SSIs [3, 7, 8,]. The practitioner must have a high level of competence and be aware of current standards, recommendations, and guidance. In addition, they should be able to apply and follow local policies and protocols in conjunction with the local infection control team [3, 7, 8].

Management of Accountable and Supplementary Items Used in Surgical or Invasive Procedures

There should be a local organisational policy and a consistent, standardised process for managing and maintaining all items used throughout a surgical invasive or interventional procedure, to prevent unintentional retained items [3, 4, 5, 11]. The surgical count forms part of the risk management process [3] to protect patients from unintended retained objects and should be undertaken for all invasive procedures [3, 4, 5, 11]. The scrub practitioner is required to have undertaken training deeming them competent at performing surgical counts, in line with local policy and national guidance and recommendations [3, 11]. Instruments that come in several parts should have each part independently identified, verified, and checked [3, 11]. It is both the scrub practitioner's and the circulator's responsibility to be satisfied that all instruments are complete, with no missing parts before and after use. They should both be knowledgeable, efficient, and experienced to reduce errors. Instrument counts must be performed immediately before the commencement of a surgical or invasive intervention [3, 11].

A swab count should be undertaken in groups of five, with the red tag being removed before counting and kept safely in a container on the instrument trolley [3, 11]. The scrub practitioner must be aware of the location of all swabs, needles, instruments, and medical devices throughout the procedure. All swabs used in the procedure must have an X-ray-detectable marker (see Figure 26.1) fixed across the width of the swab [3, 11].

It is important to remember that items must not be altered as this is a potential patient safety concern [3, 11]. Items should be counted aloud and in unison between the circulator and the scrub practitioner, one of which must be a registered practitioner [3, 11]. They should be visually recorded on a whiteboard, smart screen, or electronic theatre record, and accountable items should be documented in a patient's care plan depending on local policy and guidance [3, 11].

It is the scrub practitioner's responsibility to inform the surgeon whether the count is correct and complete; if not, they must inform the surgeon immediately [3, 11]. The surgical count should be conducted using a standardised approach and in line with the local accountable items policy [3, 11].

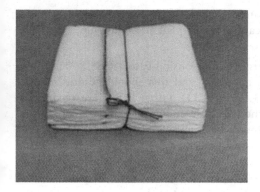

Figure 26.1 Swab with X-ray-detectable marker

The accountable items checking process is as follows:

- **Initial count:**
  - immediately before the surgical procedure commences [3, 9, 11–13];
  - on receiving additional supplementary items;

- **First closing count:**
  - at the closure of any body cavity within a cavity [3, 9, 11–13];
  - at the start of wound closure;
  - at the start of skin closure; and

- **Final count:**
  - following the completion of the surgical/invasive procedure [3, 9, 11–13].

A minimum of three counts should be undertaken [11].

Any surgical count discrepancy should be treated as follows [9, 11]:

- The scrub practitioner or circulator must promptly notify the surgeon and team of discrepancy, including type and number of items missing.
- The scrub practitioner should receive verbal recognition from surgeon.
- The circulator should call for assistance, commence a recount, and search the operating theatre if required.
- The scrub practitioner should commence a recount with the circulator and search the sterile field.
- The surgeon and assistant should pause wound closure and perform methodical wound exploration and request intraoperative imaging or an X-ray as recommended.
- The anaesthetist should stop reversal of the anaesthetic to facilitate team reconciliation of the missing item/items.
- If the missing item is retrieved/found, a recount should be performed, wound closure resumed, and the count confirmed as correct.
- If the item is not found, the count must be documented as incorrect, and alternative imaging options should be considered – CT or MRI. This should be discussed with the patient or representative (relative).

- Documentation of the reconciliation measures is taken, and the patient notified regarding the description and potential location, with a plan and follow-up.
- Notify the matron of the surgical count discrepancy.

If the surgical count is incorrect, it is the surgeon's responsibility to decide, as part of the sign-out process [4, 5], whether an X-ray is necessary and this should be documented accordingly, with corrective actions taken [3, 5, 7, 9, 11]. Often, items are reconciled, found in unusual places, concealed behind the liver, under the operating table, or mis-counted. It is the surgeon's responsibility whether to continue with closure at this stage; this incident should be recorded directly in the patient's notes and reported immediately using the organisation's electronic incident reporting system (e.g., Datix). The organisation, surgeon, and team have a duty of candour to be open and honest with the patient when something goes wrong; this is a legal and ethical requirement [14].

The above forms part of the Five Steps to Safer Surgery (team brief, sign in, time out, sign out, and team debriefing) process [4, 5].

Recommendations to Be Considered When Handling and Disposing of Sharps Safely

All sharps are considered accountable items and should be documented and managed accordingly [11]. The scrub practitioner is required to comply with current legislation, regulations, and standard precautions [15–19]. Safe protective sharps mechanisms [20] should be provided and used according to the manufacturer's instructions for use. Local organisational policies should be in place to reduce the risk of injury [3, 9, 11].

Sharps and needles in the sterile field should be managed and retained in an appropriate disposable, puncture-resistant needle container [3, 20]. If a needle or blade breaks during use, the scrub practitioner should ensure that all parts are returned and accounted for [3]. This should be reported to the Medicines and Healthcare products Regulatory Agency [21] and the manufacturer of the medical device, if it is not deemed to be a user error.

The scrub practitioner is responsible for verifying all sharps used, which includes the following (this is not an exhaustive list):

- suture needles;
- scalpels (blades);
- electrosurgical blades;
- hypodermic needles; and
- safety pins.

Needles should be accounted for by the number on the pack; if two needled sutures are indicated on the packet, two should be documented on the swab sheet. This must be verified when the pack is opened. Suture needles should be armed directly from the suture packet [12].

The following steps are recommended for sharps safety transfer:

- Sharps should be handed to the surgeon on an exchange basis only (one being returned before another is passed) [13].
- A hands-free transfer system or process to prevent needlestick injuries should be practiced, such as the creation of a neutral zone, where sharps can be placed in a receiver or receptacle for safe use and retrieval [3, 17].

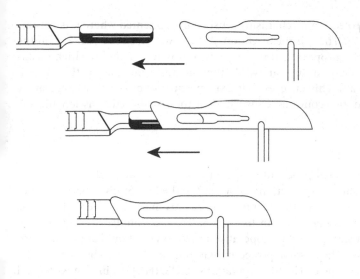

Figure 26.2 Mounting a blade

- Manual blade mounting and removal should be discouraged [13].
- Sharps must not be manipulated by hand; a heavy needle holder to attach and remove the blade can be used (see Figure 26.2) or a suitable medical device to reduce the risk of a sharp's injury [13].
- Needles must never be bent as they may break, nor should they be re-sheathed [3, 12, 17, 19].
- Needles and syringes must not be disassembled before use or disposal and should be discarded as one unit at the point of use [17].
- Whenever possible, ensure a safety device is used when handling glass amps [17].
- Always discard used sharps directly into an approved disposal container, immediately after use [3, 17].
- Whenever possible, take a sharps container to the point of use [3, 17].
- A disposable device should be used within the sterile area, away from the operating field, to contain needles and sharps, and this should be disposed of safely at the end of the procedure [3, 17].
- Never overfill sharps boxes, close securely, and change when three-quarters full [3].
- Label, date, and sign full closed sharps boxes with the name of the area and store in a secure place to await collection for final disposal [3, 17].

Needlestick and sharps injuries can be mitigated by reducing exposure and managing the risk [16, 19]. Surgical gloves can be easily penetrated by needles, blades, and sharp instruments. Double gloving has been shown to substantially reduce the risk of blood-borne virus transmission from sharps injury [22] as glove material removes 86% of blood on the outside of a needle, with the inner glove removing most of the remaining blood not already removed by the outer glove [22, 23].

Healthcare employers have a responsibility to enforce a 'zero tolerance' policy in relation to sharps injuries [15]. It requires that employers must take steps to avoid the unnecessary use of sharps. Safe sharps protection mechanisms must be implemented where it is reasonably practicable to do so [17]. The European Union Withdrawal Act 2018 [24, 25] on the 11 February 2020 brought all European Union (EU) laws onto the UK books, which means any regulations made over the past 40 years while the UK was a member of the EU will continue to apply post Brexit. This ensures that existing protections such as regulatory frameworks are maintained and continue to work even though the UK has left the EU [24, 25].

Specimen Management

During surgical and interventional procedures, specimens are routinely taken [3, 9]. It is important to discuss specimen management needs as part of the Five Steps to Safer Surgery [4] to improve efficiency and ensure the identified needs are met [9]. There should be a management system in place when human tissue [26, 27] and samples are obtained to safeguard both patients and staff [3]. All perioperative practitioners should apply standard precautions, wear the appropriate personal protective equipment (PPE) and be aware of the Control of Substances Hazardous to Health Regulations (COSHH) [28] in line with local policies to protect themselves from splash injuries from specimen fixative or body fluids [3]. It is essential that all perioperative staff are trained and educated regarding specimen management and handling, taking note of any guidance issued by their local pathology service [29] processes, to mitigate against error and risk [3, 9], as this can determine subsequent treatment of the patient [5, 6].

The scrub practitioner should be able to identify surgical specimens, and maintain and handle them appropriately in the sterile field [3, 9]. They should be able to communicate effectively to the circulating practitioner, verifying the type of specimen, and labelling and packaging required [9]. If this is incorrect, the diagnosis may not be able to be confirmed, potentially compromising a patient's health and outcomes [9]. If a specimen is lost or accidently thrown away, the surgeon must be informed immediately [9].

Specimen Types

There should be a local policy in place that reflects and considers the range of specimens likely to be collected, to facilitate efficient and safe processes required for the different types that may be retrieved [3, 9]. The type of specimens includes the following:

- histology;
- cytology;
- microbiology (local arrangement for collection should be in place);
- intraoperative investigation (e.g., frozen section), radioactive specimens (e.g., sentinel node biopsy) [30]; in the case of sentinel lymph nodes, there should be a policy in place for transportation in compliance with radiation protection and nuclear medicine department guidelines [31];
- products of conception [27];
- non-biological, forensic (e.g., bullet or blade), foreign bodies (e.g., fishbone or glass fragments), retained surgical swabs, needles, and instruments; and
- explanted medical devices (e.g., pacemaker or heart valve), explanted items (e.g., orthopaedic screws or plates), and breast implants.

Specimen Identification

This must begin at the time the specimen is removed from the patient. The surgeon should verbally verify with the scrub practitioner and circulator the following details [3]:

- the name of the specimen (e.g., breast tissue);
- the site, if relevant (e.g., breast), and presence of orientation markers; edges and margins of tissue may be tagged with 'short' and 'long suture' – this will need identifying on the label and pathology form;
- the laterality, if relevant (e.g., left);
- the investigation required (e.g., histology); and
- the medium required for transportation (e.g., formalin).

For explanted non-biological specimens, it is important first to ascertain if the implant or medical device is for bacterial pathology or mechanical examination; the following are important: identify on pathology requisition, or make a note of the serial numbers and manufacturers' codes (if available), and document on the patient's records.

The following are important to consider in the documentation labelling and packaging of specimen:

- When receiving a clinical specimen from the sterile field, the type of specimen, and transport medium, should be confirmed by the clinician/surgeon.
- Prior to the specimen being placed into a container the scrub practitioner must ask the operating surgeon to clarify the nature of each of the specimens.
- This should then be repeated clearly to the circulating practitioner who will be receiving the specimen and preparing the addressograph label.
- The circulator should place a label on the side of the container, not on the lid, for easy identification.
- The container should be placed inside a plastic bag to prevent risk of spillage during transport.
- No abbreviations should be used, and where left or right this should also be written in full.
- Remember that all specimens are biohazardous and PPE precautions should be followed.
- Fixative should cover the specimen, allowing it to float freely.
- Avoid contaminating the outside of the specimen container.
- If the specimen is fresh (dry) this will need to be sent to the laboratory quickly as it can decompose and jeopardise the pathology.

Frozen Section

If specimens are required for frozen section, this should be identified at the team brief and the histology department informed by medical staff [3]. A request form should be filled in by the surgeon before the start of the operation [3]. Specimens for frozen section do not require any transport medium and are placed in dry containers, labelled and dispatched immediately to the appropriate department, sometimes labelled for the attention of a specific pathologist who will be awaiting the specimen. It is worth noting that the specimen may be picked up directly by the pathologist if the surgeon needs to speak to them [9].

The tissue is frozen, stained, and sliced to view under microscope for diagnosis [3]. Results should be received, and a written record made, by a registered member of the surgical team. If a known malignancy exists, the surgeon may send additional frozen sections to verify whether margins are clear of tumour [29].

Care and Handling of Intraoperative Surgical Specimens

The following steps are recommended:

- The scrub practitioner should be able to anticipate and assess specimen management before the procedure and be able to discuss concerns at the (team brief) [3, 5].
- It is important to note that specimen management may be influenced by a patient's culture and personnel beliefs. For instance, in Jewish law, blood and limbs are considered part of the human being, and therefore should be buried. Limbs that are amputated require burial in the patient's future grave site [9].
- The scrub practitioner should be knowledgeable and deemed competent in how to handle and process specimens in line with local organisational policies, procedures, and national guidance [4, 5, 6]. If specimens are not handled appropriately, damaged, or lost, this may require the patient to have a second surgical procedure, result in the wrong diagnosis, and could even prevent subsequent initiation of definitive treatment [3]. It is crucial that all specimens are labelled correctly, according to the surgeon's specification and instructions [3, 12].
- The circulating practitioner should prepare the forms and select an appropriate container in relation to the size of the specimen and its purpose, based upon the information confirmed by the operating surgeon and scrub practitioner. For histopathology specimens that require fixing, the container should be large enough to ensure that the specimen floats freely, is completely covered by appropriate fixative, and is sealed for transportation [3].
- The scrub practitioner and circulator must confirm with the surgeon whether the specimen is required to be placed in a container with a transport medium, or whether it should go dry [29].
- A specimen must be transferred from the sterile field in a manner that maintains its integrity and is consistent with local policy of the organisation [3].
- The specimen should be verified with the surgeon before passing off to the circulator.
- The specimen should never be handed off on a surgical sponge [3].
- The scrub practitioner should seek consent from the surgeon to hand off the specimen of the sterile field to be placed in an appropriate container and ascertain whether fixative is required [3].
- Once confirmed, the circulator should confirm with the scrub practitioner and surgeon details required on the patient's sticker; once agreed, the sticker should be attached to the specimen pot, and the scrub practitioner should place the specimen into the container, confirming the patients details on the specimen pot.
- A written local policy should be in place for the collection and transportation of laboratory specimens. Practitioners should be aware of this policy and its contents [3, 9].
- All specimens must be collected in an aseptic manner (aseptic technique) to avoid contamination with other bacteria that may influence the laboratory result, and placed in an appropriate or sterile container as required [3, 9].

- Visual confirmation, patient identification, verification, and labelling of the specimen in the container when handing off the sterile field to the circulator should be confirmed with the surgeon and acknowledged by the circulator [3, 9].
- Labelling and requisition documentation must be correct and legible [3, 9].
- Specimens retained on the sterile field should be sequentially identified, kept moist until transferred, and monitored.
- They must not be placed on a dry absorbent service or exposed to air, as this can lead to desiccation of tissue [3, 9].
- The quality of the specimen collected has significance and implications for any microbiological diagnosis that may be reported and the subsequent prescribing of antimicrobial drugs such as antibiotics. Incorrectly collected, stored, or handled specimens can result in inappropriate or unnecessary antibiotics being prescribed [3, 9].

Waste Management

Within the perioperative environment both clinical and non-clinical waste is generated [3, 32] and is required to be managed safely. It is important that all healthcare professionals are educated in waste segregation and safe disposal, in accordance with local policy [3]. Waste removal from healthcare facilities can have an environmental impact as well as being costly to healthcare organisations. Clinical waste is known to contain both harmful micro-organisms and toxins, which can lead to disease in humans [33].

The UK's safe management of healthcare waste (HTM 07–01) government guidance [33, 34] introduced a national colour-coded system of waste receptacles so that waste can be easily identified and segregated in the waste system. Some perioperative settings have black or clear bags for non-clinical waste, such as tray wrappings and product packaging, to collect often recyclable waste at the 'setting up stage' and prior to the commencement of surgery.

Figures 26.3 and 26.4 show the colour coding systems for waste bin lins and clinical waste bags, identifying what items can be disposed of in each container or bag [34].

Yellow-lidded rigid containers or sharps containers are used for waste that may be classed as hazardous or potentially hazardous as it is contaminated with body fluids that may or may not be infectious, or where there is medicinal or chemically infected waste. Waste that is included in these categories must be placed in the appropriate receptacle and incinerated [3].

Orange bags or rigid orange-lidded yellow sharps containers are used for potentially infected clinical waste such as used dressings, swabs, bandages, and the disposal of single-use protective clothing such as gowns and gloves. Once sealed, this waste can then be sent for alternative treatment so that it is considered safe prior to disposal [3, 32].

Yellow bags or rigid purple-lidded yellow sharps containers are used for the disposal of cytotoxic drugs or cytostatic waste. Once sealed these should be sent to an authorised disposal facility for incineration [3, 32].

Red-lidded rigid containers should be used for the disposal of anatomical waste, such as recognisable body parts and maternity waste. Once sealed, this waste should be sent to an authorised site for incineration [3, 32].

Blue-lidded rigid containers can be used for waste medicines such as empty medicine bottles and unused cytotoxic or cytostatic medicines that are classed as non-hazardous. Once sealed, this waste should be sent to an authorised site for incineration [3, 32].

Bin Lid Colour	Purple	**Cytotoxic/Cytostatic: HAZARDOUS** **Waste consisting of, or contaminated with, cytotoxic and/or cytostatic products** **which requires disposal by incineration.** e.g., Blister packs, tablets in containers, unopened medicine vials, patches, gloves, gowns, aprons, wipes contaminated with cytotoxic and/or cytostatic medicines, cytotoxic waste disposal.
	Red	**Anatomical: HAZARDOUS/NON-HAZARDOUS** **Anatomical waste which requires disposal by incineration.** e.g., Body parts, organs, blood bags, blood preserves, anatomical waste.
	Yellow	**Clinical/Highly Infectious: HAZARDOUS** **Highly infectious waste which requires disposal by incineration.** e.g., Couch roll, wipes, gloves, dressings, bandages, aprons, disposable garments, infectious waste.
	Blue	**Medicinal: NON-HAZARDOUS** **Waste medicines, out of date medicines and denatured drugs which all require** **disposal by incineration.** e.g., Tablets in containers, blister packs, unopened medicine vials, liquids in bottles, inhaler cartridges, droplet bottles with pipettes.

Figure 26.3 Waste bin lid colour (used with kind permission from the Association for Perioperative Practice [35])

Bag Colour	Orange	**Clinical/Infectious: HAZARDOUS/NON-HAZARDOUS** **Infectious waste which may be treated to render safe prior to disposal or** **alternatively it can be incinerated.** e.g., Wipes, gloves, dressings, bandages, aprons.
	Yellow	**Offensive: NON-HAZARDOUS** **Non-infectious, offensive/hygiene waste which may be recycled,** **incinerated (waste for energy) or deep landfilled.** e.g., Colostomy bags, incontinence pads, nappies & wipes, gloves, disposable garments.
	Black	**BAG COLOUR – Black** **Mixed Municipal Waste: VARIOUS** **Municipal wastes and similar commercial, industrial and institutional wastes** **including separately collected fractions. Requires disposal by landfill.** e.g., Packaging, tissues, disposable cups & drinks cans, sandwich wrappers, flowers.

Figure 26.4 Clinical waste bag colour (used with permission from the Association for Perioperative Practice [35])

Yellow and black bags should be used for non-hazardous offensive or hygiene healthcare waste that does not constitute an infection or health risk. This may include items such as used catheter bags, maternity waste, or other blood products from a known screened source. Once sealed, these should be sent to a suitable energy recovery waste management site or to landfill if no such facility is available [3, 32]. Clear/black bags should be used for domestic waste and are suitable for disposal at landfill sites [3, 32, 36, 37].

Clinical waste bags should not be filled more than three-quarters full. This ensures that each bag can be adequately closed. The neck of the bag should be gathered and then twisted prior to closing with a cable tie. Alternatively, a specific heat-sealing device designated for clinical waste may be used. Staples are not a suitable closure for clinical waste bags [3]. All practitioners working within the perioperative environment should have a clear understanding and awareness regarding the disposal of both clinical and non-clinical waste. If practitioners do not feel confident within this area of practice, they should assume personal responsibility either individually or within the team to source the most up-to-date information from their line managers or the infection prevention team within their organisation [3].

Risk Assessment and Health and Safety Legislation

Healthcare organisations have a duty of care [36] to have a safe system of work, to ensure that waste is adequately managed per the COSHH regulations [28]. These regulations require organisations to manage both the risk and exposure to hazardous substances to its workforce. Education and training should be provided to reduce the risk of exposure to hazardous substances [28, 36]. A risk assessment process should be in place and all staff who dispose of waste have a responsibility to do so under the waste management policy [36].

This process should include the following guidance:

- All clinical waste should be clearly labelled with its point of origin. In addition, the container should be dated.
- Waste bags generated by individual theatre cases should be labelled in such a way that they can be identified following collection if there is a need to do so, while protecting the confidentiality of the individual patient.
- All sharps containers should conform to the BS EN ISO 23907 standards. Faulty collection containers must be identified and removed from service until the fault has been rectified.
- Sharps disposal boxes should be placed in suitable positions to ensure easy placement of contaminated items and close to the point of use.
- Sharps containers should not be placed in an area where visitors and or children can access the contents.
- Sharps disposal boxes should not be filled more than three-quarters full and should be of a design that allows them to be locked after sealing. If it may take some time for the container to be filled quickly, it is recommended that advice is sought from the designated infection control practitioner. Consideration should be given to the size of the box and the replacement interval as set out in the local policy applicable to sharps containers in community settings.
- Body fluids should not be tipped into clinical waste bags but rather placed in leak-proof containers, which are subsequently stored in rigid boxes that are clearly marked as clinical waste.

- Body fluids in suction liners or other containers may have a solidifying agent added prior to placing the container in a suitable waste receptacle.
- The bags should be removed to an area where they can be accessed if required up to completion of the procedure and if any issues regarding packaging or discrepancies present.
- Waste containers should be stored in a designated 'dirty' area. Access to this area should be restricted to staff and always locked to prevent unauthorised access to contaminated substances.
- Waste from the perioperative setting should ideally be removed without being transported through clean areas, and the design and layout of theatres should incorporate this requirement.
- Personnel involved in this process of waste removal and disposal must be provided with suitable training and personal protective clothing and equipment.
- Waste contractors should collect clinical waste from the main waste storage areas and transport it to the designated incinerators in accordance with the relevant legislation.

References

1. Perioperative Care Collaborative Position Statement. The role of the perioperative healthcare assistant in the surgical care team. Available from: www.afpp.org.uk/news/The_Perioperative_Care_Collaborative_Position_Statement.

2. Perioperative Care Collaborative Position Statement. The role of the surgical first assistant. The Perioperative Care Collaborative, 2018.

3. The Association for Perioperative Practice. *Standards and Recommendations for Safe Perioperative Practice*. Harrogate: AfPP, 2022.

4. World Health Organization. WHO guidelines for safe surgery 2009: safe surgery saves lives. Available from: http://apps.who.int/iris/bitstream/handle/10665/44185/9789241598552_eng.pdf;jsessionid=FC669EE9CA17F90C626BF4FD1D12A9DB?sequence=1.

5. NHS England. National safety standards for invasive procedures (NatSSIPs), 2015. Available from: www.england.nhs.uk/patientsafety/wp-content/uploads/sites/32/2015/09/natssips-safety-standards.pdf.

6. P. Wicker and J. O'Neil. *Caring for the Perioperative Patient*, 2nd ed. Oxford: Wiley-Blackwell, 2010.

7. The Association for Perioperative Practice. AfPP standards and recommendations: infection control. Available from: www.afpp.org.uk/news/AfPP_Standards_and_Recommendations-Infection_Control.

8. National Institute for Health and Care Excellence. Surgical site infections: prevention and treatment, 2019. Available from: www.nice.org.uk/guidance/ng125/resources/surgical-site-infections-prevention-and-treatment-pdf-66141660564421.

9. Association of periOperative Registered Nurses. Recommended practices for sponge sharps and instrument counts. *AORN Journal* 2006; **83**: 418–433.

10. H. P. Loveday, J. Wilson, R. J. Pratt, et al. epic3: national evidence-based guidelines for preventing healthcare-associated infections in NHS hospitals in England. *Journal of Hospital Infection* 2014; **86**: S1–S70.

11. Association for Perioperative Practice. Accountable items, swab, instrument, and sharps count. Available at: www.afpp.org.uk/careers/Standards-Guidance.

12. N. M. Phillips and A. Hornacky. *Berry and Kohn's Operating Room Technique*, 14th ed. St Louis, MO: Elsevier, 2020.

13. J. C. Rothrock. *Alexander's Care of the Patient in Surgery 2018*, 16th ed. St Louis, MO: Elsevier, 2018.

14. Health and Social Care Act 2008 (Regulated Activities) Regulations 2014. Duty of candour Part 3 Section 2.20.

Available from: www.legislation.gov.uk/uk
dsi/2014/9780111117613/contents.

15. European Agency for Safety and Health at
    Work. Directive 2010/32/EU – prevention
    from sharp injuries in the hospital and
    healthcare sector. Available from: https://
    osha.europa.eu/en/legislation/directives/
    council-directive-2010-32-eu-prevention-
    from-sharp-injuries-in-the-hospital-and-
    healthcare-sector.

16. Health and Safety Executive. Workplace
    health, safety and welfare regulations 1992:
    approved code of practice and guidelines,
    Available from: www.hse.gov.uk/pubns/
    priced/l24.pdf.

17. Royal College of Nursing. Sharps safety.
    Available from: www.rcn.org.uk/profes
    sional-development/publications/pub-
    004135.

18. Association of Surgical Technologist. AST
    guidelines for best practices for sharps
    safety and use of the neutral zone, 2017.
    Available from: www.ast.org/uploadedFiles/
    Main_Site/Content/About_Us/Standard_
    Sharps_Safety_Use_of_the_Neutral_Zone
    .pdf.

19. Health and Safety Executive. Health and
    safety (sharp instruments in healthcare)
    regulations 2013. Available from: www
    .hse.gov.uk/pubns/hsis7.htm.

20. Association for Perioperative Practice.
    *Accountable Items, Swab, Instrument and
    Needle Count (Clinical Guideline 8.1) in
    Standards and Recommendations for Safe
    Perioperative Practice*, 4th ed. Harrogate:
    AfPP, 2016.

21. Medicines and Healthcare products
    Regulatory Agency. Report a problem with
    a medicine or medical device. Available
    from: www.gov.uk/report-problem-
    medicine-medical-device (accessed
    January 2021).

22. NHS Employers. NHS Employers:
    managing the risks of sharps injuries
    (December 2015). Available at: www
    .pslhub.org/learn/culture/staff-safety/nhs-
    employers-managing-the-risks-of-sharps-
    injuries-december-2015-r4438/.

23. S. T. Mast, J. D. Woolwine, and
    J. L. Geberding. Efficacy of gloves in

reducing blood volumes transferred during
simulated needlestick injury. *Journal of
Infectious Diseases* 1993;**168**: 1589–1592.

24. European Union (Withdrawal) Act 2018.
    Available at: www.legislation.gov.uk/ukpg
    a/2018/16/contents/enacted.

25. Safety Management: Ensuring consistent
    standards. British Standards Institution.
    Safety Management. 2019. Available at:
    www.britsafe.org/publications/safety-
    management-magazine/safety-
    management-magazine/2018/ensuring-
    consistent-standards-after-brexit/.

26. Human Tissue Act 2004. Available from:
    www.legislation.gov.uk/ukpga/2004/30/
    contents.

27. Human Tissue Authority. Guidance on the
    disposal of pregnancy remains. Available
    from: www.hta.gov.uk/guidance-
    professionals/regulated-sectors/post-
    mortem/guidance-sensitive-handling-
    pregnancy-remains.

28. Control of Substances Hazardous to Health
    Regulations 2002 (as amended 2004).
    Available from: www.hse.gov.uk/foi/inter
    nalops/ocs/200-299/273_20.

29. The Royal College of Pathologists. Code of
    practice for histocompatibility and
    immunogenetics (H&I) services, May 2005.
    Available from: www.rcpath.org/uploads/
    assets/00cf0560-a182-4c72-
    a015c5b335e090f7/Code-of-practice-for-
    pathology-services-and-departments-May-
    2005.pdf.

30. P. L. Fitzgibbons and V. A. LiVolsi.
    Recommendations for handling
    radioactive specimens obtained by sentinel
    lymphadenectomy. *American Journal of
    Surgical Pathology* 2000; **24**: 1549–1551.

31. B. J. Coventry, P. J. Collins, J. Kollias, et al.
    Ensuring radiation safety to staff in
    lymphatic tracing and sentinel lymph node
    biopsy surgery: some recommendations.
    *Journal of Nuclear Medicine & Radiation
    Therapy* 2012; DOI 10.4172/2155-9619.
    S2-008.

32. Royal College of Nursing. The
    management of waste from health,
    social and personal care. Available from:
    www.herefordshireccg.nhs.uk/library/

infection-prevention-and-control/sharps-and-waste/1092-rcn-waste-guidelines-april-14/file.

33. Department of Health. Environment and sustainability Health Technical Memorandum 07-01: safe management of healthcare waste. Available from: www.gov.uk/government/uploads/system/uploads/attachment_data/file/167976/HTM_07-01_Final.pdf.

34. The Ionising Radiations Regulations 1999. Available from: www.legislation.gov.uk/uksi/1999/3232/pdfs/uksi_19993232_en.pdf.

35. Association for Perioperative Practice. *Theatre Etiquette: A Guide to Theatres.* Harrogate: AfPP, 2021.

36. Environment Agency 2008. *Hazardous Waste: Interpretation of the Definition and Classification of Hazardous Waste WM2*, 2nd ed., version 2.2. Bristol: The Environment Agency.

37. Landfill (England and Wales) Regulations 2002. Available from: www.legislation.gov.uk/uksi/2002/1559/contents/made.

Fundamentals of Patient Positioning for Surgery

Sarah Brady

Introduction

The ability to safely and effectively position a patient for surgery is a fundamental skill that all perioperative practitioners are required to have. The correct positioning and alignment of limbs for surgical procedures is vital [1], and all perioperative practitioners should understand their role and responsibility for safe patient positioning, and the rationale for it [2]. Safe patient positioning is always a multi-disciplinary team effort, whereby all members of the perioperative team should be present in the operating theatre at the crucial moment.

Prior to any patient being positioned for a procedure the perioperative team should have participated in a team brief or huddle [3]. During the team briefing, all patient positioning requirements should be openly discussed and planned. This includes the equipment requirements and availability, accessibility to the surgical site, staff competence, and any patient movement limitations that could affect positioning.

Good communication and the need for well-coordinated and effective manoeuvring is essential for safe positioning of the patient [2]. The anaesthetist will usually take the lead role and initiate the moving and handling procedures, although each team member has a responsibility to ensure patient safety, dignity, and stability [4].

Aims of Patient Positioning

For every patient who needs to be positioned for a surgical procedure, the aims of the perioperative team should be:

- physiological alignment;
- minimal interference with circulation;
- ensuring individual patient safety and stability;
- providing suitable access to the operative field, airway, intravenous access (and if in situ, a urinary catheter);
- maintain patient dignity and comfort; and
- avoid nerve and tissue damage to the patient.

Other issues to consider include:

- Physical stress on the perioperative team: including lifting, twisting, pushing and pulling. All such stress can be minimised by using correct moving and handling techniques and equipment.
- Time constraints: a busy operating list can put pressure on the team to rush the manoeuvre. Pre-planning and preparation can minimise delays.

- The surgeon's preference: a team who understands how their surgeon prefers the patient to be positioned for each procedure will be more efficient. There will need to be an appropriate number of team members available to move the patient. This is generally accepted to be a minimum of four team members for the most commonly occurring surgical procedures [5]. Also, consider where the surgeon will require additional equipment such as a microscope, laser, diathermy machine, and C-arm or robot to be placed.
- Length of surgery and time under anaesthesia: intraoperative passive movements may need to be performed for longer surgeries [6]. It is recommended to perform this after the 4-hour mark, although this will depend upon accessibility and the phase of the operation [7].
- General anaesthesia reduces muscle tone, therefore positions not normally attainable while the patient is awake may be inadvertently achieved, leading to compression or overstretching of a joint and related nerves [7].
- Individual patient factors: such as body weight, height, age, sex, joint mobility, previous surgery, co-morbidities, pressure areas, skin integrity (consult with pressure-area care specialists if necessary), nutritional status, patient warming, intravenous access, diathermy plate positioning, proximity to or contact with metal, tourniquet requirement and position, prosthetics, pacemakers, indwelling catheters, and stoma. All must be considered as they could each affect patient safety in different ways. Always protect skin (avoid wrinkles), muscles, and nerves, and minimise patient exposure to reduce the risk of hypothermia. Minimise changes to homeostasis, respiration, and circulation.
- Whenever possible, prepare in advance, but remember that all patients are individuals, and some novel and creative (but still risk-assessed) thinking may be required from time to time to achieve a safe position.
- Equipment should be in safe working order – all equipment should be regularly serviced according to specific healthcare trust protocols. Electronic operating tables should be fully charged, and mattresses and padding should be clean and intact, resistant to moisture, non-allergenic, and fire retardant. Any operating table, electronic or manual, should have its full range of movement checked prior to use, and attachments should be compatible and fit the table securely.
- Check skin integrity and pressure points of every patient at the end of every procedure. Document and report any issues. Be careful to ensure that patients are never dragged up or down the operating table to avoid causing shearing injuries to the skin.

Supine Position

There are several different positions used in surgery, which are detailed here and in the following sections. Of these, the supine position is the most common.

The patient is positioned on their back and their arms may be abducted on arm boards to an angle no greater than 90 degrees to avoid injury to the brachial plexus (see Figure 27.1). Arms may also be tucked or rolled into the patient's side using arm retainers and soft padding such as Gamgee. The hands should fall into their natural position where possible, which may be pronated or supinated depending upon the patient's anatomy [8]. Pressure points should be well padded to protect from pressure or nerve injury and any intravenous

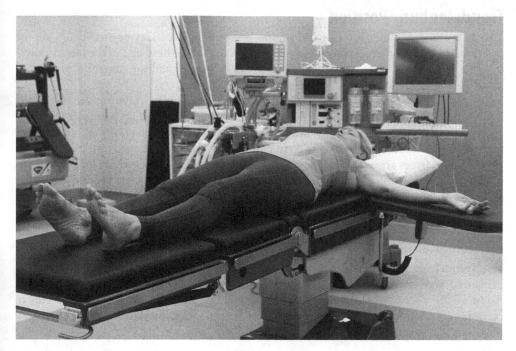

Figure 27.1 Basic supine position, prior to addition of any padding, with arms abducted on arm boards (photograph taken at Edge Hill University)

access should be secured and easily accessible. No part of the patient's anatomy should be touching any metal parts of the operating table or its attachments.

The head should be in a neutral position with the pressure points being supported and the integrity of the airway protected. The head can be supported by a pillow; alternatively, a head ring may be used for surgical access to the head or neck. A pillow can also be placed under the knees to provide relief to the lumbar vertebrae and maintain the natural curvature of the spine. This will also help prevent knee hyperextension and potential injury to the popliteal nerve [2]. Heel gel supports may be used underneath the heels (positioned at the Achilles tendon) to prevent a potential pressure injury to the heel. A pressure relieving mattress should always be used on the operating table, and for longer procedures a gel mat may also be added on top of the standard mattress, to provide further relief to the pressure points – occiput, scapula, lumbar and sacral vertebrae, heels, and elbows.

Physiological Changes in the Supine Position

There can be an initial increase in cardiac output due to the redistribution of pooled venous blood from the lower limbs. It can also cause a decrease in tidal volumes and a significant reduction in the functional residual capacity (FRC) in the anaesthetised patient. The supine position can lead to haemodynamic changes in pregnant patients (>16 weeks) caused by the gravid uterus compressing the inferior vena cava. This can lead to hypotension and reduced perfusion to the fetus [9]. This can be prevented by tilting the operating table or placing a wedge under the patient's right hip.

Trendelenburg Position

This is a common adaptation of the supine position. The patient begins in the supine position, then the operating table is gradually tilted so that the head end of the table is lower than the foot end, at an angle dictated by the type of surgery and the surgeon's preference [2]. It is commonly used in abdominal and gynaecology surgery.

Use of a pressure-relieving gel mat and safety straps can help to reduce the risk of the patient sliding down the operating table, particularly when a steep angle is required [10]. If a safety strap is used, it should not be secured too tightly as this may impede circulation; there should be space for two fingers to fit comfortably underneath the strap [5].

Common issues arising as a result of the Trendelenburg position include brachial plexus injuries, corneal abrasions, increased intraocular pressure, and oedema around the upper airway and face [10]. Debate surrounds the use of a shoulder brace for Trendelenburg positioning, and not all hospitals allow the use of this piece of equipment.

Physiological Changes in the Trendelenburg Position

The Trendelenburg position can cause cardiovascular changes, an increase in intracerebral pressure, and excessive pressure on the diaphragm from abdominal viscera [5]. Additionally, decreased blood flow and hypoxaemia of the lower limbs is a risk factor to consider [11]. As the venous return is compromised, it is also typical to see blood pooling in the upper body, causing hypertension.

Reverse Trendelenburg Position

As the name suggests, this position is the reverse of Trendelenburg, meaning that the head end of the operating table is positioned higher than the foot end. It is often used in head and neck surgery, and sometimes in bariatric surgery. Where the surgical position requires a severe tilt to be applied to the operating table, a foot plate can be used to prevent the patient from sliding down the operating table. The feet should be positioned to maintain good blood circulation and therefore dorsi or plantar flexion should be avoided [2]. Positioning of the table should be done gradually to avoid shearing injuries. Clear communication between the members of the perioperative team is vital in order to maintain patient safety.

Physiological Changes in the Reverse Trendelenburg Position

The reverse Trendelenburg position can cause haemodynamic changes such as reduced venous return and hypotension, which can result in decreased cerebral perfusion and an increased risk of venous air embolism. There is also a reduced risk of passive regurgitation [12].

Prone Position

The prone position is commonly used for surgical access to the neck, posterior head, and spine. Patients are anaesthetised in the supine position and the airway is secured before the patient is positioned into the face down position on the operating table [2]. Many specialised theatre departments may have specific equipment for turning a patient prone but, if not, it will need to be performed manually. Whichever method is used, there should always be enough team members available to move the patient safely, in a controlled manner. A minimum of four team members should be available to safely position the patient [5], although six may be preferable [13]. When turning the patient, intravenous access and any invasive lines should be protected to prevent accidental dislodgement. ECG leads, urinary catheters, bispectral index (BIS) monitors, or indeed any monitoring equipment, may need to be repositioned once the patient has been turned on to their front.

The head and airway are moved, controlled, and positioned by the anaesthetist onto a prone headrest that is specially designed to fit the face and nose comfortably, while allowing access to the airway. Commonly a reinforced endotracheal tube is used because of its reduced risk of kinking due to the spiral-wound reinforcing wire. It is important to ensure that the patient's eyes are protected as pressure can result in ophthalmic injury [5]. A simple eye ointment should be applied to the eyes and they should be protected with soft padding. It has been estimated that postoperative visual loss occurs in 0.2% of prone spinal surgery cases. Surgery lasting more than 6 hours, excessive blood loss, and poor perfusion are common contributing factors [14].

The cervical spine should be in a neutral position, with the body in a straight line. If a specialised prone mattress, such as a Montreal mattress [8], is not available then pillows should be placed under the patient, ensuring that the diaphragm is unrestricted and respiration can occur. Special attention should be taken to prevent any undue pressure to the genitalia or breasts. A team member must check that genitals are not twisted or compressed before the procedure is started [5].

The knees may be slightly flexed, with a pillow placed under the lower leg to avoid hyperextension of the knee joints, and to relieve pressure on the sciatic nerve. Arms may be rolled or tucked into the side, or moved simultaneously by two team members, in a coordinated manner, to rest at the side of the head on arm boards. These must be positioned parallel, running alongside the operating table. Arm boards should be level with the operating table, and arms should not abduct more than 90 degrees when repositioning them as this could cause a brachial plexus injury. When the arms are comfortable and secure, check that no part of the patient is in contact with any metal parts of the operating table. All pressure points should be well padded to protect from nerve or pressure injuries. Pressure injuries frequently occur in the prone position. The most at-risk areas are the dorsum of the foot, knees, pelvic area, breasts, axilla, elbows, and face [12].

Physiological Changes in the Prone Position

The prone position (see Figure 27.2) causes respiratory changes in alveolar recruitment and increased oxygenation without affecting cardiac output. Moving from the supine to prone position also leads to a relative increase in the FRC [15]. These benefits have been utilised in treating COVID-19-associated acute respiratory distress syndrome and severe hypoxaemia. It helps to facilitate more effective ventilation of the dorsal lung regions and improves ventilation–perfusion matching [16]. It is also worth remembering the challenges posed by a patient in the prone position when encountering airway management difficulties or when cardiopulmonary resuscitation is required due to the limited access available. In high-risk cases, the defibrillator pads should be applied before positioning the patient.

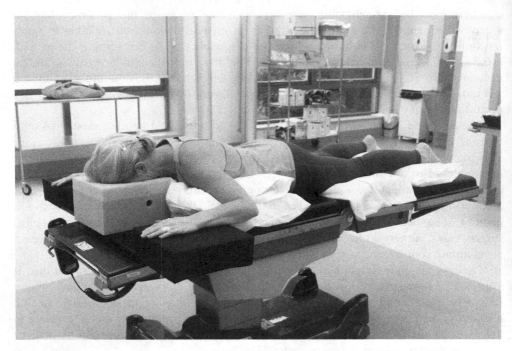

Figure 27.2 Basic prone position (photograph taken at Edge Hill University)

Lithotomy Position

The lithotomy position (see Figure 27.3) is used for a variety of colorectal, gynaeco-logical, and urological procedures. The patient begins in the supine position, but positioned lower down the table than normal, with the buttocks positioned at the break in the operating table [8]. Ensure that lithotomy boots (or poles or stirrups depending on which equipment is available) are securely attached to the table. Working simultaneously and in agreement with the anaesthetist, two team members should lift the legs (one leg each, held at the knee and ankle for safety) and place them into the boot. Moving the legs simultaneously will help to prevent lumbosacral injury [5] and alerts the anaesthetist to the possibility of haemodynamic changes occurring as a result of the changed position.

The hips and knees, for a standard lithotomy position, should be flexed up to, but not more than 90 degrees. Hips should be abducted no more than 45 degrees with neutral rotation [17], and the feet should sit in a natural position within the boot [8]. The feet should not be forced into the boot, rather the boot should be adjusted to suit the patient's natural position. This may require one team member to take the weight of the leg while the other adjusts the boot and secures it. Ideally, the legs should be placed parallel to the table, to reduce the risk of sciatic nerve injury [2].

The angle of the hips and knees may be modified depending on the type of surgery; for example, to a 45-degree angle for the Lloyd–Davies position [8]. When the position is acceptable, the foot end of the operating table is removed or lowered to provide improved surgical access. The buttocks should not be overhanging the edge of the table and patient

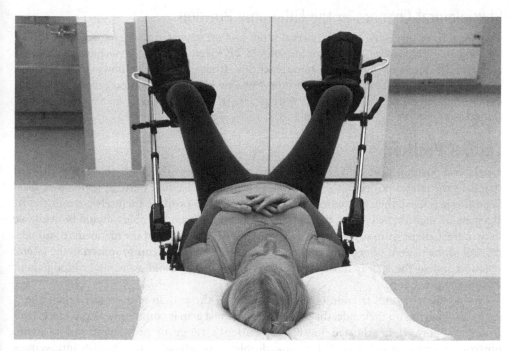

Figure 27.3 Basic lithotomy position, with arms positioned across the torso (photograph taken at Edge Hill University)

dignity should be maintained whenever possible. For instance, by not leaving the genitalia exposed unnecessarily.

The arms may be placed on arm boards, abducted to no more than 90 degrees to prevent brachial plexus injuries, or tucked in securely to the sides using elbow clips or other suitable equipment. Arms may sometimes be placed across the lower abdomen if not obstructing the surgical field. The patient's arms must not be allowed to hang off the end of the table or touch metal when the foot end of the operating table is removed or lowered [2].

There is also a risk of a pressure-related injury to the lower leg area from the external pressure of the boot or stirrup [11]; therefore, it is essential to place the foot in the correct position, at a natural angle [8]. If the lithotomy position is to be maintained for more than 4 hours, there is a risk of compartment syndrome occurring in the lower legs [8, 17]. An extended surgical time may also result in nerve injury to the peroneal nerve and so it is recommended to move the legs every 2 hours if feasible [5].

Ensure all pressure points are protected throughout the procedure. Be aware of patient digits or genitalia which may be overlapping the end of the operating table while reattaching the 'foot' end of the operating table. At the end of the procedure, two team members should lift the legs down from the boots/stirrups simultaneously, with the agreement of the anaesthetist. Check skin integrity and pressure points for signs of injury.

Physiological Changes in the Lithotomy Position

Co-morbidities involving the cardiorespiratory system may lead to dyspnoea in the lithotomy position; therefore, consideration should be given to slightly raising the torso or adjusting the angle of the table to counteract this. If necessary, use pillows or the break in the table to manipulate the patient position [5]. The lithotomy position can cause haemodynamic changes such as increased venous return and temporary increases in cardiac output [12].

Lateral Position

The lateral position is used to access the hip, thorax, kidney, shoulder, and retroperitoneal space. In the lateral position, the patient lies on one side of their body. If regional or local anaesthesia is used, then the patient can be encouraged to position themselves comfortably. If a general anaesthetic is used, then a minimum of four team members should be available to turn the patient from supine to lateral. The anaesthetist will lead the manoeuvre and take control of the patient's head and airway. Access to the airway is compromised in the lateral position and so the airway device must be well secured to avoid accidental dislodgement during the procedure.

Avoid shearing and friction burns when turning the patient and protect spinal alignment. When lying on their side, the patient's uppermost arm is commonly placed in a Carter Braine support. It is adjusted to suit the patient's range of movement and to avoid obstructing the surgical field. Where practicable, it is advisable to establish intravenous access in the uppermost arm for accessibility and safety. The bottom arm should not be compressed and, where possible, rest on an arm board. It may alternatively be rested on a pillow in a comfortable position, taking care to avoid undue brachial plexus pressure. Knees should be flexed, with padding in between bony prominences to prevent the possibility of a pressure injury to the peroneal and saphenous nerves [5]. However, the surgical position required may involve the upper knee needing to be flexed, with the lower leg extended. This scenario may well need the leg to be supported with adequate amounts of pillows or padding.

The head should be aligned with the spine, which may require the pillow to be adjusted and folded to achieve the correct height. Always check that the ear is not folded over or compressed. If lateral supports and posts are used either side of the pelvis, ensure that they are secure and the surgeon has checked their position. Padding must be adequate and should protect the genitalia [2]. The right lateral position has the patient lying with the right side down to the operating table, left side up; and left lateral sees the left side down and right side up (see Figure 27.4) [5].

Physiological Changes in the Lateral Position

In the anaesthetised patient, ventilation may be altered in the lateral position due to increased perfusion of the lower lung and hyperventilation of the upper lung [2].

Summary

Safe positioning of patients for surgery requires the participation of the whole team, and is a vital aspect of perioperative care because the anaesthetised patient is unable to protect themselves from injury due to poor positioning. Perioperative practitioners must consider

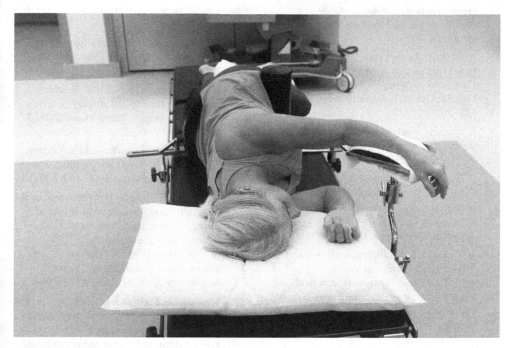

Figure 27.4 Left lateral position, with uppermost arm in Carter Braine support, and lateral posts in situ (photograph taken at Edge Hill University)

several important factors when positioning patients for surgery. These include the type and length of surgery, the patient's physical condition, ensuring physical alignment to prevent positioning injuries, and consideration of the physiological changes that occur from each position.

References

1. J. A. M. J. Van Leeuwen, F. Snorrason, and S. M. Röhrl. No radiological and clinical advantages with patient-specific positioning guides in total knee replacement. *Acta Orthopaedica* 2018; **89**: 89–94.

2. K. Woodfin, C. Johnson, R. Parker, et al. Use of a novel memory aid to educate perioperative team members on proper patient positioning technique. *AORN Journal* 2018; **107**: 325–332.

3. National Patient Safety Agency. *How to Guide. Five Steps To Safer Surgery.* London: National Patient Safety Agency, 2010.

4. Health and Care Professions Council. *Operating Department Practitioners:*

Standards of Proficiency. London: Health and Care Professions Council, 2014.

5. Association of Surgical Technologists (AST). AST standards of practice for surgical positioning. Available from: www.ast.org/uploadedfiles/Main_Site/Content/About_Us/Standard%20Surgical%20Positioning.pdf.

6. H. Bidd, R. Dulai, N. Edelman, et al. The effect of intra-operative passive movement therapy on non-surgical site pain after breast reconstruction surgery: a preliminary study. *Anaesthesia* 2014; **69**: 872–877.

7. A. Blackburn, R. Taghizadeh, D. Hughes, et al. Prevention of perioperative limb neuropathies in abdominal free flap breast

reconstruction. *Journal of Plastic, Reconstructive and Aesthetic Surgery* 2016; **69**: 48–54.

8. A. Mardell. Patient positioning for surgery. In S. Hughes, and A. Mardell (eds.), *Oxford Handbook of Perioperative Practice.* Oxford: Oxford University Press, 2011, pp. 325–333.

9. J. Warland. Back to basics: avoiding the supine position in pregnancy. *The Journal of Physiology* 2017; **595**: 1017–1018.

10. F. Souki, Y. Rodriguez-Blanco, S. Reddy Polu, et al. Survey of anaesthesiologists' practices related to steep Trendelenburg positioning in the USA. *BMC Anaesthesiology* 2018; **18**: 117.

11. K. Takechi, S. Kitamura, I. Shimizu, et al. Lower Limb Perfusion during robotic-assisted laparoscopic radical prostatectomy evaluated by near-infrared spectroscopy: an observational prospective study. *BMC Anaesthesiology* 2018; **18**: 114.

12. D. J. W. Knight, and R. P. Mahajan. Patient positioning in anaesthesia. *Continuing Education in Anaesthesia Critical Care and Pain* 2004; **4**: 160–163,

13. M. Bowers. Prone position for surgery. *Journal of Perioperative Practice* 2012; **22**: 157–162.

14. N. E. Epstein. Perioperative visual loss following prone spinal surgery: a review. *Surgical Neurology International* 2016; **7**: S347–S360.

15. H. Edgcombe, K. Carter, and S. Yarrow. Anaesthesia in the prone position. *British Journal of Anaesthesia* 2008; **100**: 165–183

16. A. Coppo, G. Bellani, D. Winterton, et al. Feasibility and physiological effects of prone positioning in non-intubated patients with acute respiratory failure due to COVID-19 (PRON-COVID): a prospective cohort study. *Lancet Respiratory Medicine* 2020; **8**: 765–774.

17. N. Stornelli, F. Wydra, J. Mitchell, et al. The dangers of lithotomy positioning in the operating room: case report of bilateral lower extremity compartment syndrome after a 90-minute surgical procedure. *Patient Safety in Surgery* 2016; **10**: 18.

Fundamentals of Perioperative Thermoregulation

28

Craig Griffiths

Introduction

The human core body temperature is around 37 °C, with a clinically acceptable range for adults of 36.5–37.5 °C being described as normothermia [1]. Temperatures can vary in accordance with the stages of the circadian cycle (daily), menstrual cycle (monthly), during pregnancy, and with ageing [2]. As a species, humans have learned to live, and undertake challenges, in extremes of temperature; for example, ultramarathon runners in the desert. To maintain a core body temperature, the body needs to ensure that heat gained equals the heat loss [3]. Surgery poses two problems: increased heat loss due to exposure to a cool theatre environment to permit surgical access; and the loss of physiological compensation due to anaesthesia. Responsibility for maintaining the patient's body temperature therefore lies with the theatre team.

Homeostasis and Body Temperature

Despite a number of physiological and environmental challenges, the body does remarkably well in maintaining a constant core temperature of around 37 °C (although 'normal' temperature differs from individual to individual). Every muscle contraction or neuron firing requires optimum conditions to take place. Hypothermia slows down these reactions, whereas a hyperthermia will cause the reactions to malfunction. These rates depend on normal enzyme functioning, and this depends on body temperature staying within a narrow range of normal. To maintain this narrow range of 'normal' the body must balance the amount of heat it produces and the amount of heat lost; a fine balance must always be maintained. There are range of physiological and behavioural responses that can be used to gain or lose heat.

To gain heat, the body responds by:

- shivering;
- using brown fat (infants);
- skin vessels constricting;
- seeking warmth;
- wearing additional clothing;
- drinking warm fluids; and
- increasing bodily activity.

In order to lose heat, the body responds by:

- skin vessels dilating;
- sweating;

- removing clothing;
- seeking shade;
- drinking cold fluids; and
- decreasing bodily activity.

Regulation of Body Temperature

Thermoregulation is an ongoing process that consists of three mechanisms – afferent sensing, central control, and efferent responses.

Afferent Sensing

Sensations of hot and cold occur in specific thermoreceptors in the nervous system. These are found in the external shell (the skin surface), the internal core (including the viscera, spine, and great veins [4]), and in the brain (preoptic area) [5]. Thermoreception describes the perception and sensation of temperature and utilises two pain fibres, two thermal fibres, and several ion channels.

Nociceptor (Pain) Fibres

The pain fibres detect extremes of heat (triggered above 45 °C) and cold (triggered below 15 °C). These reactions to 'noxious' stimuli explain why you can get the same sensation of 'burning' from extremes of cold as well as from heat. These receptors also validate testing neuraxial blocks by using an ethyl chloride cold spray on a patient [6].

There are two types of thermal fibres that detect cold and warmth up to those thresholds.

Cold Fibres

Cold fibres tend to be myelinated alpha-delta fibres and are present throughout the skin, visceral organs, and great veins where they outnumber warm fibres by two–nine times (depending on parts of the body). There is also evidence to suggest that cold is also detected from unmyelinated C fibres [7], which could account for a lingering feeling of cold that is felt after applying a cold stimulus.

Warm Fibres

Warm fibres are unmyelinated -fibres, thereby making them transmit far more slowly than their cold counterparts. Note also that warm receptors only begin firing at around 30 °C and are saturated at 45 °C where nociceptive (pain) fibres begin to trigger instead.

It is important to state that all these sensors overlap (illustrated in Figure 28.1) and that the body's ability to regulate temperature relies on sensory information across the spectrum of receptors and how the brain controls the response. The sensors are also adaptive, in that a sudden change of temperature will result in a large signal transmission, but this will dampen through continued stimulation. That is why we notice the sudden cold when we go outside or heat when we enter a hot bath, but the sensation does not continue.

Transient Receptor Potential Channels

Transient receptor potential (TRP) channels are cation channels found in cell membranes and are involved in several different areas of sensory reception with the TRPV (vanilloid) subfamily heavily involved in thermoreception [9]. As these receptors can be activated by

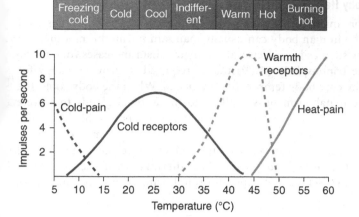

Figure 28.1 Graph showing the overlap of thermal fibre activation [8]

molecules, they are also susceptible to being 'tricked'. For instance, TRPV1 (the first known TRPV channel) is activated by temperatures over 42 °C but also by capsaicin, which is the active ingredient in chillies. This explains why certain foods and substances can cause a heating or cooling sensation.

Central Control

The control of thermoregulation involves a negative feedback loop. Signals from the efferent sensors throughout the body continuously inform the hypothalamus – in particular the preoptic area – about both the current core temperature and immediate threats to the core temperature [5]. The hypothalamus itself acts as an internal thermostat and will modulate its response to a core temperature deviating from approximately 37 °C (98.6 °F). The ways in which temperature changes can be activated are varied and involve voluntary and involuntary (mediated by the anterior or posterior hypothalamus) responses.

Efferent Responses

The response to changes in temperature mediated by the central control of the hypothalamus has several different components. As well as voluntary responses to temperature, the body also responds autonomically in order to increase or reduce temperature.

Voluntary Responses

The human body has multiple responses and reflexes that have a voluntary and involuntary component (breathing, muscle contraction, blinking, etc.), and temperature control is something that can be voluntarily controlled as well. For instance, slowing down, or having a cold drink when running on a hot day, rubbing skin to warm it up, or moving close to a heat source when cold. People can also add or remove clothing when anticipating a potential or immediate threat to their core body temperature (e.g., putting a jumper on before going outside). However, anaesthetised patients are clearly unable to utilise these voluntary responses and so their thermoregulation depends on the autonomic reactions that can increase or decrease temperature.

Maintaining or Increasing Body Heat (Thermogenesis)

Humans are endothermic organisms. This means that, unlike fish and most reptiles, they generate their own heat. The human body can usually maintain normothermia through normal metabolic processes such as by exercise, when metabolism increases (due to the extra demand of adenosine triphosphate (ATP) that is required to provide energy for muscle contractions) and the core body temperature increases. When the body cools, the hypothalamus can increase metabolism by signalling to the adrenal glands to secrete adrenaline and noradrenaline. The hypothalamus can also send signals to blood vessels, causing them to vasoconstrict to reduce heat loss from the skin. If these measures prove inadequate, then the hypothalamus can initiate the shivering response in skeletal muscles to generate heat. This occurs to prevent hypothermia when the core body temperature drops below the set core temperature following exposure to a cold environment.

Reducing Temperature

There are four ways in which the body can lose heat. The effectiveness of each depends either on the body's processes itself or the environment the body is in.

Evaporation

Evaporation is an extremely effective means of cooling the human body, primarily by sweating, and has the greatest potential for heat loss. However, this effectiveness comes at a cost as too much sweat can result in hypovolaemia and electrolyte imbalance. The evaporation of sweat also provides the only means of body cooling when the ambient temperature increases above body temperature. Heat is lost as the body heat coverts sweat to vapour, drawing heat away from the body. Sweat is secreted from both eccrine and apocrine glands that produce sweat at a certain rate depending on how much cooling is required and up to a maximum of 3-4 litres per hour.

Evaporation is also reliant on humidity. High levels of humidity in the air will decrease the effectiveness of sweating considerably, with evaporation stopping entirely at around 90% humidity. Examples of heat loss occurring through evaporation in the operating theatre include the use of alcohol-based skin preparation [10], and the exposure of body cavities and mucosal surfaces.

Radiation

Radiation is the transfer of heat to bodies or objects not in contact with the source. Typically, when people hear the term radiation they may think of the Sun or nuclear reactors but essentially it just means that anything that exists above absolute zero – 0 K (−273 °C) – radiates heat. Radiation accounts for the largest amount of heat lost by the human body (~60%) and represents the highest risk to patients with regard to hypothermia, particularly when skin is exposed for surgery or regional anaesthesia. However, at higher ambient temperatures (particularly those above the core temperature), radiation is nullified as heat begins to be gained from the environment instead.

Conduction

Conduction is the transfer of heat from objects in direct contact. This is dependent on heat transferring down the temperature gradient and becomes ineffective once both objects (e.g., the patient and the operating table) reach equilibrium. Conduction therefore has a minimal effect on heat loss because of this.

Convection

Convective heat loss is the transfer of heat from an object to moving molecules such as gas or liquid. As the gas or liquid molecules move, they take with them some of the transferred heat and are then replaced by a cooler molecule, and the process repeats until equilibrium is reached. Convection is very relevant in well-ventilated operating theatres. The effect of both turbulent and laminar flows within the operating theatre can result in a high rate of convection, particularly to exposed patients. However, as with radiation and conduction, convection is reliant on the temperature of the substance it is radiating to being lower than that of the patient. This makes these methods ineffective once equilibrium is reached or in situations of higher ambient temperatures.

Effects of Anaesthesia on Thermoregulation

Anaesthetic practices and the drugs used to achieve both general and regional anaesthesia can have a huge impact on thermoregulation. Just as drugs such as propofol have unwanted cardiovascular side effects the same can be said about thermoregulation.

General Anaesthesia

Anaesthetic drugs have the unwanted side effects of changing both the warm and cold response thresholds, effectively changing the work of the body's thermostat. This happens in several ways. Propofol and opioid analgesics [11] decrease vasoconstriction and shivering thresholds linearly. Volatile agents also have effects on these responses but in a non-linear way (affecting cold thresholds more). Therefore, there is a marked increase (from 0.3 °C to 2–4 °C) in the inter-threshold range, which is the range of core temperatures where no thermoregulatory response is triggered (see Figure 28.2). Moreover, anaesthetic agents (propofol and volatiles) also inhibit non-shivering thermogenesis and the efficacy of vasoconstriction and shivering responses, and these remain diminished until the anaesthetic agent wears off. However, the efficacy of the sweat response, albeit with a slightly increased threshold, is preserved. So patients are potentially at risk not only within the operating theatre environment (due to radiation and convection heat loss in particular) but also through the practice of general anaesthesia, which poses its own risks for the development of inadvertent intraoperative hypothermia.

Regional Anaesthesia

Given the relationship between the pain and thermal afferent sensory neurons, regional anaesthesia will impact thermoregulation. Regional blocks impair local thermoregulation such as sweating, vasoconstriction, and shivering; whereas neuraxial blockades (spinal and epidural anaesthesia), depending on siting, can disrupt a significant portion of nerve conduction (as is their intent). This disruption not only prevents the normal thermoregulation mechanisms but also the sensory signals to the brain causing the body to effectively reduce shivering thresholds by around 0.5 °C while increasing sweating threshold by 0.3 °C [12]. While this is small compared to general anaesthesia it is still a significant widening of the threshold and, in cases where both general and regional anaesthesia are used, it could potentially compound issues further.

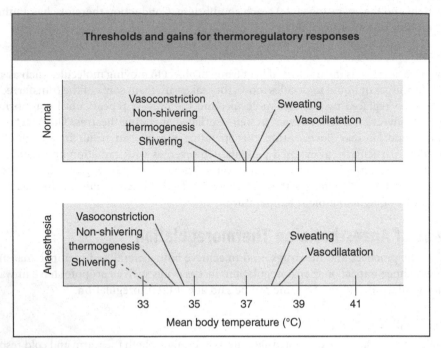

Figure 28.2 Changes to the inter-threshold range caused by anaesthesia

Inadvertent Intraoperative Hypothermia

Inadvertent intraoperative hypothermia (core temperature of below 36 °C [1]) is a common preventable surgical complication, occurring in up to 40% of patients [11]. Due to vasodilation on induction, there is a redistribution of heat from the core to the peripheries caused by the increased blood flow, and this can lead to a reduction of up to 1.5 °C within the first hour. However, this drop is less significant in patients who have been preoperatively warmed, highlighting the importance of warming patients prior to induction [13].

Inadvertent intraoperative hypothermia is associated with several complications. This includes an increased risk of a surgical site infection (due to impaired immune function), delayed wound healing, an increased risk of blood loss and need for transfusion (due to impaired platelet and clotting factor function), prolonged anaesthetic drug actions, postoperative shivering, an increased risk of postoperative cardiac events (due to the increased metabolic workload as the body attempts to warm itself by shivering), and delayed recovery. Preventing inadvertent hypothermia is vital and requires careful monitoring of the patient's temperature and employing effective warming techniques.

Malignant Hyperthermia

Malignant hyperthermia is a rare (a frequency of 1:5,000 to 1:100,000 of patients receiving general anaesthesia) and life-threatening emergency that can occur after the administration of either suxamethonium or volatile anaesthetic agents. It is the result of a mutation in the type 1 ryanodine receptor within the sarcoplasmic reticulum. Upon activation from the substances above, this faulty receptor continues to release calcium ions (Ca^{2+}). This causes a huge increase in intracellular Ca^{2+}, which in turn activates Ca^{2+} pumps to facilitate reuptake of calcium into the sarcoplasmic reticulum. This process requires energy (ATP) and therefore generates a huge metabolic drive, leading to heat production far in excess of what the body can balance through dissipation [14]. This, combined with other side effects such as hyperkalaemia and rhabdomyolysis, means that the risk of mortality is high if not promptly identified and treated. The mortality rate for malignant hyperthermia is estimated to be around 5%. Guidance for the treatment of malignant hyperthermia has been produced by the Association of Anaesthetists [15]. Initial treatment includes the following:

- Stop all trigger agents.
- Call for help (make a note of the time).
- Abandon or finish surgery as soon as possible if started.
- Administer 100% high-flow oxygen and hyperventilate.
- Remove vaporisers from the anaesthetic machine, change the breathing circuits, maintain anaesthesia with an intravenous hypnotic agent, and induce muscle relaxation with a non-depolarising muscle relaxant.
- Administer dantrolene (2.5 mg/kg immediately and repeat 1 mg/kg boluses as required) until stabilised.
- Commence active cooling – for example, reduce the theatre temperature, administer intravenous boluses of refrigerated fluids, and use ice packs.
- Continuously monitor the core and peripheral temperature, invasive blood pressure, central venous pressure, end-tidal carbon dioxide, oxygen saturation, and regular blood gases.
- Transfer the patient to a critical care unit.

Physiological Effects of Hypothermia

The effects of hypothermia can vary based on how serious the hypothermia is. A useful tool, the Swiss staging model [16], categorises hypothermia, as shown in Table 28.1.

Therapeutic hypothermia refers to the intentional cooling of a patient in order to slow their metabolism, especially of the brain. This has been used for many years in cardiac surgery for its neuroprotective properties during periods when blood flow may be interrupted [17]. However, in general, hypothermia causes disruption in all body systems with some of the major effects outlined in Table 28.2 [18].

Table 28.1 The Swiss staging model of hypothermia

Stage	Clinical findings	Typical core temperature (°C)
Stage 1	Conscious, shivering	35–32
Stage 2	Impaired consciousness, not shivering	Below 32–28
Stage 3	Unconscious, not shivering, vital signs present	Below 28–24
Stage 4	No vital signs	Below 24

Physiological Effects of Hyperthermia

Hyperthermia describes an unusually high temperature of at least 40.0 °C (104 °F) and is associated mostly with infection [19]. However, like hypothermia, hyperthermia is a spectrum. With that in mind, the Japanese Association for Acute Medicine developed a tool for the classification of hyperthermia that has shown good accuracy at predicting mortality in patients with heat-related illnesses [20]. Their classification is shown in Table 28.3, which points out potential issues caused by hyperthermia. Just as with hypothermia, it affects every organ system, as shown in Table 28.4.

Table 28.2 Effects of hypothermia on relevant physiological systems

System	Effects of hypothermia
Respiratory	Increased respiratory rate Decreased sensitivity to carbon dioxide
Cardiovascular	Bradycardia Decreased cardiac output Arrhythmias Resistance to defibrillation Vasoconstriction
Haematology and electrolytes	Increased blood viscosity Coagulopathy Acid–base changes Increase in pH
Endocrine	Decreased metabolism Decreased metabolism of carbohydrates Decreased metabolism of drugs Decreased oxygen consumption
Central nervous system	Shivering Decreased level of consciousness
Renal	'Cold' diuresis

Table 28.3 The Japanese Association for Acute Medicine heat illness classification

Stage	Clinical symptoms (simplified)	Classification
I (First aid)	Dizziness, fainting, muscle pain	Heat cramp Heat syncope
II (Admit to medical facility)	Headache, vomiting, reduced concentration	Heat exhaustion
III (Inpatient hospitalisation)	Central nervous system dysfunction Renal/hepatic dysfunction Coagulation disorder	Heat stroke

Table 28.4 Effects of hyperthermia on relevant physiological systems

System	Effects of hyperthermia
Respiratory	Increased respiratory effort Respiratory alkalosis
Cardiovascular	Tachyarrhythmias Prolonged Q-T interval Hypotension
Haematology and electrolytes	Coagulopathy Hypocalcaemia Hyperkalaemia Hypernatraemia causing brain damage
Central nervous system	Delirium and lethargy Coma Seizures
Renal	Acute renal failure Rhabdomyolysis
Gastrointestinal	Liver damage Gut ischaemia

Measurement of Body Temperature

In order to maintain normothermia for patients it is essential to know what their temperature is. Anaesthesia has a profound effect on the ability to maintain body temperature, with the core temperature potentially dropping by up to 1.5 °C in the first hour of anaesthesia. A patient's temperature should be measured before induction and then every subsequent 30 minutes until the end of surgery; continuous temperature monitoring should be used for surgery longer than 60 minutes.

Patients who are anaesthetised for longer than 30 minutes, or less than 30 minutes but at high risk for inadvertent intraoperative hypothermia, should be warmed using a forced-air warming device. A high-risk patient is one who meets two of the following criteria: American Society of Anesthesiologists Physical Status Classification grade II–V, undergoing combined regional and general anaesthesia, undergoing major or intermediate surgery, has a risk of cardiovascular complications, or arrives with a preoperative temperature below 36 °C [1].

Monitoring sites should be a direct measurement of the core temperature or accurate to within 0.5 °C and include:

- the pulmonary artery;
- the distal oesophagus;
- the deep forehead (zero heat flux);
- the tympanic membranes; and
- the nasopharynx.

Infrared tympanic membrane thermometers can be subject to variations in temperature and are not always a reliable indicator of the core body temperature [11, 21]. However, such devices are safe, easy to use, and allow a temperature measurement to be obtained quickly. If an oesophageal temperature probe is being used, optimum placement is estimated to be around T8/T9 in an adult.

Temperature Management in Theatre

When managing temperature in the operating theatre, whether heating or cooling, it is important to apply the principles of thermoregulation, summarised below.

Radiation

Often used in paediatric and neonatal patients, radiant heaters can be used to warm patients by placing them under a heater. This method is not without risks as they can overheat or burn patients if used incorrectly.

Convection

Forced-air warming blankets or mattresses use convection as a method of heating (and sometimes cooling) patients. This is the most common (and convenient) method of regulating a patient's temperature. There is a longstanding debate regarding whether forced-air warming reduces the efficacy of laminar flow ventilation and leads to increased rates of surgical site infections. However, the most recent evidence indicates that there is no clear causal relationship between the use of forced-air warmers and an increase in surgical site infections [22].

Conduction

The latest technology in thermoregulation uses conduction as a means of regulating a patient's temperature. Water-circulating mattresses and patient gowns as well as resistive heat mats are potential alternatives to convection devices as they do not disrupt air flow. However, many of these systems take time to warm up and, in the case of the water systems, carry a risk of water leakage. The National Institute for Health and Care Excellence recommends that fluids or blood products of more than 500 mL should be warmed using a fluid-warming device [1]. Warmed intravenous fluid can keep patients half a degree warmer, and reduce shivering compared with fluids administered at room temperature [23].

Summary

When looking at perioperative thermoregulation it is important to understand the mechanisms in the body that control and are affected by anaesthesia and surgery. It is also important to know the signs, symptoms, and consequences of hypo/hyperthermia in order that it is recognised and managed promptly. A fundamental principle of modern healthcare is that prevention is better than cure. The patient's temperature must be adequately monitored and managed throughout all the perioperative stages to ensure safe and effective care.

References

1. The National Institute for Health and Care Excellence. Hypothermia: prevention and management in adults having surgery clinical guideline [CG65]. Available from: www.nice.org.uk/guidance/cg65/chapter/Recommendations.

2. T. T. Chen, E. I. Maevsky, and M. L. Uchitel. Maintenance of homeostasis in the aging

hypothalamus: the central and peripheral roles of succinate. *Frontiers in Endocrinology (Lausanne)* 2015; **6**: 7.

3. E. A. Tansey and C. D. Johnson. Recent advances in thermoregulation. *Advances in Physiology Education* 2015; **39**: 139–148.

4. A. A. Romanovsky. Skin temperature: its role in thermoregulation. *Acta Physiologica* 2014; **210**: 498–507.

5. Z. D. Zhao, W. Z. Yang, and C. Gao. Hypothalamic circuit for thermoregulation. *Proceedings of the National Academy of Sciences* 2017; **114**: 2042–2047.

6. R. Ousley, C. Egan, K. Dowling, and A. M. Cyna. Assessment of block height for satisfactory spinal anaesthesia for Caesarean section. *Anaesthesia* 2012; **67**: 1356–1363.

7. M. Campero, T. K. Baumann, H. Bostock, and J. L. Ochoa. Human cutaneous C fibres activated by cooling, heating and menthol. *Journal of Physiology* 2009; **587**: 5633–5652.

8. J. E. Hall. *Guyton and Hall Textbook of Medical Physiology*, 13th ed. Philadelphia, PA: Elsevier, 2015.

9. A. Samanta, T. E. T. Hughes, and V. Y. Moiseenkova-Bell. Transient receptor potential (TRP) channels. *Subcellular Biochemistry* 2018; **87**: 141–165.

10. D. I. Sessler, A. M. Sessler, S. Hudson, et al. Heat loss during surgical skin preparation. *Anesthesiology* 1993; **78**: 1055–1064.

11. B. Bindu, A. Bindra, and G. Rath. Temperature management under general anesthesia: compulsion or option. *Journal of Anaesthesiology Clinical Pharmacology* 2017; **33**: 306–316.

12. D. I. Sessler. Temperature monitoring and perioperative thermoregulation. *Anesthesiology* 2008; **109**: 318–338.

13. J. Tanner, J. Kay, and K. Chambers. Avoiding inadvertent peri-operative hypothermia. *Nursing Times* 2016; **112**: 10–12.

14. H. Rosenberg, N. Pollock, A. Schiemann, et al. Malignant hyperthermia: a review. *Orphanet Journal of Rare Diseases* 2015; **10**: 93.

15. Association of Anaesthetists. Malignant hyperthermia crisis. Available from: https://anaesthetists.org/Home/Resources-publications/Guidelines/Malignant-hyperthermia-crisis.

16. M. Pasquier, P. N. Carron, A. Rodrigues, et al. An evaluation of the Swiss staging model for hypothermia using hospital cases and case reports from the literature. *Scandinavian Journal of Trauma, Resuscitation and Emergency Medicine* 2019; **27**: 60.

17. H. Saad and M. Aladawy. Temperature management in cardiac surgery. *Global Cardiology Science and Practice* 2013; **2013**: 44–62.

18. K. H. Polderman. Mechanisms of action, physiological effects, and complications of hypothermia. *Critical Care Medicine* 2009; **37**: S186–S202.

19. S. S. Evans, E. A. Repasky, and D. T. Fisher. Fever and the thermal regulation of immunity: the immune system feels the heat. *Nature Reviews Immunology* 2015; **15**: 335–349.

20. Y. Kondo, T. Hifumi, J. Shimazaki, et al. Comparison between the Bouchama and Japanese Association for Acute Medicine heatstroke criteria with regard to the diagnosis and prediction of mortality of heatstroke patients: a multicenter observational study. *International Journal of Environmental Research and Public Health* 2019; **16**: 3433.

21. R. Graveling, L. MacCalman, and H. Cowie. The use of infra-red (tympanic) temperature as a guide to signs of heat stress in industry. Available from: www.hse.gov.uk/research/rrpdf/rr989.pdf.

22. W. Ackermann, Q. Fan, A. J. Parekh, et al. Forced-air warming and resistive heating devices. Updated perspectives on safety and surgical site infections. *Frontiers in Surgery* 2018; **5**: 64.

23. G. Campbell, P. Alderson, A. F. Smith, and S. Warttig. Warming of intravenous and irrigation fluids for preventing inadvertent perioperative hypothermia. *Cochrane Database of Systematic Reviews* 2015; **4**: CD009891.

Fundamentals of Fluid and Electrolyte Balance during Surgery

Chris Wood and Rebecca Parker

Introduction

Optimum perioperative fluid management improves both perioperative morbidity and mortality [1]. This is achieved by a multi-professional team approach. Clinical team members should have a good understanding of intravenous fluid composition, physiological compartments, intravascular control mechanisms, and clinical assessment signs to reflect common fluid states. The goal of perioperative fluid management is to maintain a normal circulating volume and is known as euvolaemia. This chapter will cover important aspects of fluid therapy throughout the perioperative period.

Definitions

By definition, a fluid is any substance that has no fixed shape (can be made to flow or to fill a shape) and therefore includes gases and liquids, but this chapter focuses on the importance of liquids. The human body contains a range of bodily fluids that are directly involved in fluid balance (blood, intracellular fluid, extracellular fluid, urine, and lymph) and those with a specialised function (synovial, pleural, and cerebrospinal fluids).

An electrolyte refers to a solution containing charged ions, which can therefore conduct electricity. Electrolyte solutions may contain a range of ions such as sodium, chloride, potassium, and calcium. Concentrations are described in milliequivalents (mEq). A milliequivalent is the equivalent amount of a substance that will react with a certain number of hydrogen ions. The concentration of each electrolyte in a solution will be printed on the bag in both milliequivalents/litre and concentration in percentage. Thus, 0.9% sodium chloride contains 153.8 mEq/L or 0.9 g/100 mL of sodium chloride, respectively.

Fluid Movement

Total body water describes the total fluid volume within a human; this can be divided into the intra- and extracellular compartments. The extracellular compartment is made up of the intravascular and interstitial compartments, separated by a single continuous barrier (endothelial cell membrane) (Figure 29.1).

The interstitial compartment is the central volume between the intravascular and intracellular spaces, containing a large, mesh-like structure insoluble to proteins and fibres [2]. The composition is comparable to plasma but with a lower protein and cell count; however, this will vary depending on a range of factors including the location of the endothelium, the surface area, and Starling's forces applied. Starling's forces determine the degree of fluid movement across a capillary wall (Figure 29.2) [3]. Two Starlings forces are described across a capillary bed (a collection of capillaries in a tissue).

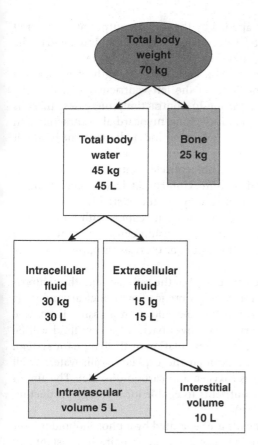

Figure 29.1 Fluid compartments (estimated for a 70-kg male): the total body water is composed of the intracellular and extracellular compartments; the extracellular division is formed from the intravascular and interstitial volumes

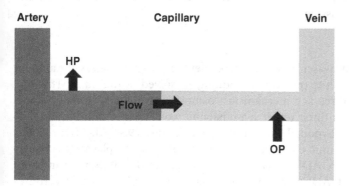

Figure 29.2 Capillary Starling forces: fluid flow is defined by oncotic pressure (OP) and hydrostatic pressure (HP); flow from an artery to a vein is via a capillary bed

First, the hydrostatic pressure is the force applied by the cardiac output at the arterial side of the capillary, which pushes fluid out of the vessel. The cardiac output is defined by the stroke volume (defined by the Frank–Starling law) multiplied by the heart rate.

The Frank–Starling relationship describes the link between the length of myocardial fibres and the force generated during contraction. As the left-ventricular end-diastolic volume (volume of blood in the left ventricle prior to contraction) increases, there is a greater crossover of myocardial filaments, thus increasing myocardial contractility. In other words, the more dilated (stretched) the ventricle is at the end of diastole, the harder it will contract during systole. Conversely, as the filling pressure decreases (for example, by hypovolaemia due to bleeding or fluid depletion), the ventricle contracts less forcefully, reducing the cardiac output and therefore blood pressure. Unfortunately, this relationship is limited, and at higher levels of filling the ventricle may be too distended to contract efficiently and the cardiac output is not enhanced. It may even reduce, with blood being pumped inadequately, resulting in heart failure. This relationship can be manipulated to ensure the circulating fluid volume (via fluid administration or diuresis) is optimal in order to optimise the cardiac output.

Secondly, oncotic pressure is highest at the venous end of the capillary and the composition of plasma proteins 'pulls' fluid back into the vessel. A range of pathological conditions can affect the hydrostatic and oncotic pressures. If the total filtration pressure is positive (meaning more fluid moves out of the capillary than moves back in) excess fluid will be found in the interstitium. Excess fluid is returned to the circulation by the lymphatic system. Three groups of substances can rapidly diffuse through the capillary wall; water, small molecules (lactic acid and creatinine), and gases (oxygen and carbon dioxide). The aim of this process is to supply local tissues with key nutrients to enable local energy production (i.e., skeletal muscle to aid muscular contraction).

The intracellular and interstitial compartments are separated by a phospholipid bilayer (thin membrane composed of two layers of lipid molecules). Fluid remains in constant flux between all three compartments (Figure 29.3). The phospholipid bilayer bordering the intracellular environment supports transmembrane proteins which regulate the intracellular composition. Hydrophobic and small uncharged polar molecules diffuse through, while large uncharged polar molecules (glucose) and charged ions (sodium, potassium, and calcium) are prevented from passing [4].

Fluid Regulation

Fluid regulation within the intravascular space is dependent on two parameters: the amount of water and the amount of solute (principally sodium) dissolved in the water. The total body water is regulated by three key mechanisms: osmosis (movement of water across a semi-permeable membrane), thirst under hypothalamic control, and antidiuretic hormone (ADH) secretion via the hypothalamic pituitary axis (Figure 29.4) [5]. ADH remains the key mechanism. Hypothalamic osmoreceptors detect increases in plasma osmolarity (and low volume), leading to ADH release from the posterior pituitary gland and a conscious awareness of thirst. ADH travels intravascularly to the kidney where it activates vasopressin receptor 2 (V2 R), increasing the permeability to water and in turn leading to an increased absorption within the collecting duct via aquaporin channels [6].

Sodium is lost through a range of mechanisms (urine, sweat, and faeces) and increased by the adrenal hormone aldosterone. Aldosterone is released under the control of the

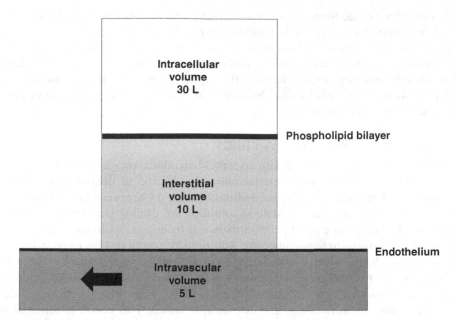

Figure 29.3 Fluid movement throughout compartments: volumes are estimates for a 70-kg male; water has free movement while sodium is transported across the endothelium

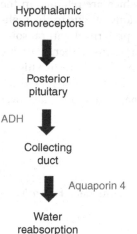

Figure 29.4 Hypothalamic pituitary axis: control of plasma osmolarity by ADH secretion; ADH acts on the collecting duct in the renal apparatus to mediate activation of aquaporin 4, which is transported to the basal membrane to enable water conservation, thus lowering the plasma osmolarity

renin–angiotensin–aldosterone system. A reduction in sodium delivery or perfusion of the renal tubule results in active secretion of renin from renal juxtaglomerular epithelioid cells [7]. Renin converts angiotensin to angiotensin one, which is subsequently converted to angiotensin two in the lungs by the angiotensin converting enzyme. Angiotensin two has a broad range of cardiovascular effects: it increases sympathetic tone, aldosterone, and

ADH. The release of aldosterone from the adrenal gland increases sodium absorption and water retention in the distal collecting tubules within the kidney.

Sodium is only one essential ion in the human body. Other key regulatory electrolytes include potassium, calcium, magnesium, and phosphate. Potassium is an intracellular ion, which is tightly regulated in order to maintain physiological function (e.g., neuromuscular activity, control of intracellular fluid balance, and acid–base regulation) and to prevent toxicity and myocardial instability.

Composition of Intravenous Fluids

Intravenous fluids can be grouped into crystalloid solutions, colloid solutions, and blood products. When resuscitation and maintenance is required in dehydration, crystalloid solutions (e.g., Hartmann's solution and sodium chloride 0.9%) remain the first-line agents, although other more balanced crystalloid solutions are gaining popularity. Hartmann's solution can be helpful to correct pH disturbance as its organic molecules include lactate, which the liver converts to bicarbonate [8]. Additionally, it contains electrolytes, including potassium and calcium, which can be helpful to provide physiological balance (Table 29.1).

It is important to note that a 5% dextrose solution should not be used in resuscitation as the glucose component is rapidly metabolised, leading to the widespread movement of water throughout the intracellular and extracellular spaces. This results in minimal fluid retention in the intravascular space (Figure 29.3). In contrast, infusion of electrolyte solutions increases the plasma osmolality and thus fluid retention within the extracellular space.

The other group of intravenous fluids are colloid solutions, which are retained in the vascular compartment for longer than simple crystalloid preparations [9] due to the high-molecular-weight molecules in the solution. Albumin is the most prescribed natural solution and gelatine solutions are the most popular synthetic preparations. Other synthetic preparations such as hydroxyethyl starch have been withdrawn from the UK due to a higher incidence of renal dysfunction [10]. Simple crystalloid solutions are frequently used for resuscitation in non-anaemic patients due to the lower risk of anaphylaxis and the lower unit cost [11].

Table 29.1 Composition of commonly used intravenous fluids

	Na$^+$ mmol/L	Cl$^-$ mmol/L	K$^+$ mmol/L	Ca^{2+} mmol/L	Additional	mOsm/L*
0.9% sodium chloride	154	154				308
Hartmann's	131	111	5	2	29 mmol/L Lactate	281
5% Glucose					50 g glucose	278

* mOsm = milliosmole, the number of moles of solute that contribute to the osmotic pressure of a solution.

Preoperative Assessment of Fluid Status

The preoperative visit should include an assessment of fluid status based upon a patient's history, clinical signs, and available investigations.

The history broadly encompasses three areas: symptoms suggestive of current fluid status, past medical history, and current medications. Symptoms suggestive of hypervolaemia or fluid overload involve both the respiratory (shortness of breath, cough, wheeze) and cardiovascular (abdominal swelling and limb oedema) systems. Conversely, symptoms suggestive of hypovolaemia include non-specific symptoms (headaches, tiredness, confusion), cardiovascular symptoms (palpitations, dizziness), and evidence of ongoing loss from the gastrointestinal (vomiting and diarrhoea) and renal tracts (polyuria). A past medical history should focus on three organs involved in fluid regulation including the heart (ventricular and valvular dysfunction), kidney (acute and chronic impairment), and, finally, liver dysfunction (acute liver decompensation or chronic cirrhotic liver disease). Current medications exert their effect on the cardiac (beta, calcium, and alpha blockers) and renal (angiotensin-converting enzyme inhibitors and diuretics) systems by exploiting normal physiological processes. Key medications should be noted and optimised.

The examination is focused on the cardiorespiratory system. Signs suggestive of hypovolaemia are non-specific and include delayed capillary refill time, cool peripheries, tachycardia, hypotension, and dry mucus membranes. Conversely, signs of hypervolaemia include warm peripheries, tachycardia, hypertension, elevated jugular venous pressure, lung crepitations, elevated respiratory rate, low oxygen saturation, third heart sound, ascites, and peripheral oedema.

Investigations involve blood tests, imaging, and functional assessments. Routine blood tests include full blood count, urea and electrolytes, and liver function tests. Radiological investigation of the thorax is broadly divided into X-rays and CT. The latter provides sensitive information about cardiorespiratory anatomy and volume status, but a simple chest X-ray may allow the identification of signs of fluid overload (pleural effusions, upper-lobe venous diversion, interstitial and alveolar oedema). Echocardiography can assess ventricular and valvular function, which may support a diagnosis of cardiac dysfunction or reflect underlying complications of lung disease.

Preoperatively, various blood products (packed red blood cells, fresh frozen plasma, cryoprecipitate, and platelets) may be prescribed to improve oxygen delivery or correct coagulopathy. The haematological function must be assessed before the infusion of blood products as administration in some at-risk groups is associated with increased morbidity and mortality [12].

Once an assessment of fluid balance has been made the patient can be optimised and this may include intravenous hydration or fluid offloading by diuretic and renal replacement therapies [13]. This allows the patient to arrive in the anaesthetic room in a euvolaemic state.

Intraoperative Care

Surgical (duration, intra-cavity, or open procedures) and patient factors (co-morbidities and underlying aetiology) will determine the anaesthetic setup requirements. High-risk cases will often require invasive monitoring (catheter, arterial line, central line, cardiac output monitoring) to enable ongoing fluid assessment.

Intraoperative fluid losses vary depending on the surgery (duration, technique, complexity, and ongoing haemorrhage), anaesthetic (anaesthetic agent used, central and peripheral sympathetic blockade, and histamine-releasing agents) and patient (activation of stress response, temperature, coagulation profile, and body surface area) factors [14, 15].

The physiological stress response is mediated by both anaesthetic (pressor response to laryngoscopy) and surgical (skin incision) factors [16]. This results in the activation of both the sympathetic nervous system and the hypothalamic–pituitary axis, increasing the plasma concentrations of key hormones (growth hormone, cortisol, prolactin, vasopressin), enabling the mobilisation of energy substrates (carbohydrates, proteins, and lipids) and fluid preservation.

Anaesthetic Agents and Cardiovascular Function

The most common intravenous (propofol and thiopentone) and volatile (sevoflurane, isoflurane, and desflurane) agents have similar effects on the cardiorespiratory system. They all precipitate hypotension by reducing systemic vascular resistance and myocardia contractility [17]. These effects can be enhanced by increasing intra-thoracic pressure during intermittent positive-pressure ventilation, which can lead to a reduction in venous return and thus impaired cardiac output. Similarly, both groups of agents reduce minute ventilation, leading to hypercapnia and apnoea. Ketamine, unlike other intravenous agents, activates the sympathetic nervous system, mediating hypertension and tachycardia, and thus is an important agent for maintaining cardiovascular stability [18].

Intraoperative Fluid Assessment

Intravascular volume assessment can be estimated broadly by three mechanisms; static parameters, dynamic parameters, and, finally, goal direct therapies [19].

Static parameters are the least sensitive predictors of volume status when used individually. Measures include blood pressure, heart rate, respiratory rate, urine output, and central venous pressure (CVP) monitoring. Multiple intraoperative factors affect physiological parameters (blood pressure and heart rate) including the degree of stress response, pharmacological blockade (beta blockers), and anaesthetic position (lithotomy, Lloyd–Davies). As a result, these are poor markers when used independently. Similarly, urine output (<0.5 mL/ kg per hour) can be used as a surrogate for hypovolaemia; however, volatile agents may independently reduce urine output. Finally, the CVP has frequently been shown to be poorly correlated to volume status.

Dynamic assessment has advanced over recent years. Cardiac output assessment can be performed by invasive, semi-invasive, and non-invasive measures. The gold standard tool remains the pulmonary artery catheter; however, due to its invasive nature and risk profile, it is infrequently used outside of the cardiothoracic setting. Semi-invasive measures include: assessment of respiratory variation (pulse pressure variation), pulse contour analysis (e.g., the Vigileo™ monitor), and stroke volume estimates (oesophageal Doppler) [20]. Finally, non-invasive assessment includes transthoracic impedance cardiography.

Goal-Directed Therapy

Historically, fluids were administered liberally during anaesthetic practice; however, it is now known that excess fluid administration can be harmful. Goal-directed therapy utilises cardiovascular volume status assessment, as gained from cardiac output monitoring, and can be used to optimise fluid administration. The therapy allows for an individualised fluid infusion strategy based on a patient's fluid responsiveness (improved cardiac function or blood pressure following a defined fluid bolus). Theoretically, goal-directed therapy sounds promising; however, improvements in long-term morbidity and mortality remain controversial [21, 22]. The therapy is associated with a reduction in the duration of hospital admission and intensive care stay [23, 24].

Intraoperative Fluid Delivery

The main determinant of fluid flow into a patient will be dictated by various cannula (width and length) and fluid (viscosity) parameters (Table 29.2). The size of cannula or other needle is classified by the wire gauge (G) system. This system was developed for the manufacturing of cables. It is denoted by the number of times the wire is passed through the draw plate. The fewer times it is passed through the draw plate, the larger the cable and hence the larger cannula size (the diameter of a 16 G cannula is larger than a 22 G). Fluid is delivered to the cannula by giving sets; a standard set contains a 15-micron filter, while larger blood-giving sets incorporate a 200-micron filter. The flow rate through the cannula can be increased by pressuring the bag or using dedicated rapid infusion devices (e.g., a Belmont* Rapid Infuser).

Fluids should be warmed to prevent hypothermia. Intraoperative hypothermia is associated with multi-system effects (Table 29.3). Those of importance significance include coagulopathy and thus an increased risk of bleeding [25], wound infection, cardiovascular events, postoperative pain, reduced drug metabolism and increased length of hospital stay [26–28]. A broad range of warming devices are commercially available on the market. Methods can be categorised into three groups; warm the bag of fluid, warm the giving set (3M Ranger™) and finally; independent warming units can be used (Level 1* H-1200 Fast Flow Fluid Warmer).

Following on from Fluids

Additional interventions can be provided in patients who remain hypotensive despite an adequate circulating volume. Treatments are aimed at improving one of three cardiac measures; enhance cardiac rate (chronotrope), contractility (inotrope), or peripheral

Table 29.2 Various intravenous cannula sizes identified by colour

Cannula gauge	Colour	Maximum flow rates (mL/min)
14 G	Orange	240
16 G	Grey	180
18 G	Green	90
20 G	Pink	60
22 G	Blue	35

Maximum flow rates determined under standardised conditions (distilled water preheated to 22 °C, connected to a cannula by a standard 110-cm tubing with a 4-mm internal diameter. Pressurised by 10 kPa to aid flow).

Table 29.3 Complications of intraoperative hypothermia based on bodily system

System	Effect
Respiratory	Decreased respiratory rate
Cardiovascular	Arrhythmias
	Increased heart rate, contractility and cardiac output
Metabolic	Metabolic acidosis
	Decreased basal metabolic rate by 7% per °C if not shivering
	Hyperglycaemia
	Decreased drug metabolism
Hematological	Decreased coagulation and platelet activation
	Increased blood viscosity
	Left shift of oxyhaemoglobin dissociation curve
Neurological	Decreased cerebral blood flow, cerebral metabolic rate for oxygen
Renal	Decreased glomerular filtration rate
	Increased sodium, water, and glucose reabsorption
Gastrointestinal	Ileus

vascular resistance (PVR) [29]. A decision to start a specific agent should depend on the underlying aetiology of ongoing hypotension. Hypotension precipitated by septic shock is related to a reduction in the PVR, hence; agents which enhance the PVR, such as noradrenaline, are essential. Conversely, cardiac decompensation secondary to heart failure require an inotropic agent (such as adrenaline or dobutamine) to enhance the function [30].

Postoperative Fluid Management

On arrival to recovery, the patient should be euvolaemic, with appropriate haemoglobin targets reflecting their co-morbidities. The following should be assessed: intraoperative fluid losses, ongoing losses (via body cavities and drainage bags), and sensible and insensible fluid losses; finally, there should be a clinical assessment of ongoing cardiovascular variables. Urine output is a marker of volume status. Similarly to the intraoperative period, an elevated concentration of vasopressin resulting from the stress response may result in postoperative oliguria. Oliguria is defined as a low urinary output (<30 mL/h) and can be the first indication of an acute kidney injury. Postoperative oliguria is not always linked to acute kidney injury in the absence of other clinical signs which suggest euvolaemia [31]. Depending on the nature of the procedure, the patient may require ongoing intravenous infusions or, often for day case procedures, oral intake may be more appropriate.

Benefits of Enhanced Fluid Management

Postoperative euvolaemia states are associated with a range of benefits including improved wound healing, cardiopulmonary function, gastrointestinal motility, and reduced third-space fluid loss (defined by fluid losses into spaces that are not visible, for example the bowel lumen in bowel obstruction) [32–34]. Excess fluid accumulation leads to widespread organ

Table 29.4 Indications for burns referral to tertiary centre

Category	Indication
Burn characteristics	≥3% Total body surface area (adults) Circumferential Full thickness Specific locations: hands/face/genitals/face
Burn class	Electrical Chemical Inhalational
Associated conditions	Pregnancy Immunosuppression
Paediatric	Non-accidental injury ≥2% Total body surface area

dysfunction, particularly affecting the cardiorespiratory and gastrointestinal systems. Bowel oedema impairs absorption and function, increasing the risk of bacterial translocation [35]. Pulmonary oedema causes ventilation–perfusion mismatch (the ability of the lung alveoli to match oxygen delivery with blood flow), increasing the arterial–alveolar oxygen gradient [36]. This gradient, measures the difference between the oxygen partial pressure in the lung alveoli and arterial blood. Diseases of the lung which reduce oxygen diffusion (emphysema) lead to lower arterial oxygen partial pressures.

Special Circumstances

There are a range of conditions associated with increased fluid loss. Burns to the skin is one example. They can be caused by a range of different energy sources (electrical, thermal, chemical, and radiation). Patients with severe burns are at risk of significant fluid loss with the peak effect occurring at 8 hours for up to 24 hours. Systemic inflammatory response syndrome leads to widespread release of vasoactive mediators (histamine and cytokines), enhancing capillary permeability, resulting in third spacing and fluid loss [37]. Without aggressive fluid replacement, large burns may lead to hypovolaemic shock. Therapeutic goals include the following: patient assessment to estimate the degree and percentage burns, implementation of fluid resuscitation by the Parkland formula (4 mL × total body surface area (%) × body weight (kg)), with 50% given within the first 8 hours from the time of injury and the following 50% over 16 hours [38]. Finally, pain should be managed and dead tissue removed to manage the infection risk. Criteria have been set to enable early referral to specialised burns centres to improve patient outcome (see Table 29.4) [39].

References

1. J. M. Silva Jr, A. M. R. R. de Oliveira, F. A. M. Nogueira, et al. The effect of excess fluid balance on the mortality rate of surgical patients: a multicenter prospective study. *Critical Care* 2013; **17**: R288.

2. K. Aukland and R. K. Reed. Interstitial-lymphatic mechanisms in the control of extracellular fluid volume. *Physiological Reviews* 1993; **73**: 1–78.

3. A. Haggerty and M. Nirmalan. Capillary dynamics, interstitial fluid and the lymphatic system. *Anaesthesia and Intensive Care Medicine* 2019; **20**: 182–189.

4. N. J. Yang and M. J. Hinner. Getting across the cell membrane: an overview for small molecules, peptides, and proteins. In A. Gautier and M. J. Hinnerda (eds.), *Site-Specific Protein Labeling: Methods and Protocols.* New York: Springer, 2015, pp. 29–53.

5. M. Lozić, O. Šarenac, D. Murphy, and N. Japundžić-Žigon. Vasopressin, central autonomic control and blood pressure regulation. *Current Hypertension Reports* 2018; **20**: 11.

6. M. Boone and P. M. T. Deen. Physiology and pathophysiology of the vasopressin-regulated renal water reabsorption. *Pflügers Archiv European Journal of Physiology* 2008; **456**: 1005–1024.

7. T. Yang and C. Xu. Physiology and pathophysiology of the intrarenal renin-angiotensin system: an update. *Journal of the American Society of Nephrology* 2017; **28**: 1040–1049.

8. M. Varrier and M. Ostermann. Fluid composition and clinical effects. *Critical Care Clinics* 2015; **31**: 823–837.

9. S. Mitra and P. Khandelwal. Are all colloids the same? How to select the right colloid? *Indian Journal of Anaesthesia* 2009; **53**: 592–607.

10. C. Boer, S. M. Bossers, and N. J. Koning. Choice of fluid type: physiological concepts and perioperative indications. *British Journal of Anaesthesia* 2018; **120**: 384–396.

11. S. R. Lewis, M. W. Pritchard, D. J. Evans, et al. Colloids versus crystalloids for fluid resuscitation in critically ill people. *Cochrane Database of Systematic Reviews* 2018; **8**: CD000567.

12. M. Elmi, A. Mahar, D. Kagedan, et al. The impact of blood transfusion on perioperative outcomes following gastric cancer resection: an analysis of the American College of Surgeons National Surgical Quality Improvement Program database. *Canadian Journal of Surgery* 2016; **59**: 322–329.

13. S. Finfer, J. Myburgh, and R. Bellomo. Intravenous fluid therapy in critically ill adults. *Nature Reviews Nephrology* 2018; **14**: 541–557.

14. M. Jacob, D. Chappell, and M. Rehm. The 'third space': fact or fiction? *Best Practice and Research: Clinical Anaesthesiology* 2009; **23**: 145–157.

15. L. O. Lamke, G. E. Nilsson, and H. L. Reithner. Water loss by evaporation from the abdominal cavity during surgery. *Survey of Anesthesiology* 1979; **23**: 222.

16. G. Russell and S. Lightman. The human stress response. *Nature Reviews Endocrinology* 2019; **15**: 525–534.

17. K. S. Khan, I. Hayes, and D. J. Buggy. Pharmacology of anaesthetic agents I: intravenous anaesthetic agents. *Continuing Education in Anaesthesia, Critical Care and Pain* 2014; **14**: 100–105.

18. P. Y. Tsui and M. C. Chu. Ketamine: an old drug revitalized in pain medicine. *BJA Education* 2017; **17**: 84–87.

19. A. A. Al-Ghamdi. Intraoperative fluid management: past and future, where is the evidence? *Saudi Journal of Anaesthesia* 2018; **12**: 311–317.

20. D. C. Mackenzie and V. E. Noble. Assessing volume status and fluid responsiveness in the emergency department. *Clinical and Experimental Emergency Medicine* 2014; **1**: 67–77.

21. N. Herzog, J-B. Dablin, C. Giacardi, et al. Goal-directed therapy in the perioperative management: is a complete hemodynamics bundle of care better? *Critical Care* 2021; **25**: 105.

22. A. Messina, C. Robba, L. Calabrò, et al. Association between perioperative fluid administration and postoperative outcomes: a 20-year systematic review and a meta-analysis of randomized goal-directed trials in major visceral/noncardiac surgery. *Critical Care* 2021; **25**: 43.

23. J. Jin, S. Min, D. Liu, et al. Clinical and economic impact of goal-directed fluid therapy during elective gastrointestinal surgery. *Perioperative Medicine* 2018; **7**: 1–8.

24. K. E. Rollins and D. N. Lobo. Intraoperative goal-directed fluid therapy in elective major abdominal surgery. *Annals of Surgery* 2016; **263**: 465–76.

25. S. Rajagopalan, E. Mascha, J. Na, et al. The effects of mild perioperative hypothermia on blood loss and transfusion requirement. *Anesthesiology* 2008; **108**: 71–77.

26. A. Kurz, D. I. Sessler, and R. Lenhardt. Perioperative normothermia to reduce the incidence of surgical-wound infection and shorten hospitalization. *New England Journal of Medicine* 1996; **334**: 1209–1215.

27. R. Lenhardt, E. Marker, V. Goll, et al. Mild intraoperative hypothermia prolongs postanesthetic recovery. *Anesthesiology* 1997; **87**: 1318–1323.

28. S. M. Frank, L. E. Fleisher, M. J. Breslow, et al. Perioperative maintenance of normothermia reduces the incidence of morbid cardiac events: a randomized clinical trial. *American Journal of Rhinology* 1997; **277**: 1127–1134.

29. A. Belletti, M. L. Castro, S. Silvetti, et al. The effect of inotropes and vasopressors on mortality: a meta-analysis of randomized clinical trials. *British Journal of Anaesthesia* 2015; **115**: 656–675.

30. J. T. DesJardin and J. R. Teerlink. Inotropic therapies in heart failure and cardiogenic shock: an educational review. *European Heart Journal: Acute Cardiovascular Care* 2021; **10**: 676–686.

31. R. H. Thiele, K. Raghunathan, C. S. Brudney, et al. American Society for Enhanced Recovery (ASER) and Perioperative Quality Initiative (POQI) joint consensus statement on perioperative fluid management within an enhanced recovery pathway for colorectal surgery. *Perioperative Medicine* 2016; **5**: 24.

32. K. Jonsson, J. A. Jensen, W. H. Goodson 3rd, et al. Tissue oxygenation, anemia, and perfusion in relation to wound healing in surgical patients. *Annals of Surgery* 1991; **214**: 605–613.

33. R. H. Thiele, K. M. Rea, F. E. Turrentine, et al. Standardization of care: impact of an enhanced recovery protocol on length of stay, complications, and direct costs after colorectal surgery. *Journal of the American College of Surgeons* 2015; **220**: 430–443.

34. D. N. Lobo, K. A. Bostock, K. R. Neal, et al. Effect of salt and water balance on recovery of gastrointestinal function after elective colonic resection: a randomised controlled trial. *Lancet* 2002; **359**: 1812–1818.

35. A. Reintam Blaser, J-C. Preiser, S. Fruhwald, et al. Gastrointestinal dysfunction in the critically ill: a systematic scoping review and research agenda proposed by the Section of Metabolism, Endocrinology and Nutrition of the European Society of Intensive Care Medicine. *Critical Care* 2020; **24**: 224.

36. M. Sarkar, N. Niranjan, P. K. Banyal. Mechanisms of hypoxemia. *Lung India* 2017; **34**: 47–60.

37. J. A. Farina, M. J. Rosique, and R. G. Rosique. Curbing inflammation in burn patients. *International Journal of Inflammation* 2013; **2013**: 715645.

38. P. Guilabert, G. Usúa, N. Martín, et al. Fluid resuscitation management in patients with burns: update. *British Journal of Anaesthesia* 2016; **117**: 284–296.

39. National Network for Burn Care. National Burn Care Referral Guidance Available from: www.britishburnassociation.org/wp-content/uploads/2018/02/National-Burn-Care-Referral-Guidance-2012.pdf.

Chapter 30

The Physiology of Blood and Its Administration

Suzanne Arulogun and Paul Wheeler

Introduction

An understanding of the physiological role of blood and its role in the supply of oxygen to tissues is important for the perioperative care of the patient. A thorough approach to administration of blood components is vital in this setting. This chapter addresses the special properties of the red blood cells in promoting oxygen carriage, the methods of safe blood component transfusion, and consideration of hazards of transfusion.

The Physiology of Blood

The vascular system and the blood which flows within it can be regarded as the communication and nutrient highway of the body. Blood consists of a fluid phase (plasma) and cells of the haematopoietic system. Plasma contains numerous elements, chemical messengers and protective proteins, including coagulation factors. The cellular part of the blood consists of red blood cells (discussed in more detail below), platelets, which are essential for normal haemostasis, and white blood cells, which are the travelling immune system responsible for host defence.

Red Blood Cells

Red blood cells have a normal lifespan of 120 days and are densely packed with haemoglobin. The red cell shape (forming a biconcave disc) and its lack of a nucleus allow the red cell to be deformable, giving it the ability to squeeze through the microcirculation where the vessels are less than half the red cell diameter.

One of the key functions of blood is the transport of oxygen (mainly by the haemoglobin in the red cells) to the tissues and removal of carbon dioxide from them. Red blood cells are produced in the bone marrow, originating from pluripotent stem cells, and are released in a carefully controlled manner so that the production of new red cells (about 2×10^{11} per day) balances the rate of destruction. The rate of production can be increased considerably (up to about eight times the normal rate); this occurs when demand is increased because of anoxia, haemorrhage, haemolysis, or at increased altitudes. Red cell production is controlled by many factors such as the supply of essential constituents and cofactors (including iron, vitamin B_{12}, and folate), specific hormones and cytokines (in particular, erythropoietin), and others such as growth hormone, thyroxine, corticosteroids, and androgens. Erythropoietin is produced mainly in the kidneys, with some produced in the liver, and it enhances red cell production in response to tissue anoxia.

The Physiology of Haemoglobin and Oxygen Affinity

Red cells are densely packed with haemoglobin, a unique chemical that binds oxygen and facilitates the delivery of oxygen to tissues as red cells circulate through the body. Haemoglobin is a tetramer, with each haemoglobin molecule comprising four polypeptide globin subunits, two alpha and two beta polypeptide chains. At the centre of each globin chain resides a haem group, which contains an iron atom; the oxygen molecule reversibly binds to this iron atom. Each haemoglobin molecule therefore contains four haem groups. These are not all oxygenated or deoxygenated together, but rather the oxygenation of one will affect the rate of oxygenation of the others. When one haem is oxygenated, the attraction for oxygen of the other three haems on the molecule is increased.

There are many factors that influence the affinity of haemoglobin for oxygen. A higher oxygen affinity state means it is more difficult for haemoglobin to unload oxygen to the tissues, and therefore oxygen delivery to tissues is impaired; this can be caused by reduced concentrations of 2,3-disphosphoglycerate (as is the case with transfusion of stored blood and severe septicaemia or acidosis). In tissues where there is greater need for oxygen binding to haemoglobin (e.g., within the lungs), the lower pH, lower carbon dioxide, and higher partial pressure of oxygen within those tissues increase oxygen affinity, thereby maximising the saturation of haemoglobin with oxygen. Conversely, a lower oxygen affinity state means that there is increased oxygen delivery to the tissues. Factors that cause lower oxygen affinity (such as anaemia, increased body temperature, and increased carbon dioxide) occur particularly in tissues where there are high rates of metabolism; for example, in muscles during exercise. This means that, when the need of oxygen is increased, the haemoglobin is more likely to unload more of the oxygen it is carrying.

White Blood Cells

White blood cells, or leucocytes, account for less than 1% of the total blood volume and are a vital part of the body's defence against infection. Types of white blood cells include neutrophils, lymphocytes (including B and T lymphocytes), monocytes, eosinophils, and basophils. In a donor unit of blood, the number of neutrophils is inadequate to contribute to the defence system when transfused into a recipient. The presence of white blood cells in donor blood may be deleterious under some circumstances. They may be immunogenic to the recipient (i.e., provoking an antibody reaction), especially in individuals who are repeatedly transfused; these antibodies can increase the likelihood of both febrile transfusion reactions (see below) and sensitisation to other red cell antigens. Furthermore, donor lymphocytes may be viable in a recipient for a prolonged period and, if the recipient is immunosuppressed, may attack the recipient (or host); this can give rise to transfusion-associated graft-versus-host disease (TA-GVHD), a rare but almost invariably fatal complication of transfusion. Because of these considerations, all blood components undergo a filtration process after collection to remove the white cells (i.e., leukoreduction or leukodepletion). Blood components can also be irradiated to inactivate any white cells that remain after this filtration process, prior to being administered to at-risk or immunosuppressed recipients (e.g., bone marrow transplant patients, premature infants, and patients receiving certain types of chemotherapy).

Blood Transfusion

Blood transfusion is the infusion of a blood component or blood product from one person (the donor) into another person (the recipient). Blood components are therapeutic constituents of blood (red cells, platelets, fresh frozen plasma (FFP), cryoprecipitate or granulocytes), whereas blood products are derived from the whole blood or plasma (e.g., albumin and anti-D immunoglobulin). While transfusion is usually safe and effective, a high standard of practice is required at each step, from selection of donors, processing, selection, and matching of products through to infusion into the correctly identified recipient to avoid dangerous errors. Careful documentation is required at every stage to provide a complete audit trail from donor to recipient.

History of Blood Transfusion

Although there are accounts of transfusion of blood from animals into humans as early as 1667, the first successful transfusion of blood from one person to another is attributed to James Blundell in 1818. He subsequently performed at least 10 transfusions, about half of which were successful. Landsteiner identified ABO antibodies in 1900, leading to the important identification of the ABO blood group system. This was not fully exploited until 1907 when Ottenberg was the first to use compatibility testing, that is, crossmatching, a process involving the addition of recipient plasma to donor red cells to check for clumping or destruction of red cells (this is the sign of an antibody–antigen reaction that indicates incompatibility). Anticoagulation of blood was essential and, in 1914–15, citrate was introduced, which permitted the use of stored blood during the First World War. In subsequent years, the anticoagulant solution was refined and reduced in volume and other constituents were added to enhance the quality and the storage life of blood. The advent of plastic bags and tubing from 1949 enabled blood to be separated into components – a major advance in the 1950s.

Blood Groups and Blood Group Antibodies

The surface of the red blood cell is covered by many chemicals that are genetically distinct and antigenic, which means that, if they are transfused into an individual who has not been previously exposed to them, antibodies may develop. More than 300 such antigens have been described but fortunately only a small number have the potential to cause clinically significant antibody formation and antibody–antigen reactions. There are about 16 major groups of antigens, the most important of which are the ABO and Rh (formerly termed Rhesus) groups; all blood donations are typed for these. A number of other antigens can also give rise to problems because of the development of antibodies. Antibodies to blood group antigens may be 'naturally occurring' (as with the ABO system) or stimulated by exposure to the antigen (e.g., Rh antibodies).

Naturally Occurring Antibodies

The importance of the ABO system lies in the presence of naturally occurring antibodies. Individuals of one group will develop antibodies to the antigens not present (see Table 30.1).

These antibodies are either not present or only present in low titres at birth, but soon increase. When an individual is transfused with blood of an ABO group against which they possess naturally occurring antibodies (e.g., group A blood given to a group

Table 30.1 ABO blood groups, corresponding antibodies, and UK frequency (as of December 2018)

Blood group	Red cell antigen	Naturally occurring antibodies	Frequency in UK (%)
O	None	Anti-A and Anti-B	48%
A	A	Anti-B	38%
B	B	Anti-A	10%
AB	A and B	None	3%

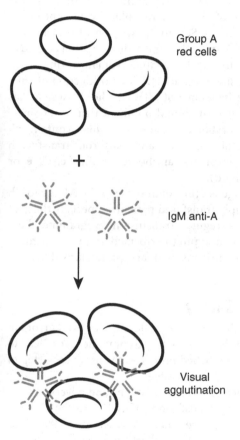

Group A red cells

IgM anti-A

Visual agglutination

Figure 30.1 Reaction of anti-A with a group A-positive red cell: in ABO blood grouping, immunoglobulin M (IgM) antibodies (for example, anti-A) will directly agglutinate red cells carrying the appropriate antigen (reprinted from A. Davey and C. S. Ince (eds.), *Fundamentals of Operating Department Practice*. Cambridge: Cambridge University Press, 2000, p. 232)

O individual) the recipient's antibodies react with the donor red cells, causing rapid destruction of the transfused cells (see Figure 30.1). This results in a transfusion reaction that may be associated with severe consequences such as renal failure and, at worst, death (10%). Because of these antibodies, ABO compatibility is essential for safe blood transfusion.

Immune Antibodies

These antibodies develop after an immune challenge, such as a blood transfusion or pregnancy (via the transfer of fetal red cells across the placenta). The most important antibodies develop in the Rh system; 'D' is the most important antigen in the Rh system, and about 15% of the population are negative for Rh(D). Approximately 50% of D-negative individuals transfused with D-positive blood will develop anti-D antibodies, meaning the D antigen is highly immunogenic (i.e., able to provoke an immune response). The development of anti-D antibodies becomes problematic if the individual is subsequently transfused with D-positive red cells, or if another pregnancy occurs with a D-positive fetus; in the latter situation, maternal anti-D antibodies can cross the placenta causing agglutination and haemolysis of the fetal red blood cells, known as haemolytic disease of the fetus and newborn (HDFN). Sensitisation against the D antigen can be prevented by avoiding transfusion of D-negative individuals with D-positive blood, and by giving anti-D immunoglobulin to any D-negative woman during pregnancy and immediately after the birth of a D-positive infant [1]. The introduction of anti-D prophylaxis in 1969 has greatly reduced the incidence of HDFN. The Rh system has five antigens: c, C, e, and E, as well as D. As such, it should be noted that 'emergency' group O, D-negative blood is not safe for everybody – these units may contain Rh antigens that the recipient may harbour antibodies against – and dangerous transfusion reactions may still occur (e.g., mediated by recipients' antibodies against c, C, e or E antigens that may be present in the donor blood).

Antibodies can develop to other red cell antigens other than those of the ABO and Rh systems and are most commonly found in multiply transfused patients, especially those of different racial origin. Before embarking on a regular transfusion programme these patients should have more extensive red cell phenotyping performed so that transfused blood can be matched against other red cell antigens that are particularly likely to provoke antibodies.

Blood Transfusion Procedures and Safety

When correctly practised, blood transfusion in the UK is very safe [2]. However, errors in requesting, blood sampling, collection, and administration of blood components can lead to significant risks for patients. As such, there are established processes to ensure each step of the entire transfusion process is undertaken as safely as possible.

Haemovigilance is the 'systematic surveillance of adverse reactions and adverse events related to transfusion', with the aim of improving transfusion safety [3]. In the UK, the Serious Hazards of Transfusion (SHOT) haemovigilance scheme was set up in 1996. This independent, professionally led, voluntary reporting system collects anonymised information on adverse events and reactions in transfusion. When a major adverse event has been identified, the hospital blood bank or haematology medical staff complete an online SHOT reporting form. The adverse events will be analysed and collated with the intention of making recommendations to further improve transfusion safety.

Selection of 'Safe' Blood Donors and Screening

Blood donors are healthy people between the ages of 17 and 66 years (or 70 if they have donated before) who can donate approximately 450 mL up to once every 12 weeks (for male donors) and 16 weeks (for female donors). Donors are asked not to donate if they are unwell or are in certain high-risk groups with the potential of transmitting infection, for example, those with a prior history of intravenous drug use, sex workers, HIV positive individuals, and carriers of hepatitis B or C [4].

Donated blood is also tested for potentially transmissible and serious infections. Each donor at every donation is currently tested for evidence of infection with HIV, hepatitis B, C, and E, and syphilis. Additional tests may include human T-lymphotropic virus (with a donor's first donation and in selected subsequent donations), malaria antibodies, and cytomegalovirus (CMV) antibodies.

Processing and Storage of Blood at the Blood Centre and Hospital

Currently, blood is collected into sterile plastic bags with satellite packs attached. Each bag contains an anticoagulant solution composed of citrate, phosphate, dextrose, and adenine. After centrifugation, depending upon the satellite system and requirements, a unit of whole blood is usually separated into component parts (e.g., plasma-reduced blood, plasma, and platelet concentrate). Collected blood must be stored under carefully controlled conditions in a special blood bank refrigerator (with an alarm and temperature chart recorder) to keep the temperature at 4 °C (±2 °C). Under these conditions, the storage life will be 35 days and bacterial growth is minimised. Units of blood must never be stored in a domestic refrigerator on the wards – the temperature in these is not adequately controlled and can vary between +8 °C and +10 °C at the front to freezing at the rear. Blood that is too warm is a culture medium, promoting bacterial growth, and freezing leads to lysis of the red cells, with disastrous consequences for the recipient.

Correct Procedures for Blood Transfusion

Transfusion in the UK is generally safe. According to the SHOT data for the last 5 years, the risk of death from transfusion is 0.87 per 100,000 components issued [3]. Delays in transfusion and pulmonary complications (mainly transfusion-associated circulatory overload) were the main causes of reported transfusion-related deaths in 2019. Nowadays, ABO incompatibility is a rare, but very important, cause of transfusion-related death; about 1 in 10 ABO-incompatible transfusions is fatal. These occur from two main mistakes of identification: the blood samples taken from the potential recipient are wrongly labelled (usually because more than one patient has been bled at a time); and the unit of blood is transfused into the wrong patient. The second error most often occurs in the operating theatre when the patient is unconscious and unable to identify themselves. Mistakes of identification are very rarely made within hospital transfusion laboratories. Overall, errors continue to account for majority of reports to SHOT; in 2019, 84.1% of all reports were due to errors [3].

A flowchart summary of the key action points in the process of blood component administration is shown in Figure 30.2 [5]. Attention to detail in the practice of blood component transfusion is essential, with the following two points being particularly important:

1. When taking samples from a patient for transfusion, the patient must be correctly identified, and the procedure carried out as a single uninterrupted operation. The individual collecting the blood sample must label the tube with the patient's name, date

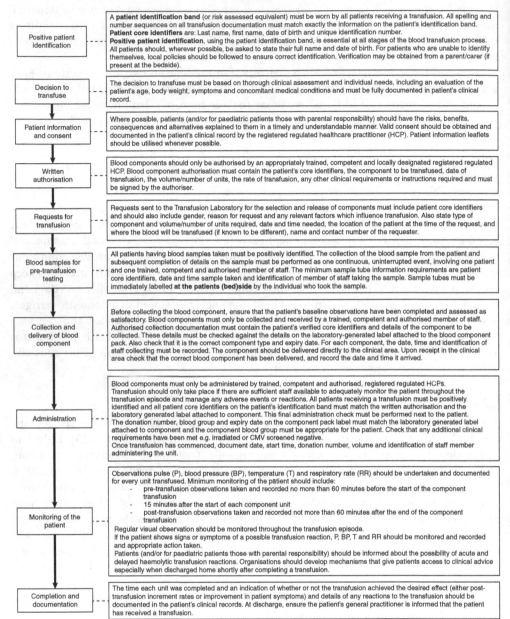

Figure 30.2 Summary of key procedures in the safe administration of blood components (used with permission from John Wiley & Sons)

of birth, and unique identification number (hospital number), as well as the date/time the blood sample was taken, and their own identification. Never prelabel the tubes and never let another person label the tubes for you. The details on the request form must match those on the sample. If the details are incomplete or do not match, the hospital transfusion laboratory will not process your request. Other clearly defined arrangements (i.e., some method of unique numbering of samples) should exist for unidentifiable casualties and major incidents.

2. When a blood component is to be transfused, the final administration check must always be conducted next to the patient by the trained healthcare professional who is going to administer the component. National guidelines no longer require double independent checking.

A patient who has never been transfused before at a particular centre/hospital requires two independent/separate blood samples collected – the second is used for a group check – before blood components can be issued. A prior group check, electronically recorded in the hospital's laboratory information system, can be used for patients who have previously had a group and screen performed at that centre.

In addition to the above, it is important that formal records are kept, including the volume of product infused, the duration of the infusion, and the unique donation number of every blood component transfused. The latter is vital if a problem is subsequently identified with a donor (e.g., seroconversion to HIV or hepatitis), which necessitates tracking of patients to whom their components have been given. Blood should not be removed from the blood bank until it is about to be transfused and it should not be out of the controlled temperature for more than 30 minutes before being set up. The maximum time from removal of blood from the controlled environment to completion of transfusion being 4 hours. These limits are set by the transfusion service to reduce the risks of infection. Every hospital should have a written procedure for blood transfusion and an ongoing training programme for all staff involved, to reduce the risks of error.

Valid informed consent for blood transfusion must be obtained and documented appropriately in the patient's clinical record by the healthcare practitioner. Patients who have received a blood transfusion and who were not able to give valid consent prior to transfusion should be retrospectively provided with information about transfusion and risks.

The 'Crossmatch'

The compatibility test (or 'crossmatch') tests the donor red cells against the serum of the recipient. A hospital transfusion laboratory first screens a potential recipient's serum for red cell antibodies when a sample is sent for a 'group and antibody screen'. If no irregular antibodies are detected by this screening, the crossmatch is very unlikely to be incompatible; in this circumstance, the crossmatch can be electronically performed (i.e., the blood component is electronically matched to the patient, based on electronically recorded group/antigen details about the patient), and blood components electronically issued without performing a routine crossmatch. In an emergency, it is usually safe to issue group-compatible units (i.e., of the same ABO and Rh group) if the recipient has a negative antibody screen.

Crossmatched blood may be pre-ordered for elective surgery, in case of intraoperative blood loss, but often this is not required. Unused blood may be returned to stock and re-crossmatched for another patient, to reduce wastage. In addition, it is evident that there are considerable variations in practice between teams performing the same surgical procedures (for example, the number of orthopaedic patients transfused after total hip replacement varies from 60% to 93% in different series). In many hospitals, recommended maximum blood-ordering schedules have been set in place, after discussion with anaesthetists and surgeons (often via a hospital blood transfusion committee) to rationalize crossmatching policies. These are not rigid but are designed to improve efficiency and to reduce unnecessary crossmatching and wastage.

Blood Components for Transfusion

Red Cell Components

Red blood cells are transfused to restore the oxygen carrying capacity in individuals with symptomatic anaemia and blood loss where alternative treatment is ineffective or inappropriate. A transfusion of red cells is generally considered when a person's haemoglobin falls to 70 g/L or less. Units of red cells are leucodepleted and plasma reduced. Each unit of red cells is obtained from a standard donation of 470 mL (range of 427.5–522.5 mL) of blood from a single donor, added into 66.5 mL of citrate phosphate dextrose anticoagulant. During processing, the majority of plasma is removed and replaced by additive solution comprising saline, adenine, glucose, and mannitol (SAG-M). A standard red cell component in additive solution contains red cells (haematocrit 0.50–0.70 and haemoglobin content > 40 g/unit), 5–30 mL of plasma, and 100 mL of SAG-M solution in a total volume of 220–340 mL. Red cells in additive solution can also be collected by apheresis. Standard red cells contain no functional platelets, granulocytes, or coagulation factors [6]. Red cells can be stored at 2–6 °C for up to 35 days from donation.

Fresh Frozen Plasma

Standard UK donor-derived FFP is separated within 6 hours of collection from whole units of donated blood by centrifugation, and frozen soon after collection to maintain the activity of blood-clotting factors. This product is only indicated for the replacement of coagulation factors in bleeding patients; the use of FFP for prophylaxis in patients who have abnormal coagulation tests but without documented bleeding (including patients with liver disease) is not supported by evidence [7]. Units of FFP contain 200–300 mL of plasma, and have a shelf life of up to 3 years if stored below −25 °C. The starting dose is 10–15 mL/kg and it must be group compatible (i.e., it must not contain antibodies that could lyse the recipient's red cells).

Solvent detergent (SD)-treated FFP (Octaplas®) is widely available in the UK and is prepared from pooling donations that are sourced and imported from overseas. The SD process inactivates bacteria and most encapsulated viruses, including hepatitis B and C and HIV. Units of SD-FFP contain a standardised volume of 200 mL of plasma and can be stored below −18 °C for up to 4 years. All types of FFP must be thawed in the transfusion laboratory before use and administered within 24 hours of thawing.

Cryoprecipitate

Cryoprecipitate is made by thawing UK donor FFP at 4 °C and collecting the precipitate that forms at this temperature. The collected product is then stored frozen at below −25 °C with a shelf life of 36 months. A unit of cryoprecipitate comprises pooled products from five donations (approximately 200–300 mL in total volume). It is rich in factor VIII, von Willebrand factor, and fibrinogen. In the 1960s and 1970s, this product was the mainstay of treatment for haemophilia A and von Willebrand's disease. Nowadays, heat-treated, plasma-derived, or genetically engineered factor concentrates are the treatment of choice for these inherited bleeding disorders. Cryoprecipitate has limited use: it is indicated in the treatment of disseminated intravascular coagulation (DIC) and for the management of conditions where there is low fibrinogen. It may also be of benefit in the microvascular bleeding syndrome associated with massive transfusion.

Platelets

Platelets for transfusion are separated from whole donor units at the blood transfusion centre and left suspended in a small volume of fresh plasma. Platelet concentrates are stored at 20–24 °C in plastic bags that permit gas exchange, are kept constantly moving on an agitator, and have a shelf life of 5–7 days. Platelets do not remain viable under the normal storage conditions for red cells (4 °C). Each donor unit should have at least 55×10^9 platelets and an adult 'unit' of platelet concentrate normally includes 5–6 units pooled together. Aside from separating and pooling platelets from donor units of whole blood, platelet concentrates may also be obtained from single donors via an apheresis procedure, in which whole blood is removed from the donor, platelets are separated and collected by a machine, and the remaining blood (red cells and most of the plasma) is returned to the donor. This reduces the number of donors per platelet concentrate and hence the risk of viral transmission.

Adverse Effects of Blood Transfusion

All patients receiving a transfusion of blood or blood products should be monitored before and during the infusion to detect any adverse events. If any occur, the infusion should be stopped, appropriate investigations and remedial action taken, and all clinical information should be clearly documented in the patient's case record. Adverse transfusion events and reactions are divided into immediate (occurring within 24 hours of transfusion) and delayed (occurring >24 hours of transfusion).

Immediate Reactions

Acute transfusion reactions include: haemolytic reactions, anaphylaxis and allergic reactions, febrile non-haemolytic transfusion reactions (FNHTRs), transfusion-associated sepsis, and pulmonary complications, especially transfusion-associated circulatory overload (TACO). Acute haemolytic transfusion reactions (e.g., due to ABO incompatibility) are among the most serious transfusion reactions but are fortunately rare (<0.02% of transfusions) [3]. The infusion of group A red cells into a group O donor (who has naturally occurring anti-A antibodies) is the most dangerous scenario. The IgM antibodies cause intravascular destruction of the red cells and, in the most severe form, may be evident after only 5–10 mL of blood have been infused. The patient may complain of chills, loin or back pain, dyspnoea or chest pain, and may show flushing, tachycardia, and hypotension. The damaged red blood cells may trigger the coagulation system, leading to DIC. Many of these symptoms and signs will be masked in the anaesthetised patient. Later, the patient may develop haemoglobinuria or renal failure, and death may ensue.

Anaphylaxis may develop due to plasma components. This can also occur with infusion of fresh frozen plasma or cryoprecipitate and rarely may be due to anti-immunoglobulin A (IgA) antibodies in the recipient. A significant number of the general population (one in 600 in the UK) have isolated IgA deficiency and may therefore be sensitised by previous transfusion [8]. Urticaria (itchy skin weals) may occur related to an allergy to various plasma components. It is usually treated with antihistamines.

FNHTRs are common, occurring in approximately 1% of transfusions. They are due to cytokine release from recipient neutrophils and macrophages, triggered by recipient antibodies to donor antigens. These occur most often in previously transfused individuals or women who have had previous pregnancies.

In very rare circumstances, red cells may be infected by some strains of Gram-negative bacteria (e.g., *Pseudomonas* species) that proliferate preferentially at the cold storage temperatures and use citrate as an energy source, leading to coagulation of the blood and transfusion-associated septic shock and hypotension. The outcome is often fatal. As such, each unit of blood should be visually inspected before being transfused; infected units usually show evidence of haemolysis or partial coagulation. Platelet concentrates may also become infected because of their higher storage temperature, most commonly with staphylococcal species, but fatal infections with *Salmonella* and *Escherichia coli* have been reported. It is therefore essential to obtain blood cultures in any patient who develops fever during transfusions. Bacterial infections from platelet concentrates have been greatly reduced by the introduction of bacterial screening systems.

TACO can occur when patients receive large volumes of blood components. Symptoms include dyspnoea, tachycardia, and hypertension. Certain underlying co-morbidities (such as heart failure), as well as faster rates of infusion, may increase an individual's risk of developing TACO.

Delayed Reactions

Delayed haemolysis of transfused cells occurs in about 0.2% of transfusions. Such reactions are rarely fatal and are usually due to immunoglobulin G (IgG) antibodies, which lead to extravascular destruction over several days. The haemoglobin concentration falls over 3–10 days and jaundice may develop, together with a fever. The antiglobulin test will be positive, indicating the presence of an antibody on the red cells. In a mild case, the reaction may be missed. Any patient who has had a blood transfusion should be carefully observed over the following 10 days. These reactions are more common in regularly transfused patients, particularly those with haemoglobinopathies.

TA-GVHD and post-transfusion purpura and are rare (<0.01% of transfusions) but potentially life-threatening delayed complications of transfusion. TA-GVHD has almost been eliminated by the introduction of leucocyte depletion in 1999. The latter occurs when individuals who are negative for particular platelet surface antigens develop antibodies to the surface antigens of transfused platelets. If they are previously sensitised, there is an abrupt onset of purpura and bleeding as the patient's own platelets are consumed by the antibody (the reasons for this are not fully understood). Treatment is with intravenous immunoglobulin or plasma exchange.

Transmission of viral or other infections may become manifest weeks, months, or years later. Transfusion-transmitted viral infections, such as HIV and hepatitis B and C, are now very rare (less than 1 case per 1 million units transfused) due to routine screening of all donated blood for these viruses. Although the risk of these infections has been much reduced, there is still a chance of unexpected infection; therefore, no blood component or blood product should be infused without a clear clinical indication, which has been recorded in the patient medical records.

Massive Transfusion

When a patient has acute and severe blood loss a considerable proportion of the circulating blood volume may be lost. A major haemorrhage is usually taken to mean loss of the patient's total blood volume in 24 hours (or loss of 50% of the patient's blood volume in 3 hours or loss of 150 mL/min), although such definitions are often not helpful clinically. Early recognition of significant blood loss is paramount. A major haemorrhage is most commonly related to trauma, obstetric emergencies, or complicated surgery. In addition to the coagulation disturbances that can result, some of these patients will have pre-existing coagulopathies (liver disease, shock with DIC), predisposing them to excessive blood loss. Hospitals must have established major haemorrhage protocols for the activation of the transfusion laboratory and notification of relevant team members (including senior medical staff). Often there is enough time to obtain group-compatible units, which can often be available within 5–10 minutes if the patient's blood group is already known [9].

Maintenance of Adequate Circulating Volume and Oxygen Carriage

Because of the large volumes of fluid required, two large-bore venous cannula (e.g., 14 gauge) should be introduced. In the short term, a loss of up to 20% of the blood volume (the first litre in an adult) can be corrected by rapid infusion of crystalloid solutions. The maintenance of an acceptable urine output, as measured by an indwelling urinary catheter, is a good guide to the success of the resuscitation. Red cells contain the haemoglobin necessary for the transport of oxygen to the tissues. The haemoglobin concentration or the haematocrit (the proportion of red blood cells in a whole blood sample) is used to determine the need for red cell transfusion.

Surgical Control of the Bleeding

It is important that senior medical help is readily available because the UK's Confidential Enquiry into Perioperative Deaths (CEPOD) has identified massive bleeding as a major cause of avoidable perioperative mortality.

Watch the Coagulation Profile

Due to the risk of dilutional coagulopathies developing, FFP is included with red cells in a massive transfusion pack. Additional blood products such as platelet concentrates and/or cryoprecipitate may also be given, depending on the volume of transfusion required and with guidance from laboratory results. It is therefore important to send adequate initial and repeat samples for estimations of haemoglobin, platelet count, crossmatch, and coagulation profiles.

Rapid, large-volume blood transfusion can lead to other complications. If the rate of infusion is more than 50 mL/kg per hour (or more than 500 mL per 10 minutes) a blood warmer should be used to minimise hypothermia. The patient should be monitored for hyperkalaemia, acidosis, and hypocalcaemia (the latter is rarely a problem and formula replacement of calcium may be dangerous). Bleeding problems may be exacerbated by the development of microvascular bleeding manifested as bleeding from mucous membranes, catheter and venepuncture sites, oozing from raw surfaces, and petechiae and larger expanding bruises. Thrombocytopaenia, with platelets often less than 50×10^9/L, can occur due to both dilution by transfusion and increased consumption; management is with platelet concentrates. Other coagulation factors are rarely depleted significantly and should be monitored with regular coagulation profiles. Cryoprecipitate should be given if the fibrinogen falls below 1 g/L [7].

Transfusion Alternatives

Cell salvage can produce a rapid supply of washed, salvaged red cells which can be reinfused to a bleeding patient. This is suitable for surgery where the site is bacteriologically clean and free from tumour. Several machines are now available (e.g., Haemonetics cell saver systems). The blood is sucked into an anticoagulant solution and filtered prior to reinfusion. In some systems, the blood is washed and resuspended before reinfusion. The most advanced machines can process about one unit of packed red cells every 3 minutes, which makes them suitable for major surgery, with a considerable saving of donated blood (see Chapter 25).

References

1. H. Qureshi, E. Massey, D. Kirwan, et al. BCSH guideline for the use of anti-D immunoglobulin for the prevention of haemolytic disease of the fetus and newborn. *Transfusion Medicine* 2014; **24**: 8–20.

2. D. Norfolk. Transfusion handbook, 5th edition: Joint United Kingdom (UK) Blood Transfusion and Tissue Transplantation Services Professional Advisory Committee. Available from www.transfusionguidelines .org/transfusion-handbook/publication-information.pdf.

3. S. Narayan (ed.), M. Bellamy, D. Poles, et al., on behalf of the Serious Hazards of Transfusion (SHOT) steering group. The annual SHOT report 2019. Available from: www.shotuk.org/wp-content/uploads/ myimages/SHOT-REPORT-2019-Final-Bookmarked-v2.pdf.

4. Joint United Kingdom (UK) Blood Transfusion and Tissue Transplantation Services Professional Advisory Committee. Guidelines for the Blood Transfusion Services in the United Kingdom (the Red Book). Available from: www .transfusionguidelines.org.uk.

5. S. Robinson, A. Harris, S. Atkinson, et al. The administration of blood components: a British Society for Haematology guideline. *Transfusion Medicine* 2018; **28**: 3–21.

6. M. Ray. NHSBT portfolio of blood components and guidance for their clinical use Available from: https://nhsbtdbe .blob.core.windows.net/umbraco-assets-corp/16494/spn223v10.pdf.

7. L. Green, P. Bolton-Maggs, C. Beattie, et al. British Society of Haematology guidelines on the spectrum of fresh frozen plasma and cryoprecipitate products: their handling and use in various patient groups in the absence of major bleeding. *British Journal of Haematology* 2018; **181**: 54–67.

8. PID UK. Selective IgA deficiency patient information sheet. Available from: https:// mft.nhs.uk/app/uploads/sites/7/2018/04/ SelectiveIgAdeficiencypatientsheet.pdf.

9. B. J. Hunt, S. Allard, D. Keeling, et al. A practical guideline for the haematological management of major haemorrhage. *British Journal of Haematology* 2015; **170**: 788–803.

Fundamentals of Wound Healing, Dressings, and Drains

Steve Moutrey

Introduction

It is important that perioperative practitioners understand the physiological process of wound healing as it plays a key role in the patient's ability to maintain homeostasis and recover from surgery. A wound is any break in the continuity of the skin. Understanding the process of wound healing provides insight into understanding wound assessment and the choice of appropriate dressings and drains. The principles outlined in this chapter apply equally to wounds caused by trauma, surgical incisions, intravenous cannulation, and invasive haemodynamic monitoring.

What Is Wound Healing?

Irrespective of the cause, healing is an automatic, coordinated, and self-regulating physiological process that has enabled human beings to survive disease and trauma for hundreds of thousands of years. This process is essential for restoring skin integrity and protecting the body from infection and further harm [1]. The physiological response rapidly initiates the four phases of wound healing:

- haemostasis;
- inflammation;
- proliferation; and
- maturation or remodelling.

The four distinct phases have classically been referred to as the healing cascade and are essential for repair and healing. Repair and healing describe the restoration of tissue architecture and function of diseased or damaged tissues [2]. The length of time required for tissue repair and healing depends on the nature of the wound. For instance, superficial wounds, all things being equal, heal quickly, while wounds that affect the deeper layers of connective tissue take much longer to repair and heal. However, the efficacy of normal wound healing can be affected by several factors, such as the type of tissue injury and the patient.

Primary, Secondary, and Tertiary Intention

There are two predominant ways that a wound heals – by primary or secondary intentions. Surgical incisions tend to be clean, involve minimal tissue loss, and the edges of the wound can be brought together by sutures or staples and heal very quickly with minimal scarring [3]. This is an example of healing by primary intention or primary closure. It is important that the tissue edges are not under tension; the role of the suture is to provide approximation without tension, to facilitate the normal process of inflammation and new vessel growth [4].

In some cases, a surgical wound may be left open to heal by the process of granulation and epithelisation, which is known as secondary intention. For these types of wounds, it may not be possible to bring the edges together due to extensive tissue loss and so granulation tissue must fill the defect left open [5]. Healing by secondary intention is therefore much slower but can have several benefits following certain kinds of surgery. For example, following surgery for pilonidal sinus, patients whose wounds were healed by secondary intention were less likely to get the disease again compared to those who had it sutured closed [6].

For some wounds, it is necessary to delay wound closure due to the presence of infection or inflammation and this is known as tertiary intention. Most commonly, this is for 4–6 days and is subsequently closed after granulation tissue has formed [7].

Phases of Wound Healing

The normal wound healing process involves four distinct but overlapping processes (see Figure 31.1):

- Day 1: Haemostasis occurs, leading to the flow of blood stopping from the wound and the activation of clotting factors.
- Days 1–4: Inflammation prevents infection and further blood loss by vasoconstriction.
- Days 4–21: Proliferation leads to the development of new blood vessels, connective tissue, and collagen, and the wound begins to reduce in size.
- Days 21–2 years: Maturation describes the remodelling of the collagen and complete closure of the wound [7].

Haemostasis Phase

Haemostasis is the process of the wound being closed by the clotting process. First, the blood vessels constrict to restrict blood flow to the wound site. Second, platelets stick together to seal the break in the wall of the blood vessel. Finally, coagulation occurs and reinforces the platelet plug with threads of fibrin, which are like a molecular binding agent. The haemostasis stage of wound healing must occur quickly to prevent exsanguination. The platelets adhere to the sub-endothelium surface within seconds of the rupture of a blood vessel's epithelial wall. After that, the first fibrin strands begin to adhere in about 60 seconds. As the fibrin mesh begins, the blood is transformed from liquid to gel through pro-coagulants and the release of prothrombin. The formation of a thrombus or clot keeps the platelets and blood cells trapped in the wound area [8].

Inflammatory Phase

Inflammation begins right after the injury when the injured blood vessels leak transudate (made of water, salt, and proteins), causing localised swelling. The inflammation phase can last for up to 2 weeks in normal wounds [8]. The fluid engorgement allows healing and repair cells to move to the site of the wound. During the inflammatory phase, damaged cells and pathogens are removed from the wound area. White blood cells, growth factors, nutrients, and enzymes create the swelling, heat, pain, and redness commonly observed during this phase of wound healing. Inflammation is a natural part of the wound healing process, but it can be prolonged in chronic non-healing wounds.

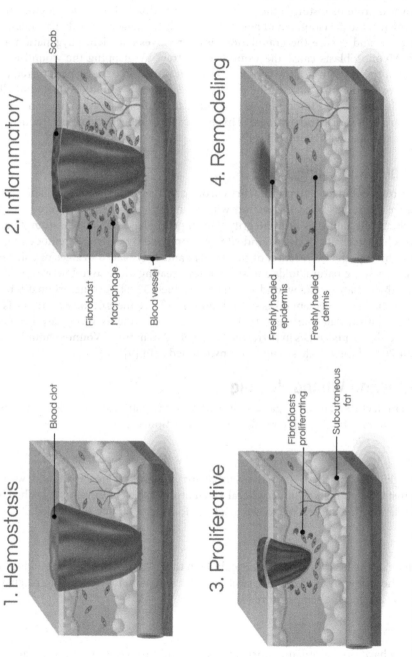

Figure 31.1 Four stages of wound healing

1. Hemostasis

Blood clot

2. Inflammatory

Scab

Fibroblast

Macrophage

Blood vessel

3. Proliferative

Fibroblasts proliferating

Subcutaneous fat

4. Remodeling

Freshly healed epidermis

Freshly healed dermis

Proliferative Phase

The proliferative phase of wound healing is when the wound is rebuilt, with new tissue made up of collagen and proteins restoring the structure and function to the tissue. Angiogenesis also occurs, which is the development of new blood vessels to replace those damaged and to restore circulation and ensure the granulation tissue receives sufficient oxygenation and nutrients [8]. Myofibroblasts cause the wound to contract by gripping the wound edges and pulling them together. In healthy wound healing, granulation tissue is pink or red and uneven in texture. In the final stage of the proliferative phase of wound healing, epithelial cells resurface the injury. It is important to remember that epithelialisation happens faster when wounds are kept moist and hydrated. This phase fills in the wound defect, reduces its size, and covers the area with epithelial cells.

Maturation or Remodelling Phase

Maturation or remodelling usually commences around 20 days after the injury. The previous proliferative phase has filled the wound with granulation tissue and covered it with epithelium, which re-establishes skin integrity. During this phase, the tensile strength and the functional characteristics of the wound site are improved by extensive remodelling of the new tissue through the destruction of the earlier randomly placed bridges of collagen. The new tissue lies along natural folds and stress lines, creating more useful networks. Two weeks after epithelialisation, the wound will have regained 30–50% of its original tensile strength, but further improvement takes several months. The redness of the wound starts to fade, leaving a whitish, flat, hairline scar. In a minority of patients this phase becomes exaggerated, and the scar becomes hypertrophic and keloid in nature. Wounds should go on to reach about 70% of the tensile strength of unwounded skin [9].

Factors Affecting Wound Healing

There are several factors that can negatively impact wound healing and the risk of postoperative wound complications, each considered in this section.

Oxygenation

Adequate oxygenation of the tissues is essential for effective tissue repair and wound healing. For instance, patients with peripheral vascular disease have slower wound healing because it influences the amount of oxygen available for normal tissue activity [5].

Infection

Infection will delay the healing process, particularly in the inflammatory phase, and is often recognised by the classic signs of redness, swelling, heat and pain, together with a discharge accompanied by an elevated temperature [8].

Age

Elderly patients have slower inflammatory, migratory and proliferation responses and are more likely to have chronic or degenerative disease. Therefore, not only will wound healing be slower and less effective, but they are also at higher risk of postoperative wound complications [5].

Obesity

The decreased vascularity of adipose tissue can decrease the delivery of nutrients and cellular elements required for effective wound healing. Not only can wound healing be delayed, but there is also an increased risk of other postoperative wound complications such as infection and dehiscence [10].

Diabetes

Diabetes is associated with an increased risk of wound complications and an increased tendency for infection. It leads to a delayed cellular response to tissue injury, reduced cellular function at the wound site, and reduced wound strength [7].

Hypothermia

It is important that normothermia is maintained throughout the patient's journey. This is because inadvertent perioperative hypothermia – a core temperature below 36 °C – is associated with delayed wound healing and an increased risk of a surgical site infection. To mitigate these negative outcomes, patients' temperatures should be routinely monitored, and active warming utilised to maintain normothermia [11].

Wound Dressings

Function of Wound Dressings

Wound dressings are used to create and maintain an appropriate environment that promotes wound repair and healing. Following the end of a surgical procedure it is common for the surgical wound to be covered by a dressing to provide a barrier from contamination, and to reduce the risk of a surgical site infection. Wound dressings function as an important component of postoperative wound management; however, there remains a lack of definitive evidence that their use is associated with a reduction in surgical site infections [12]. Because no two wounds are the same, it is important to consider several important factors when deciding which dressing to use; these include the site, position, size, and depth of the wound, and the level of exudate [13]. The wound dressing should be comfortable for the patient so that there is minimal awareness of the dressing, and provide protection from the pulling of any sutures/staples on clothing or bedding. It should also stay securely in place during movement and must also be absorbent if there is likely to be leaking – of blood, serum, or other body fluids – from the wound.

Types of Wound Dressing

There are a vast range of wound dressings available, each with their own advantages and disadvantages. The primary criteria for the choice of dressing will be patient need, but the final choice is often reducible to surgeon preference and financial cost. A summary of some of the different kinds of wound dressings is detailed below.

Hydrocolloid Dressings

These are self-adhesive dressings that facilitate rehydration and autolytic debridement, absorb exudate, are waterproof, flexible, and can be used for surgical wounds, minor burns, and abrasions. Hydrocolloid dressings contain a gel-forming agent that keeps the wound clean and protects it from infection but should not be used on infected wounds.

Hydrogel Dressings

These dressings contain 90% water in a gel base that helps to facilitate moist wound healing through autolytic debridement. Hydrogel dressings can be used for a range of wounds, such as minor burns, radiation burns, graft and donor sites, and pressure ulcers. However, they are not recommended for wounds with heavy exudate.

Alginate Dressings

These offer effective protection for wounds that have high amounts of drainage, partial thickness burns, trauma wounds, pressure ulcers, and for packing wounds required to heal by granulation. Alginate dressings absorb excess liquid and create a gel that promotes wound healing. They contain sodium and seaweed fibres that can absorb high amounts of fluid and require changing regularly due to the amount of fluid that they can absorb.

Collagen Dressings

These are used for chronic wounds or pressure sores, transplant sites, surgical wounds, ulcers, burns, or injuries with a large surface area. Collagen dressings act as a scaffolding for new cells to grow and encourage wound healing. They do so by helping to remove dead tissue, aiding the growth of new blood vessels, and helping to bring the wound edges together.

Foam Dressings

These work well for wounds of varying degrees of severity, and injuries that exude odours. Foam absorbs exudate from the wound and promotes faster healing. Foam dressings also allow water vapour to enter, keeping the area moist and preventing bacteria from entering the wound site.

Transparent Dressings

These are useful for when healthcare professionals want to monitor wound healing, as it makes identifying complications easier. For this reason, transparent dressings are often used on surgical wounds, burns and ulcers, and on intravenous sites. These dressings are breathable but impermeable to bacteria and help to keep the wound clean and dry. They are also flexible, which makes them comfortable to wear.

Gauze Dressings

These are the most used form of wound dressing and often used to protect open wounds or areas of broken skin. Gauze dressings are suitable for minor injuries such as grazes, cuts, or areas of delicate skin and have the benefit of being inexpensive, easily accessible, and easy to apply [13].

Negative Pressure Wound Therapy

Negative pressure wound therapy (NPWT) is provided through a sealed dressing that is attached to a vacuum source; the vacuum draws fluid from the wound while encouraging blood flow. Used to promote healing in acute or chronic wounds, it also significantly reduces surgical site infections and wound dehiscence in many surgical wound types. The

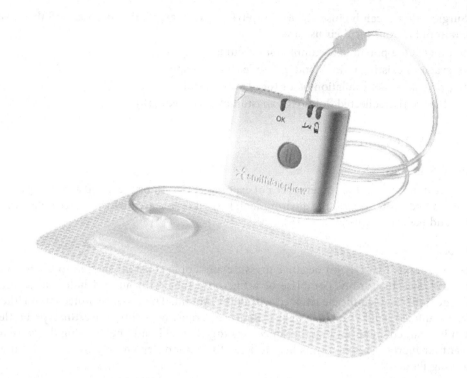

Figure 31.2 PICO suction unit and dressing

PICO is a portable battery-operated NPWT system attached directly to the wound dressing and consists of four layers (see Figure 31.2). The first is a silicone adhesive contact layer and the other layers consist of an airlock layer to distribute pressure evenly across the dressing, an absorbent layer to remove exudate and bacteria, and a top layer acting as a barrier allowing moisture to evaporate. The purpose of a PICO is to promote healing and prevent surgical site infections, particularly in patients at risk of developing complications [14].

Surgical Drains

These are devices used in surgery and act as a deliberate channel or conduit to drain established or potential collections of blood, serous fluid, pus, intestinal secretions, or air from a wound or operative site to prevent complications or treat already established pathology. Surgical drains will normally evacuate their contents from the body by either active or passive action. The type of drain will normally be selected by the surgeon, but a thorough knowledge must be possessed by the perioperative practitioner to aid preparation, selection, and care. During post-anaesthetic care, the drain needs to be checked, measured, and observed as it may have an impact on the patient's fluid management. Drains should be removed as soon as its purpose has been served and per the operative notes. The general rule is that if a drain has produced less than 1 mL/h in the previous 24 hours then it will be safe to remove [15]. Drains should always be managed aseptically to reduce the risk of introducing pathogens to the wound site and in line with the surgeon's recommendations.

Surgical drains can be inserted for prophylactic or therapeutic purposes and the most common indications for their use are:

- to prevent the potential accumulation of fluid;
- to evacuate existing fluid: blood, pus, bile, and exudate;
- to prevent the accumulation of air (dead space); and
- to characterise collected fluid (e.g., anastomotic leakage) [15].

Drain Classification

Closed Drains

These are drains where the contents are not exposed to the atmosphere and avoids exposure of the drained contents with the environment. Closed drains are further sub-classified into active and passive categories.

Active Drains

These are drains that rely on negative pressure and apply constant suction to the wound site. Modern active drains comprise of a fine-bore tube with an end hole and several drainage holes that should be situated within the wound. The tube is connected to either a pre-vacuumed solid container (e.g., a Redivac™ drain) or a soft concertinatype bottle, which is 'charged' by squashing the concertina together by hand, then closing the valve to prevent air ingress. Active drains help to keep the wound dry and are highly efficient at removing fluid.

Passive Drains

These generally allow fluid to be drained passively by gravity, body movement, or capillary action. Passive drains can drain into a collection device or into an absorbent dressing. The siting of these drains needs to be carefully selected, as the patient's movement may disrupt its efficiency and dislodge it. These drains are typically made from silicone or polyvinyl chloride plastic. An example of an open passive drain is the Penrose™ drain.

Open Drains

The drained contents are exposed to the atmosphere and are usually collected in gauze or a bandage. Open drains are not usually sutured in but may have a safety pin at the end to prevent the drain from being pulled into the wound.

References

1. H. Sorg, D. J. Tilkorn, S. Hager, et al. Skin wound healing: an update on the current knowledge and concepts. *European Surgical Research* 2017; **58**: 81–94.

2. K. P. Krafts. Tissue repair: the hidden drama. *Organogenesis* 2010; **6**: 225–233.

3. M. Martin. Physiology of wound healing. In M. Flanagan (ed.), *Wound Healing and Skin Integrity: Principles and Practice*. Chichester: Wiley-Blackwell, 2013.

4. D. Son and A. Harijan. Overview of surgical scar prevention and management. *Journal of Korean Medical Science* 2014; **29**: 751–757.

5. A. Young and C.-E. McNaught. The physiology of wound healing. *Surgery* 2011; **29**: 475–479.

6. A. AL-Khamis, I. McCallum, P. M. King, and J. Bruce. Healing by primary versus secondary intention after surgical treatment

for pilonidal sinus. *Cochrane Database of Systematic Reviews* 2010; **1**: CD006213.

7. S. Chhabra, N. Chhabra, A. Kaur, et al. Wound healing concepts in clinical practice of OMFS. *Journal of Oral and Maxillofacial Surgery* 2017; **16**: 403–423.

8. G. Schultz, G. Chin, L. Moldawer, R. Diegelmann. Principles of wound healing. In R. Fitridge and M. Thompson (eds.), *Mechanisms of Vascular Disease: A Reference Book for Vascular Specialists*. Adelaide: University of Adelaide Press, 2011.

9. G. Han and R. Ceilley. Chronic wound healing: a review of current management and treatments. *Advances in Therapy* 2017; **34**: 599–610.

10. S. Guo and L. A. DiPietro. Factors affecting wound healing. *Journal of Dental Research* 2010; **89**: 219–229.

11. J. Tanner, J. Kay, and K. Chambers. Avoiding inadvertent peri-operative hypothermia. *Nursing Times* 2016; **112**: 10–12.

12. C. J. Walter, J. C. Dumville, C. A Sharp, and T. Page. Systematic review and meta-analysis of wound dressings in the prevention of surgical-site infections in surgical wounds healing by primary intention. *British Journal of Surgery* 2012; **99**: 1185–1194.

13. K. Yao, L. Bae, and W. P. Yew. Post-operative wound management. *Australian Family Physician* 2013; **42**: 867–870.

14. C. Payne and D. Edwards. Application of the single use negative pressure wound therapy device (PICO) on a heterogeneous group of surgical and traumatic wounds. *Eplasty* 2014; 14: e20.

15. R. Durai R, A. Mownah, and P. C. H. Ng. Use of drains in surgery: a review. *Journal of Perioperative Practice* 2009; **19**: 180–186.

Chapter 32

Understanding Sutures and Skin Closure

Steve Moutrey and Paul Bond

Introduction

There is evidence of the use of sutures from as far back as 3000 BCE, in ancient Egypt, where the use of plant fibres, hair, tendons, and wool threads have been discovered from mummified remains. The first detailed descriptions of suturing techniques were from the Indian surgeon Sushruta and these date from 500 BCE. He documented the use of sheep intestine as suture material for several different kinds of surgery [1]. Surgical sutures are medical devices used to hold body tissue together following injury or surgery. The application generally involves using a needle with an attached length of suture thread. Suture thread can be made from numerous materials. The original sutures were made from biological materials, such as catgut, cotton, and silk. Today, most sutures are made of synthetic polymer fibres, with silk being the only biological material still in use.

Suture Characteristics

Optimal suture qualities include:
- having high uniform tensile strength, permitting the use of finer sizes;
- having high tensile strength retention in vivo, holding the wound securely throughout the critical healing period, followed by rapid absorption;
- having a consistent uniform diameter;
- being sterile;
- being pliable for ease of handling and knot security;
- having freedom from irritating substances or impurities for optimum tissue acceptance; and
- having a predictable performance.

Sutures are split into four groups: monofilament, multifilament/braided, absorbable, and non-absorbable (see Table 32.1 for details).

Monofilament Sutures

This type of suture is made of a single strand, which is relatively more resistant to microorganisms. Monofilament sutures provide a better passage through tissue as they have a low friction factor compared to braided sutures. Great care must be taken when handling and tying a monofilament suture as any crushing or crimping of the suture can weaken it, which leads to a premature suture failure.

Table 32.1 Suture materials

Suture type	Absorbable	Non-absorbable	Monofilament	Multifilament/ braided	Plus suture
Vicryl	✓			✓	✓
PDS	✓		✓		✓
Monocryl	✓		✓		✓
Nylon		✓	✓		
Prolene		✓	✓		
Silk		✓		✓	

Multifilament/Braided Sutures

Multifilament or braided sutures tend to provide better knotting and knot security, as they are easier to handle, being more flexible and softer. Multifilament/braided sutures can also provide a focal point for infection as bacteria can infiltrate between the fibres. Some multifilament/braided sutures are often coated with various compounds to provide ease of use and some with an antibacterial coating, which helps to prevent suture infections.

Absorbable Sutures

The body breaks down the suture material over time by body enzymes (if natural) or by hydrolysis (if synthetic) [2]. The time for this breakdown depends on the suture material, the location of insertion, and the individual patient. If a patient has an ongoing infection or a protein deficiency this can increase the absorption rate of a suture.

Non-absorbable Sutures

Non-absorbable sutures remain in place until they are removed and are not degraded by the body; they also have extremely low tissue reactivity and provide longer-term tissue approximation. Non-absorbable sutures can be used on the skin, and removed later, or used inside the body where they will be retained. Common uses include vessel repair/anastomosis, bowel repair, hernia repair, tendon repair, and skin closure [2].

New Guidance

In June 2021, the UK's National Institute for Health and Care Excellence issued medical technologies guidance which recommends the adoption of Plus sutures, the first absorbable sutures with antibacterial protection. Plus sutures are a range of synthetic, absorbable sutures impregnated or coated with triclosan, a purified medical-grade antimicrobial. Clinical evidence shows that using Plus sutures instead of standard absorbable sutures can reduce the risk of surgical site infections by 30% and result in a significant cost saving on average of £13.62 per patient [3].

Suture Size

The diameter of the suture will affect its handling properties and tensile strength. The larger the size ascribed to the suture, the smaller the diameter is; for example, a 7/0 suture is

Table 32.2 Suture sizes

Suture size: smallest to largest	Uses
10/0	Typically used in the most delicate surgeries. Common in both Ophthalmic surgery and for repairing small, damaged nerves, often due to lacerations in the hand
9/0	As 10/0
8/0	As 10/0
7/0	Used for repairing small vessels and arteries or for delicate facial plastic surgery
6/0	Common for use in vascular graft suturing such as in carotid endarterectomy
5/0	Used for larger vessel repair such as an abdominal aortic aneurysm or skin closure
4/0	As 5/0
3/0	Skin closure when there is a lot of tension on the tissue, closure of muscle layers, or repair of bowel in general surgery
2/0	Fascia/subcutaneous tissue closure (e.g., external oblique in hernia repair)
0	For the closing of the fascia layer in abdominal surgery, the joint capsule in knee and hip surgery, or deep layers in back surgery
1	For repair of tendons or high-tension structures in larger orthopaedic surgeries

smaller than a 4/0 suture (see Table 32.2). When choosing a suture size, the smallest size possible should be chosen, while considering the natural strength of the tissue [2].

Needles

The shape, length, and size of the needle used in surgery varies. They may be straight or curved, larger handheld needles or very fine small needles with various curvatures, requiring the use of a needle holder to manipulate. Therefore, there are several shapes of surgical needles. These shapes include; straight, ¼ circle, ⅜ circle, ½ circle, ⅝ circle, compound-curve half curve (also known as ski); half curved at both ends of a straight segment (also known as canoe); and 'J' curve – commonly used for laparoscopic surgery (see Figure 32.1).

Needles may also be classified by their point shape and makeup. Examples are as follows:

- **Taper points**: the needle body is round and tapers smoothly to a point, and is used on easily penetrated tissues – it minimises the potential of tearing fascia.
- **Blunt points**: these are sharp enough to penetrate fascia and muscle but not skin. They are used for suturing friable tissue such as the liver. Using a blunt needle virtually eliminates accidental glove puncture.

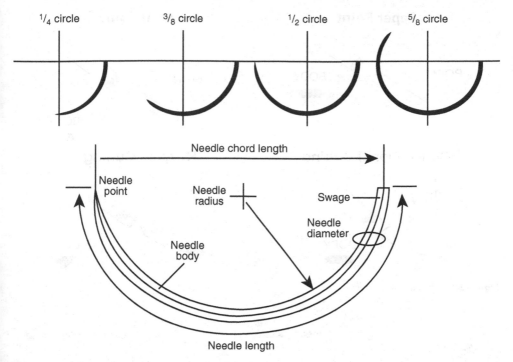

Figure 32.1 Anatomy of the needle

- **Conventional cutting**: the needle body is triangular and has a sharpened cutting edge on the inside curve. This is normally used for general skin closure.
- **Reverse cutting**: the reverse cutting needle is similar to a conventional cutting needle except that the cutting edge faces down instead of up. This may decrease the likelihood of sutures pulling through tissue in some cases.

These are illustrated in Figure 32.2. Several additional key suture details can be found on the suture packaging (see Figure 32.3).

Tissue Penetration

The shape and cross-section of the needle tip will denote its preferred use and how it will penetrate the tissue being sutured. Round-bodied needles with a pinpoint tip will usually be used on soft or delicate tissues. Spatula needles are designed for mainly ophthalmic procedures as the needle will separate through the thin layers of the sclera or corneal tissue, which is quite hard and requires a sharper cutting type needle to allow penetration.

Conventional cutting needles have a sharp cutting edge on the inside curvature of the needle, which forms a triangular point allowing better penetration of tougher tissue. The reverse cutting needle used for the same purpose has a triangular shape with an extra cutting edge on the outside cutting curvature of the needle – best used for suturing skin as the suture strand will not cut through towards the edge of the wound. Minimal trauma and early regeneration of tissue are the primary concerns. Finally, atraumatic needles may be permanently swaged to the suture, or they may be designed to come off the suture with a sharp straight tug. These are

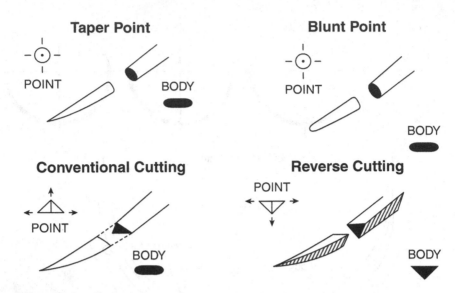

Figure 32.2 Needle point shapes

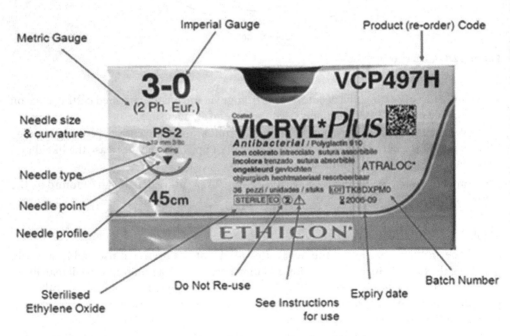

Figure 32.3 Suture packet information (used with kind permission from Ethicon)

commonly used for interrupted sutures, where each suture is only passed once and then tied. When positioning the needle in the needle holder, care must be taken to grasp the main body of the needle in the jaws of the needle holder and not grasp the end where the suture has been

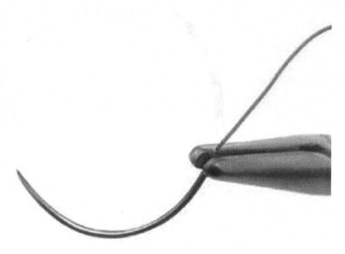

Figure 32.4 Incorrect way to grasp a needle

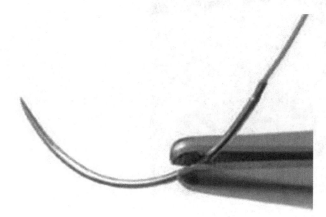

Figure 32.5 The correct way to grasp a needle

attached – the swage (see Figures 32.4 and 32.5). This swaged area is the weakest part of the needle and may break or bend when the suture is being applied to the tissue or skin.

Eyed needles are still used, commonly in gynaecology; an example of these are Mayo needles, which are used to rethread sutures already placed after initial insertion through a structure. Eyed needles are more traumatic as two thicknesses of suture material and a large eye needs to be pulled through tissue, whereas the swaged needles are much less traumatic as they have a smooth transition from needle to suture (see Figure 32.6).

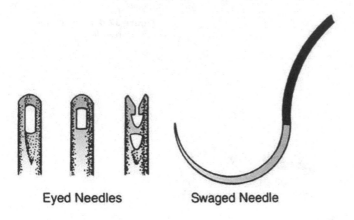

Figure 32.6 Eyed and swaged needle

Eyed Needles   Swaged Needle

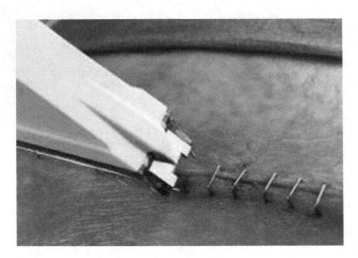

Figure 32.7 Application of skin staples

Surgical Staples

Some traditional sutures, ligatures, and suturing techniques have been replaced with metal clips and staples. These have now been utilised in both wound closure (skin) and internally to replace sutures for bowel anastomosis, for example. The skin staples or clips are the most universally used (see Figure 32.7). Staples are made from high-quality stainless steel and are available in different sizes, delivery systems, numbers, and widths. These were originally loaded into re-usable, re-loadable delivery systems, which have now been replaced by a single-use stapling device that allows multi-fire, with a set number of staples loaded into the device. The advantage of staples is that they are individually placed and therefore can be removed individually to drain a haematoma or infection/pus build-up without fully opening the wound. They can be less reactive to the skin than closure with sutures and reduce subsequent scarring. The primary use of skin closure staples is for the closure of wounds on

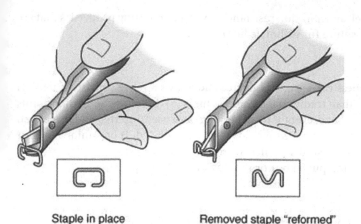

Figure 32.8 Removing staples

Staple in place　　　　　　Removed staple "reformed"

the scalp and limb extremities, where these wounds are under higher tension; they are also used in securing split-skin grafts in place.

The advantages of staples are as follows:

- increased speed of closure [4];
- improved wound edge eversion;
- reduced tissue/skin reaction; and
- decreased risk of infection.

Their disadvantages are:

- it sometimes requires an experienced assistant to evert skin edges and approximate these during the closure;
- they are less precise wound closure;
- they are more expensive than a suture;
- they are not usually used over a bony prominence, fine tissue, or highly mobile areas.

Removal of Staples

Staples are removed with a specially designed extractor, which slips under the staple; when operated, the staple is bent in the middle, pulling the claws of the staples up and out of the wound. This should be a painless procedure (see Figure 32.8).

Specialist Sutures and Skin Closure Products

New sutures are frequently being developed – a huge range of various sutures are now available to the surgeon. It is therefore essential for the practitioner to understand the various sutures, their differences, structure, and indications for use. This enhances the practitioner's ability to both advise and procure over their use. Several non-invasive skin closure products and techniques have also been developed to enhance wound healing.

FiberWire®

This is a structure that is constructed of a multi-strand ultra-high molecular weight polyethylene core with a braided outer covering of polyester that gives FiberWire® suture its superior strength, soft feel, and abrasion resistance. Excellent knotting properties that are extremely secure – a useful suture for orthopaedic surgery.

Stratafix™

This suture provides a knotless tissue control device and allows a more consistent tension with more points of fixation than traditional tension sutures [5]. It has spiral, anchor points along the length of the suture that prevent it from moving once used/inserted and there is no need for the assistant to follow as the suture holds itself once placed. It has unique anchor points all along the length of the suture, which works in a similar principle to a fishhook barb, and prevents it from being pulled out or moving once placed [6].

Skin Glue

Surgical skin glue is a compound glue made from the chemical cyanoacrylate. This same compound makes up 'superglue', which is available for commercial use. The only difference is that skin/surgical glue has a different formulation to prevent the stinging and irritability that would be present by using 'superglue' on the skin [7]. Skin glue can be used by itself, or with sutures and wound adhesive strips. It is primarily used on small straight incisions, where the wound edges can easily be approximated, and not over mobile areas such as joints. Some surgeons use glue on small skin incisions instead of applying another formal dressing by using a fine strip of glue over the wound to seal it, once it has been closed. A glued wound closure should produce less scarring as there are no suture track marks from this closure method.

References

1. T. M. Muffly, A. P. Tizzano, and M. D. Walters. The history and evolution of sutures in pelvic surgery. *Journal of the Royal Society of Medicine* 2011; **104**: 107–112.

2. M. Byrne and A. Aly. The surgical suture. *Aesthetic Surgery Journal* 2019; **39**: S67–S72.

3. National Institute for Health and Care Excellence. Plus sutures for preventing surgical site infection. Available from: www .nice.org.uk/guidance/mtg59/resources/ plus-sutures-for-preventing-surgical-site-infection-pdf-64372124642245.

4. M. P. Kochar and S. P. Singh. Incised surgical wound closure with sutures and staples: a controlled experimental study.

International Surgery Journal 2015; **2**: 69–372.

5. E. I. Smith, S. T. DiSegna, P. Y. Shukla, and E. G. Matzkin. Barbed versus traditional sutures: closure time, cost, and wound related outcomes in total joint arthroplasty. *Journal of Arthroplasty* 2014; **29**: 283–287

6. B. R. Levine, N. Ting, and C. J. Della Valle. Use of a barbed suture in the closure of hip and knee arthroplasty wounds. *Orthopaedics* 2011; **34**: e473–e475.

7. B. Thomas, M. Bruns, and J. Worthington. Using tissue adhesive for wound repair: a practical guide to dermabond. *American Family Physician* 2000; **61**: 1383–1388.

33

Perioperative Care of the Paediatric Patient

Faye Lowry and Daniel Rodger

Introduction

Providing safe and effective care for children requires a clear underpinning knowledge of their unique needs. It is important to note that a common misconception is that children are just little adults [1]. Conscious consideration of age-dependent characteristics such as anatomical, physiological, and behavioural changes is essential in the delivery of paediatric patient care. The rationale for adaptations to the delivery of care is to ensure children receive anaesthesia and surgery in a safe and appropriate environment. This chapter addresses differentials in the anatomy and physiology of children and adults, modifications of practice, and other special considerations.

Anatomical and Physiological Variations

It is important to differentiate between a neonate, infant, child, and adolescent. A neonate is defined as being less than 4 weeks old, an infant is less than 1 year of age, a child is more than 1 year old and has not yet reached puberty, and an adolescent is between puberty and maturity (see Table 33.1).

There are numerous anatomical and physiological differences a perioperative practitioner must know to safely assist an anaesthetist or surgeon. When combined, these differences can pose challenges throughout the entire perioperative pathway and can require adaptation from the approach used in adult practice.

The Airway and Lungs

Challenges in paediatric anaesthesia are more prevalent in children of around the age of years and under. These patients often present with notable anatomical differences in the upper airway [2], including a large head (relative to body size), prominent occiput, small mandible, and short neck, which can be barriers to basic airway management. Establishing a neutral position of the head is the recommended manoeuvre in the first instance. Head and shoulder supports are common adjuncts to assist with and maintain an open airway;

Table 33.1 Age groups

Neonate	The first 28 days of *ex utero* life
Infant	1–12 months of age
Child	1–12 years of age
Adolescent	13–17 years of age

these are often gel or foam materials to protect the integrity of the skin and reduce the incidence of pressure sores [3]. For children over 1 year old, a head tilt chin lift is an effective airway opening manoeuvre. If there is any suspicion of trauma or injury to the cervical spine, a jaw thrust is the required manoeuvre, regardless of the patient's age [4].

Infants are prone to upper-airway obstruction due to the increased size of the tongue relative to the airway. Infants under the age of 6 months are obligate nasal breathers, meaning they have a preference or reflex to breath nasally. If nasal congestion is noted, there may be challenges when using nasal cannula for oxygen delivery or passing a nasogastric tube. Tonsils and adenoids are often enlarged and a common cause of upper-airway obstruction, often requiring a jaw thrust and continuous positive airway pressure (CPAP).

The larynx is positioned anteriorly, meaning that direct laryngoscopy can be more complex in children and infants. The large tongue often sweeps to the right side of the laryngoscope blade and a floppy 'U'-shaped epiglottis commonly falls back if the laryngoscope is not placed on the laryngeal surface, affecting the quality of visualising the vocal cords for intubation [2]. The trachea is more conical in shape with the cricoid ring being the narrowest part of the upper airway. Tracheal rings and cartilage are notably softer, requiring much less cricoid pressure if assisting for a rapid sequence induction. The larynx in infants and children lies at the level of C3/C4 and advances to C5/C6 as they reach puberty [2, 5].

Mature alveoli are not uniformly present until 36 weeks gestation, leading to a common occurrence of chronic chest infections in children born prematurely [6]. Infants have an increased oxygen demand due to a relatively high basal metabolic rate and therefore an increased respiratory rate to compensate, and they have a limited ability to increase their tidal volume. Children have a reduced respiratory reserve due to cartilaginous ribs and fewer fatigue-resistant fibres. Because the chest wall is much more compliant than in an adult the functional residual capacity and therefore oxygen reserve is relatively low. Neonates and infants consume oxygen reserves much more quickly than an adult so a rapid decrease in oxygen saturation and cyanosis (usually occurring at an oxygen saturation of 85% or less) are sometimes observed following induction of anaesthesia. If there is a delay in the recognition and treatment of hypoxia, bradycardia will often follow, precipitating a cardiac arrest. An immature pons and medulla have been identified as a common cause of respiratory depression in the paediatric patient. There is also an increased incidence of right main-bronchus intubation (rather than the left main-bronchus intubation seen in adults) due to the short trachea bifurcating at the same angle for the left and right main bronchi [4, 7].

It is not unusual for the heart rate of an infant to range between 110 and 160 beats per minute (bpm). As a child reaches puberty, their heart rate will decrease to between 60 and 100 bpm. Like an infant's respiratory rate, a child's heart rate is also much higher than that of an adult due to the increased basal metabolic rate required to maintain normothermia. Blood pressure increases as the child grows with age because cardiac muscle mass is smaller in neonates and infants resulting in a lower peak pressure [8]. Normal parameters for age in relation to heart rate and blood pressure are shown in Table 33.2 [9].

Thermoregulation

General anaesthesia compromises the ability to thermoregulate during the perioperative phase and this is compounded by a cold operating-theatre environment. Therefore, an

Table 33.2 Normal age-specific parameters

Age	Heart rate (bpm)	Blood pressure (mmHg)	Circulatory volumes (mL/kg)
<1 year	110–160	65/40	80–90
2–5 years	95–140	95/55	75–80
5–12 years	80–100	115/60	70–75
>12 years	60–100	120/70	65–70

active warming device with continuous temperature monitoring should be routinely used for paediatric patients. Neonates and infants, for instance, have thinner subcutaneous fat, a large surface area-to-body mass ratio, and an inability to shiver so they normally generate heat to maintain normothermia by moving, crying, and non-shivering thermogenesis (in the first 6 months of life) [10]. Non-shivering thermogenesis describes a mechanism of heat production that does not involve the contraction of skeletal muscles and occurs during the first 6 months of postnatal life. Other means of mitigating inadvertent hypothermia in neonates and infants include increasing the ambient temperature in the theatre to about 25 °C, a woollen cap for the head, infusion of warmed intravenous fluids, and using an overhead warmer where appropriate. Neonates should be returned to their incubators as soon as possible following surgery.

Developmental Psychology

Before the twentieth century, little regard was given to the mind of a child and their unique developmental needs. We now know that admission to hospital may have profound psychological effects on children. The type of disturbance will depend upon the child's age, social and family factors, and their hospital 'experience'. All staff who care for children in hospital should realise the important role they can play in minimising psychological trauma. Infants younger than 6 months of age are not usually upset by short-term separation from parents, though prolonged separation may impair parent–child bonding. Separation anxiety is a developmental milestone that does not develop until about 6 months of age. This is due to the onset of object permanence – the understanding that things and people exist even if they are not present (not in the room or close by).

Older infants and preschool children are more likely to be distressed by a hospital stay, primarily because of the separation from their family. School-age children are usually less upset at separation and may be more concerned with the surgical procedure and its possible mutilating effect, while adolescents fear the loss of control and the possibility of not being able to cope with their illness. Approximately 50–75% of children develop preoperative anxiety before undergoing surgery [11]. Preoperative anxiety in children usually manifests as verbal or physical resistance, crying, screaming, becoming quiet and withdrawn, or expressing fear or sadness. There are a range of non-pharmacological and pharmacological methods available that can be utilised to reduce preoperative anxiety.

Preoperative Assessment

Preoperative assessment, induction of anaesthesia, and recovery of the paediatric patient are notable for the presence of parents or carers, who are often visibly anxious. Good rapport is created by communicating effectively with the child and their carer(s) and considered a subjective measure of the quality of anaesthetic care, setting the tone for the entirety of the perioperative journey [12]. Children should ideally be welcomed, assessed, and recovered in a dedicated paediatric setting. The designated area for preoperative assessment is often brightly coloured, with age-appropriate entertainment including games, toys, and music available. Where possible, a separate area should be available for adolescents, both pre- and postoperatively. Play specialists and translators can enhance the quality of the perioperative experience of the child and carers alike. In non-specialist hospitals, children are cared for in a predominantly adult environment but the same principles for the care of the paediatric patient should still apply.

Preoperative assessment of the child is undertaken in the same way as adult practice. The length of assessment is dependent on the urgency and complexity of the surgery. Special considerations for the family history are noted to unearth if any further investigations are required prior to surgery, such as parental adverse events related to anaesthesia or sudden cardiac death in the family [7]. Home circumstances may also trigger a risk assessment and alter the care or length of hospital stay postoperatively [7]. The preoperative assessment facilitates an opportunity for the anaesthetist to build a rapport with the child and their parent or carers prior to surgery. It is essential during interactions with the child that perioperative practitioners communicate in a way that the child can understand, to reduce anxiety in an often unfamiliar environment. Sitting down and engaging in eye contact at the child's level can increase the efficiency of communication and overall quality of the interaction. At this stage, an assessment can be made of any anxiety the child is displaying that could negatively affect their perioperative care.

The preoperative visit can in some cases help to reduce anxiety but in children with heightened anxiety or additional needs, a premedication may be indicated. Premedication is usually unnecessary for infants and young children having day-care surgery, but some anxious older children may benefit from sedative premedication given orally. Midazolam is the most common drug of choice due to its short onset of action in as little as 15 minutes. The drug is taken orally and is bitter in taste, which can be masked in a small volume of sweetened clear fluid [13]. Before prescribing a premedication for a child, alternative methods of reducing anxiety should be explored, such as written information and visits to the perioperative environment.

It is common practice to invite a parent or carer to be present at the induction of anaesthesia; this can sometimes help reduce anxiety for both the child and parent. Play therapy can be used during the perioperative phase, where distraction techniques are used to actively engage the child with toys and videos to reduce anxiety specifically for the child, support parents, and build a rapport between the perioperative team and the patient [14]. Trained play therapists are an invaluable addition to the multidisciplinary team. Therapists will often readily identify the small number of children for whom elective premedication may be beneficial [14].

Preoperative Fasting

Infants and children should not be subjected to unnecessarily prolonged fasting. Historically, guidance for fasting advocates 6 hours for solids, 4 hours for breast milk, and 2 hours for clear fluids, respectively [12]. More recently it has been shown that it is safe for children to drink clear fluids up to 1 hour before general anaesthesia, with no increased risk of pulmonary aspiration [15], with some even advocating water up until the patient is sent for. Contraindications to shortening preoperative fasting should be decided by the anaesthetist but include patients with gastro-oesophageal reflux and renal failure [7].

Regional Anaesthesia

The use of regional anaesthesia as an adjunct to general anaesthesia has the potential to decrease requirements of anaesthetic during the perioperative phase and opioids in the postoperative phase [16]. For shorter procedures, such as a hernia repair, single injection techniques are used although these do not always provide effective pain relief for the intended amount of time. To prolong the effects of regional anaesthesia, an adjunct drug can be used in combination with the local anaesthetic to improve the quality and length of the block [17]. Until recently, the transference of anatomical landmarks for regional anaesthesia from adults to children was considered the same, but on a smaller scale; this has transpired to be untrue and can lead to errors and adverse outcomes that include nerve damage [18].

Inhalational Induction

Although an intravenous induction may be ideal clinically, especially when rapid control of the airway is required, it is common for young children to undergo an inhalational rather than intravenous induction as cannulation may be technically difficult, especially in the absence of patient cooperation [19]. It is painless, safe, provides a slower loss of protective reflexes, can be given in increments, has rapid recovery if abandoned, and has few absolute contraindications other than a family or patient history of malignant hyperthermia [20].

The most commonly used agent for volatile induction is sevoflurane because it is less pungent than isoflurane and desflurane and causes minimal airway irritation. The main disadvantages of an inhalational induction are that that it is slower than intravenous induction and precludes rapid sequence induction. Although the loss of airway reflexes is gradual, it is not always easily reversible, which may result in obstruction [21]. Furthermore, there is also a degree of risk associated with being unable to rapidly administer emergency drugs without intravenous access, complicating the treatment of laryngospasm or brady-cardia. For this reason, intravenous access should be secured immediately following loss of consciousness.

Intravenous Access

Difficulty gaining peripheral intravenous access occurs in more than 30% of children requiring cannulation [22]. Common challenges to obtaining intravenous access in children are the smaller vessel size, increased subcutaneous fat, they are less cooperative, and, in more recent years, a rise in paediatric obesity [23, 24]. Where appropriate, play specialists can assist, and distraction techniques employed that can involve toys, smartphones, and tablets to aid with the successful cannulation of a child [25]. An ultrasound device can also be a useful and has become a commonly used aid for difficult intravenous cannulation access in infants and young children. When using an ultrasound device, it is important to use enough gel with minimal skin pressure to avoid collapsing the blood vessels.

General Anaesthesia

The anatomical and physiological differences between children and adults heavily influence the practice of anaesthesia and support the rationale of paediatric anaesthesia being defined as a subspecialty [26]. Children are at greater risk of drug errors due to pharmacological variations, meaning that drug doses are calculated on surrogate markers such as weight, age, or calculated body surface area. In emergency circumstances, a child's weight must often be estimated [27]. Innovative advances in technology have paved the way for smartphone and tablet applications that provide a wealth of useful information, such as calculations for paediatric drug doses [28].

Anaesthetic Equipment

Most of the basic equipment used in paediatric anaesthesia is like that used in adults but smaller. This includes face masks, endotracheal tubes, supraglottic airway devices, blood pressure cuffs, ECG dots, and pulse oximeters. Despite advances in equipment and technology the Ayre's T-piece (Mapleson E) circuit and Jackson–Rees modification (Mapleson F) continue to be widely used in paediatric anaesthesia. The Ayre's T-piece is a valveless breathing system used in smaller children up to 25 kg, with the addition of an open-ended reservoir bag on the Jackson–Rees modification [29].

Supraglottic airways devices such as laryngeal mask airways (LMAs) are commonly used to maintain anaesthesia in children for short and minor surgical procedures, but they also have a role in the management of a difficult airway. LMAs come in a range of sizes and can be safely used in term neonates, infants, children, and adolescents. However, complications are more likely when using sizes 1 and 1.5 LMAs [30]. Supraglottic airway devices are a good intermediate airway because they can tolerate pressures that enable positive-pressure ventilation. An LMA can also be used as a conduit to facilitate fibre-optic intubation or as a rescue device following a failed intubation.

Anatomical and physiological differences in children mean direct laryngoscopy can be challenging. Direct laryngoscopy remains the primary choice for tracheal intubation of children, using a straight laryngoscope blade for neonates and infants, traditionally graduating to a curved Macintosh blade as the child grows with age. Some anaesthetists prefer a straight blade such as a Miller blade in paediatrics, and especially in neonates. However, in infants and children less than 2 years of age, an optimal laryngeal view can be observed with either a Miller or Macintosh laryngoscope blade [31].

The literature on rapid sequence induction for the paediatric patient is varied. Pre-oxygenation is recommended but is often challenging in infants and young children due to non-compliance [32] and may compound preoperative anxiety and stress. Cricoid pressure continues to be used in practice, despite debate about the application of force required and its overall efficacy [32]. Fibre-optic flexible scopes were the primary method of managing a difficult airway in previous years. However, innovative developments have seen an increase in the use of a videolaryngoscopes suitable for the paediatric patient [33].

Cuffed versus Uncuffed Endotracheal Tubes

Historically, cuffed endotracheal tubes were only used in the care of children in intensive care. In more recent years, specially designed cuffed endotracheal tubes (e.g., Microcuff® tubes) for use in infants and children have been developed. These permit a tracheal seal at lower pressures by utilising a high-volume low-pressure cuff that helps to reduce the risk of tissue damage. It is important to routinely use a cuff pressure-measuring device to avoid hyperinflation, maintaining it below 20 cmH$_2$O. Additional benefits include a reduction in re-intubation due to a leak, a reduction in team exposure to waste anaesthetic gases due to a leak, and avoiding the additional trauma caused by repeat laryngoscopies [34].

The recommended size and depth of endotracheal tubes are as follows:

- For children between 2 years and 10 years of age, the formula for endotracheal tube size is: the child's age (years)/4 + 4 cm.
- Cuffed endotracheal tubes should be 0.5 times smaller, to account for the diameter of the cuff and the formula is: the child's age (years)/4 + 3.5 cm.
- The depth of the endotracheal tube is measured at the lips, and for children over 2 years of age the formula is: the child's age (years)/2 + 12 cm.

Laryngospasm

Laryngospasm occurs more frequently in children than adults and is the most common life-threatening airway emergency in children. Laryngospasm describes the spasm of the vocal cords that causes the complete or partial closure of the glottis and obstruction of airflow to the trachea and lungs. This can be caused by stimulation during an inappropriate depth of anaesthesia such as during extubation, stimulation from laryngoscopy, or when an irritant is in contact with the vocal cords, such as blood and mucous [35].

It is vital to recognise laryngospasm promptly and treat it as quickly as possible. If the glottis is only partially obstructed, there may be a characteristic crowing noise, but if it is completely obstructed this will not be present and the airway will be silent. Depending on the degree of obstruction, paradoxical chest movement, intercostal recession, and tracheal tug will be visible and lead to a rapid decrease in oxygen saturation if left uncorrected. Primary treatment is:

- removing any triggering stimulation, including any supraglottic airway device;
- application of CPAP with 100% oxygen;
- if ventilation cannot be resumed, administer intravenous propofol 0.5 mg/kg;
- if laryngospasm continues, administer intravenous suxamethonium 1–2 mg/kg or, if intravenous access is unavailable, 4 mg/kg intramuscular [36].

Differences in Surgical Technique and Pathology

Basic surgical principles are the same for all age groups but, particularly in neonates and infants, extra care should be taken to prevent excessive blood loss and unnecessary trauma to tissues. Paediatric surgery mainly differs from adult surgery because of the distinctive nature of the pathology encountered in paediatric practice. Degenerative pathology is rarely seen, and relatively little tumour work is undertaken. Most of the paediatric surgery performed is elective, such as hernia repairs and the correction of undescended testicles. Common emergency procedures include pyloromyotomy for pyloric stenosis and appendicectomy [37].

Postoperative Effects of General Anaesthesia

Emergence delirium is described as the perceptual and psychomotor disturbances experienced during the post-anaesthetic period and is more prevalent in children aged 2–5 years [36]. It can cause uncontrolled thrashing movements, uncontrollable crying, distress, or confusion, and the child becomes uncooperative. There is a wide variation of emergence delirium for postoperative paediatric patients, with a sevoflurane identified as a major contributory factor. Propofol is thought to reduce the incidence of emergence delirium and supports the rationale for opting for an intravenous induction where this is feasible [36].

Postoperative nausea and vomiting (PONV) is approximately twice as common in children as in adults and contributes to postoperative morbidity, complications, and parental frustration [38]. The incidence of PONV increases in relation to the length of surgery, and intravenous induction of anaesthesia has shown to reduce the incidence of PONV in the postoperative phase [38].

Assessing postoperative pain in infants can be challenging and is best assessed using physiological parameters such as heart rate and blood pressure alongside behavioural indices such as facial expression, crying, and their overall demeanour. Older children may be able to use a visual analogue scale such as a five-point series of faces that have different colours and expressions. Whatever the child's age, and where possible, it is always worthwhile asking the parent or carer to contribute towards the assessment of their pain.

References

1. V. Chidambaran, A. Costandi, and A. D'Mello. Propofol: a review of its role in pediatric anesthesia and sedation. *CNS Drugs* 2015; **29**: 543–563.

2. V. Lesch. Anatomy, physiology and psychology. In E. Doyle (ed.), *Paediatric Anaesthesia*. Cambridge: Cambridge University Press, 2007, pp. 3–25.

3. J. Peyton, M. C. Gummerson, R. J. Ramamurthi, et al. Physics and anesthesia equipment. In K. Matthes, A. E. Laubach, and T. A. Anderson (eds.), *Pediatric Anesthesiology: A Comprehensive Board Review*. Oxford: Oxford University Press, 2015, pp. 21–41.

4. T. Goodman and C. Spry. *Essentials of Perioperative Nursing*. Burlington, MA: Jones & Bartlett Learning, 2016.

5. Advanced Paediatric Life Support Group. *Advanced Paediatric Life Support: A Practical Approach to Emergencies*. Chichester: Wiley-Blackwell, 2016.

6. A. A. Colin, C. McEvoy, and R. G. Castile. Respiratory morbidity and lung function in preterm infants of 32 to 36 weeks' gestational age. *Pediatrics* 2010; **126**: 115–128.

7. K. Nelson, C. Nicholls, and V. C. Muckler. Pediatric review and perioperative considerations. *Journal of Pediatric Nursing* 2018; **33**: 265–274.

8. R. S. Holzman. Fundamental differences between children and adults. In R. S. Holzman, T. J. Mancuso, and D. M. Polaner (eds.), *A Practical Approach to Pediatric Anesthesia*. Philadelphia, PA: Wolters Kluwer, 2016, pp. 22–44.

9. A. N. Borucki and H. Ellinas. Anatomy. In K. Matthes, A. E. Laubach, and T. A. Anderson (eds.), *Pediatric Anesthesiology: A Comprehensive Board Review*. Oxford: Oxford University Press, 2015, pp. 3–20.

10. S. Whyte and S. Butterworth. Paediatric cases. In J. Sturgess, J, Davies, and K. Valchanov (eds.), *A Surgeon's Guide to Anaesthesia and Peri-operative Care*. Cambridge: Cambridge University Press, 2014, pp. 168–180.

11. B. Kassai, M. Rabilloud, E. Dantony, et al. Introduction of a paediatric anaesthesia comic information leaflet reduced preoperative anxiety in children. *British Journal of Anaesthesia* 2016; **117**: 95–102.

12. M. Harvey and T. Geary. Preoperative assessment and preparation for safe paediatric anaesthesia. *Anaesthesia and Intensive Care Medicine* 2018; **19**: 401–408.

13. J. A. Short and J. K Jordan. Preoperative assessment and preparations for anaesthesia in children. *Anaesthesia and Intensive Care Medicine* 2015; **16**: 381–388.

14. R. Nandi. Pre-operative assessment for paediatric anaesthesia. In I. James and I. Walker (eds.), *Core Topics in Paediatric Anaesthesia*. Cambridge: Cambridge University Press, 2013, pp. 51–59.

15. M. Thomas, C. Morrison, R. Newton, et al. Consensus statement on clear fluids fasting for elective pediatric general anesthesia. *Pediatric Anesthesia* 2018; **28**: 411–414.

16. V. Ponde. Recent trends in paediatric regional anaesthesia. *Indian Journal of Anaesthesia* 2019; **63**: 746–753.

17. P. Lönnqvist. Adjuncts should always be used in pediatric regional anesthesia. *Pediatric Anesthesia* 2015; **25**: 100–106.

18. S. Byun and N. Pather. Pediatric regional anesthesia: a review of the relevance of surface anatomy and landmarks used for peripheral nerve blockades in infants and children. *Clinical Anatomy* 2019; **32**: 803–823.

19. N. M. Dave. Premedication and induction of anaesthesia in paediatric patients. *Indian Journal of Anaesthesia* 2019; **63**: 713–720.

20. J. D. Brioni, S. Varughese, R. Ahmed, et al. A clinical review of inhalation anesthesia with sevoflurane: from early research to emerging topics. *Journal of Anesthesia* 2017; **31**: 764–778.

21. T. Engelhardt and M. Weiss. A child with a difficult airway: what do I do next? *Current Opinion in Anaesthesiology* 2012; **25**: 326–332

22. M. A. Rodríguez-Calero, I. Blanco-Mavillard, J. M. Morales-Asencio, et al. Defining risk factors associated with difficult peripheral venous cannulation: a systematic review and meta-analysis. *Heart and Lung* 2020; **49**: 273–286.

23. N. Greene, S. Bhananker, R. Ramaiah. Vascular access, fluid resuscitation, and blood transfusion in pediatric trauma. *International Journal of Critical Illness and Injury Science* 2012; **2**: 135–142.

24. A. Hruby and F. B. Hu. The epidemiology of obesity: a big picture. *Pharmacoeconomics* 2015; **33**: 673–689.

25. D. Leslie, S. Froom, and C. Gildersleve. Equipment and monitoring for paediatric anaesthesia. *Anaesthesia and Intensive Care Medicine* 2015; **16**: 389–394.

26. I. Sen, N. Dave, N. Bhardwaj, et al. Specialised training in paediatric anaesthesia: need of the hour. *Indian Journal of Anaesthesia* 2021; **65**: 17–22.

27. T. G. Hansen. Developmental paediatric anaesthetic pharmacology. *Anaesthesia and Intensive Care Medicine* 2015; **16**: 417–422.

28. R. Bhansali and J. Armstrong. Smartphone applications for pediatric anesthesia. *Pediatric Anesthesia* 2012; **22**: 400–404.

29. L. Oswald, E. J Smith, M. Mathew, et al. The Ayre's T-piece turns 80: a 21st century review. *Pediatric Anesthesia* 2018; **28**: 694–696.

30. B. Patel and R. Bingham. Laryngeal mask airway and other supraglottic airway devices in paediatric practice. *Continuing Education in Anaesthesia Critical Care and Pain* 2009; **9**: 6–9.

31. Y. Passi, M. Sathyamoorthy, J. Lerman, et al. Comparison of the laryngoscopy views with the size 1 Miller and Macintosh laryngoscope blades lifting the epiglottis or the base of the tongue in infants and children <2 yr of age. *British Journal of Anaesthesia* 2014; **113**: 869–874.

32. R. Newton and H. Hack. Place of rapid sequence induction in paediatric anaesthesia. *BJA Education* 2016; **16**: 120–123.

33. R. Park, J. M. Peyton, J. E. Fiadjoe, et al. The efficacy of GlideScope® videolaryngoscopy compared with direct laryngoscopy in children who are difficult to intubate: an analysis from the paediatric difficult intubation registry. *British Journal of Anaesthesia* 2017; **119**: 84–992.

34. C. R. Bailey. Time to stop using uncuffed tracheal tubes in children? *Anaesthesia* 2018; **73**: 147–150.

35. S. Collins, P. Schedler, B. Veasey, et al. Prevention and treatment of laryngospasm

in the pediatric patient: a literature review. *AANA Journal* 2019; **87**: 145–151.

36. L. L. Reduque and S. T. Verghese. Paediatric emergence delirium. *Continuing Education in Anaesthesia Critical Care and Pain* 2013; **13**: 39–41.

37. Royal College of Surgeons of England. Paediatric surgery. Available from: www.rcseng.ac.uk/news-and-events/media-centre/media-background-briefings-and-statistics/paediatric-surgery/ (accessed 5 August 2021).

38. A. L. Kovac. Management of postoperative nausea and vomiting in children. *Pediatr-Drugs* 2007; **9**: 47–69.

Perioperative Pain Management

Senthil Jayaseelan

Chapter

34

What Is Pain?

The International Association for the Study of Pain (IASP) defines pain as 'an unpleasant sensory and emotional experience associated with, or resembling that associated with, actual or potential tissue damage' [1]. Pain expression is like a signature unique to each individual and it is strongly influenced by biological, psychological, and social factors. Pain in turn affects a person's mood, ability to function, and interactions with others.

How Can Pain Be Classified?

Pain can be classified according to the duration as well as the pathophysiology. Depending on the duration, pain can be acute (lasting for 3 months or less) or chronic (lasting more than 3 months). Patients with chronic pain can also present with acute exacerbation of existing pain or for a different reason with acute pain.

Depending on the pathophysiology, pain can be nociceptive, neuropathic, or mixed. Nociceptive pain is caused by tissue injury or inflammation. This usually happens after trauma or surgery to a body part or in inflammatory conditions such as arthritis. This type of pain is well localised to the body part affected and is usually felt as aching, throbbing, or squeezing or sharp discomfort.

Neuropathic pain is caused by a lesion or disease of the somatosensory nervous system. Patients can experience shooting or burning discomfort, often associated with numbness or tingling. This type of pain is not well localised and can be caused by various conditions such as painful diabetic neuropathy, shingles, and multiple sclerosis.

In many cases, both nociceptive and neuropathic conditions co-exist. A typical example is degenerative disc disease of the lumbar spine, giving rise to nociceptive back pain and neuropathic lower limb pain because of nerve irritation.

Why Should Pain Be Managed?

There are many advantages in managing pain effectively. It not only benefits the patient but also the patient's family and wider society [2]. In the immediate postoperative setting, good pain management enables quicker mobilisation and early recovery. This also helps in reducing complications like chest infections, myocardial ischaemia, urinary tract infections, and deep vein thrombosis [3]. This in turn facilitates early discharge from hospital and reduces healthcare costs. Effective management of acute pain also helps in reducing the incidence of developing chronic pain.

How Can We Assess Pain?

A patient's self-report of pain is the most reliable and useful indicator in the assessment because pain is a subjective experience. Occasionally, objective measures of pain behaviour are used in special situations to measure pain for people with cognitive impairment and in younger children.

When eliciting a pain history from a patient, it is very important to know the site, onset, character, radiation of pain to other areas of the body, associated symptoms, time course (i.e., does the pain follow a pattern in relation to time), exacerbating/relieving factors, and severity (easy-to-remember mnemonic: SOCRATES).

In the acute postoperative setting, it is very important to assess a patient's pain frequently and this should be done in conjunction with the measurement of other vital parameters. It is important to assess pain at both rest and on movement, including during breathing or coughing. Measurements of pain should be done before and after administration of analgesics.

Pain can be measured using unidimensional and multidimensional scales – multidimensional scales are predominantly used in chronic pain assessments. The commonly used self-report measurements in acute pain for adults are verbal rating scale, visual analogue scale, and numerical rating scale. In children, the commonly used self-report measurement of acute pain is the Wong–Baker Faces Pain Rating scale (Figure 34.1).

In patients who cannot self report pain, the CRIES scale can be used for infants, the COMFORT scale for children in intensive care or perioperative setting, and the Doloplus-2 or the Abbey pain scales for patients with cognitive impairment.

The following scales are also commonly used in adults:

- In the Verbal Rating Scale (VRS), patients are asked to describe their pain as none, mild, moderate, or severe.
- In the Numerical Rating Scale (NRS), patients are asked to rate their pain between 0 (when there is no pain) to 10 (worst pain imaginable).
- In the Visual Analogue Scale (VAS), patients are asked to mark a point on a 10-centimetre horizontal line, with the left-hand end representing no pain and the right-hand end representing the worst pain imaginable (Figure 34.2).

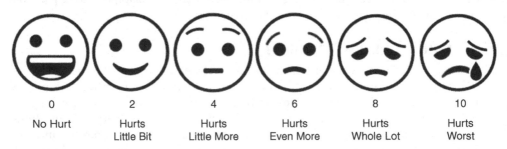

0	2	4	6	8	10
No Hurt	Hurts Little Bit	Hurts Little More	Hurts Even More	Hurts Whole Lot	Hurts Worst

Figure 34.1 Wong–Baker Faces Pain Rating scale (licenced under CC BY-SA 4.0)

0 (no pain)   10 (worst pain imaginable)

Figure 34.2 Visual Analogue Scale

The area of pain needs to be examined as part of the general examination of the patient to rule out any new pathology. In the acute postoperative setting, the predominant pain type is nociceptive, but patients can also experience neuropathic pain and, as a result show, mixed pain character.

Multidimensional scales are usually used in chronic pain assessments. The McGill Pain Questionnaire assesses pain under three main dimensions: sensory (discriminative}, motivational (affective), and cognitive (evaluative). Another example of a multidimensional tool is the Brief Pain Inventory, which has been validated for pain assessment in a variety of chronic pain conditions.

Recognition and assessment of pain are important to treat pain effectively and to improve outcomes, particularly in the perioperative setting. This will also help the health-care providers to choose the right form of treatment that can be used to help reduce the suffering secondary to pain.

Pain Physiology and Its Practical Application

To treat pain effectively, it is important to understand how pain is perceived by a patient because not every painful stimulus elicits a pain response. There are multiple steps in the pathway between the site of injury/nociceptive focus and the brain, which play an important role in the final output or the pain perception.

Transduction

In this step, the inciting event (injury/surgery) causes the release of inflammatory substances (substance P, prostaglandins etc.) in the tissues which activate the A-delta and C fibres in the periphery.

Transmission

The pain signal travels along the A-delta and C fibres to the dorsal horn of the spinal cord (first relay station) where they connect with the second-order neurons. The second-order nerves from there cross over to the other side of the spinal cord and travel up the spinothalamic tract to reach the thalamus (the second relay station). From there, the third-order neurons connect to the cortex, brainstem, and the limbic system.

Perception

The cortex, limbic system, and brainstem all contribute to pain perception. The cortex is responsible for the localisation of pain. The limbic system is responsible for the emotional component attached to pain and the brain stem is responsible for the reflex responses to pain and the coordination of pain modulation.

Modulation

The pain signal reaching the dorsal horn in the spinal cord can be modulated (the signal strength amplified or diminished) by signals from other peripheral nerves. There is also a descending inhibitory pathway from the brain stem to the spinal dorsal horn, which acts to inhibit the pain signals coming from the periphery. This balance between ascending and descending pathways is described in the gate theory developed by Melzack and Wall [4].

Different pain management strategies (pharmacological and non-pharmacological) work on the above steps in the pathway mentioned above. So, in successful management of pain, a multimodal approach is needed, which can address different parts of this pathway. Pain perception also depends on multiple factors including psychological factors, personality, social factors, cultural issues, and beliefs about pain. The presence of other illnesses can also influence perception.

Management of Pain

When treating pain, it is important to consider both non-pharmacological and pharmacological treatments.

Non-Pharmacological Management

Psychological

Simple explanation and reassurance play a very important role in allaying anxiety and fear. In some cases, involvement of psychologists in counselling can be very useful, especially in patients who have had major life changing events or in those with chronic pain issues.

Physical

Simple treatments like acupuncture, transcutaneous electrical nerve stimulation and physiotherapy are very useful in managing musculoskeletal pain. Surgery can also be part of the treatment of pain; for instance, the removal of an inflamed appendix or gallbladder, or drainage of an abscess.

Pharmacological Management

Pain management using medicines is a very useful and effective treatment strategy. Different medicines work on different parts of the pain pathway and because of this, we can combine pharmacological agents to help address the patient's discomfort and to reduce side effects from a higher dose of a single medication.

General Principles in Pharmacological Management

The World Health Organization (WHO) ladder is widely known in pain management. However, this was developed for management of pain in cancer as the pain gets worse over time. The WHO ladder recommends regular, oral administration of drugs starting from the use of simple analgesics in mild pain, weaker opioids with simple analgesics in moderate pain and use of strong opioids with simple analgesics in severe pain.

The above strategy does not work well in acute severe pain that is observed in postoperative settings. In this scenario, the WHO ladder will need to be reversed, starting at the at the top of the ladder and step down as the pain improves:

(1) severe pain – use of strong opioids (e.g., morphine) with simple analgesics (e.g., paracetamol);

(2) moderate pain – use of weaker opioids (e.g., codeine, tramadol) with simple analgesics; and

(3) mild pain – use of simple analgesics.

Pain Medications

Simple Analgesics

Paracetamol

Paracetamol is an effective analgesic for a broad range of conditions, especially when it is administered intravenously. The exact mechanism of paracetamol's action is unclear, but it is proposed that it inhibits prostaglandin synthesis in the central nervous system and may be involved in the activation of descending serotonergic pathways. Paracetamol can be given orally, intravenously, or rectally. The maximum dose is 4 grams in 24 hours in adults above 50 kg. The dose needs to be adjusted according to body weight in children and adults below 50 kg. Paracetamol is a safe drug that can be used in mild pain and can be combined with other medications for treating moderate to severe pain; it is also an effective antipyretic [5].

Non-Steroidal Anti-Inflammatory Drugs

Non-steroidal anti-inflammatory drugs (NSAIDs) are widely used in the treatment of mild to moderate pain. NSAIDs inhibit the cyclo-oxygenase 2 (COX-2) enzyme. COX-2 enzymes aid in the production of prostaglandins. Prostaglandins are lipid compounds, which are largely hormonal in effect and have varying effects on different tissues, one of which can be associated with inflammation and pain. NSAIDs inhibit the production of COX-2. Side effects of NSAIDs are gastrointestinal irritation, kidney injury, fluid retention, exacerbation of asthma/chronic obstructive pulmonary disease, bleeding risk, and hypotension. There are specific side effects (increased risk of myocardial infarction/stroke) with certain COX-2 inhibitors.

Opioids

Opioids work on the opioid receptors by closing the voltage-gated calcium channels. This is part of a wider processes which inhibits neurotransmitter release between neurons. Examples of weaker opioids include codeine and tramadol, and stronger opioids include fentanyl, morphine, and oxycodone.

All opioids work on the opioid receptors as agonists. Tramadol also inhibits the re-uptake of noradrenaline and 5-hydroxytryptamine (serotonin), thereby increasing the descending inhibitory signals in the spinal cord. Depending on the type of drug, opioids are available for enteral and parenteral use. The common side effects of opioids include nausea and vomiting, constipation, sedation, histamine release, muscle rigidity, meiosis, urinary retention, and pruritus.

The commonly used opioids in perioperative care in the UK are morphine, oxycodone, fentanyl, alfentanil, and remifentanil. They are administered through various routes such as oral, intramuscular, intravenous, and transdermal, depending on the clinical situation and type of the drug. One of the common routes of morphine/oxycodone administration post operatively in major surgeries is via a patient controlled analgesia (PCA) system (Figure 34.3). With PCA, a specified dose of the drug is delivered through an intravenous cannula when the patient activates the device by pressing a button. There is 'lock-out' period built in as a safety feature to prevent overdose.

Adjunct Drugs

There are certain drugs which can be useful as agents which by their mechanism of action can aid reduction of pain and also work on specific types of pain such as neuropathic pain. These drugs can be combined with other drugs mentioned above to reduce the side effects related to the use of a higher dosage of single medication.

Antidepressants

Drugs such as tricyclic antidepressants (amitriptyline, nortriptyline, imipramine) and selective serotonin re-uptake inhibitors (venlafaxine, duloxetine) can be useful in increasing the descending inhibitory signals in the spinal cord thereby reducing neuropathic pain.

Anticonvulsants

Drugs such as pregabalin and gabapentin reduce neurotransmitter release, which in turn reduces abnormal firing of pain nerves. Medications such as sodium valproate,

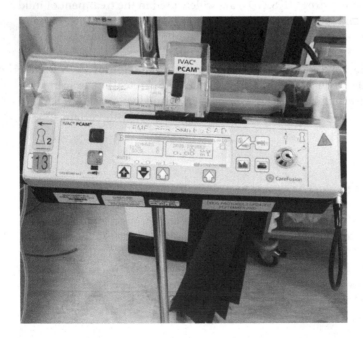

Figure 34.3 PCA machine with preloaded morphine syringe

carbamazepine, and phenytoin target the sodium channels and prevent them from returning to an active state, which reduces abnormal nerve transmission.

Ketamine

The N-methyl-D-aspartate (NMDA) receptor is involved in long-term signal potentiation. This receptor is inhibited by ketamine, which is widely used in anaesthetic and pain management (acute and chronic).

Clonidine

Clonidine is an agonist. It stimulates alpha-2 receptors, resulting in reduced sympathetic outflow. In the spinal cord clonidine augments endogenous opiate release involved in spinal nociceptive processing. Side effects of clonidine include drowsiness, fatigue, hypotension, and bradycardia. Rebound hypertension can occur if clonidine is stopped abruptly.

Local Anaesthetics

Local anaesthetics are widely used in blocking pain signals. They are used in peripheral nerve blocks or as an infiltration around the surgical site. They are also used in spinal and epidural anaesthesia. Local anaesthetics work by blocking the sodium channels. They are classified, based on the linkage between the lipophilic group and hydrophilic group in their structure, as esters (procaine, amethocaine, and cocaine) and amides (lidocaine, bupivacaine, ropivacaine, and prilocaine).

The dosage of local anaesthetics used depends on the body weight. The absorption of local anaesthetic varies with the site of administration and usage of vasoconstrictors. Higher levels of local anaesthetic in the blood can lead to central nervous system (circumoral tingling, visual disturbances, convulsions) and cardiovascular (arrythmias, hypotension, cardiac arrest) side effects.

Nerve Blocks in Acute Pain

Nerve blocks using local anaesthetics can be very useful in the perioperative setting in reducing the surgical stress response, intraoperative and postoperative analgesic requirements, avoiding general anaesthesia altogether, sometimes, and facilitating early discharge from the hospital [6].

Specific nerve blocks include brachial plexus block for upper limb procedures; erector spinae blocks and thoracic paravertebral blocks for rib fractures, and transversus abdominis plane blocks for anterior abdominal wall procedures such as Caesarean section. Central neuraxial blockade, which includes spinal, caudal, and epidural injections, can be used as a sole anaesthetic technique or in combination with general anaesthesia to provide excellent analgesia in the perioperative period.

Principles of Acute Pain Management in Chronic Pain Patients on Long-Term Opioids

The identification of patients on long-term opioids is an important part of preoperative assessment as they have higher analgesic requirements compared with other patients.

Multidisciplinary involvement including the surgical, anaesthetic, and pain teams is vital in proper planning of the perioperative care of such patients. The patient's background opioids will need to be prescribed to prevent withdrawal. Paracetamol and NSAIDs (if applicable) should be prescribed for their opioid-sparing effects. Regional anaesthetic techniques should be used whenever possible. Local policies must be in place for the use of opioids in neuraxial blocks, and they need to be clearly communicated to the staff looking after such patients and should be strictly followed. A short-term PCA using opioids can be considered for postoperative pain management. Whenever feasible, the pain team in the hospital should be involved as early as possible in their care. When discharging such patients to the community, clear communication to the patient's general practitioner about the drugs and dosages, including a weaning plan, is mandatory.

Chronic Post-Surgical Pain

The International Association for the Study of Pain defines this as persistent pain after surgery of greater than 3 months' duration. The reported incidence ranges between 5% and 50% [7]. There are many reasons for the development of chronic post-surgical pain (CPSP). The pathogenic mechanisms can be grouped into preoperative, intraoperative, and postoperative risk factors.

Preoperative Risk Factors

Preoperative factors include genetic (variation in pain sensitivity), psychosocial (presence of anxiety, depression, and passive coping), and the presence of long-term pain in the planned surgical area.

Intraoperative Risk Factors

Procedures involving surgical fields where major nerves cross (thoracotomy, amputation, breast surgery, and groin hernia repair) can lead to a higher incidence of CPSP. Intraoperative nerve injury can be a significant risk factor.

Postoperative Risk Factors

Increased postoperative pain is considered an independent risk factor for CPSP. Postoperative chemotherapy and radiotherapy can also lead to the development of long-term pain issues. Disease recurrence (e.g., malignancy, hernia) can also contribute to persistent pain.

How Can the Incidence of Chronic Post-Surgical Pain Be Reduced?

The identification of risk factors during the preoperative assessment, using specific nerve-sparing techniques (nerve identification, avoidance of involvement in sutures, mesh inflammation), laparoscopic techniques, and aggressive administration of multimodal analgesia intraoperatively and postoperatively can go a long way in reducing the incidence of persistent postoperative pain.

References

1. S. N. Raja, D. B. Carr, M. Cohen, et al. The revised International Association for the Study of Pain definition of pain: concepts, challenges, and compromises. *Pain* 2020; **161**: 1976–1982.

2. W. Morriss, R. Goucke, L. Huggins, et al. Essential pain management: workshop manual, 2nd edition, 2017. Available from: https://fpm.ac.uk/sites/fpm/files/docu ments/2020-02/EPM%20UK%20Workshop %20Manual%20.pdf.

3. N. E. Epstein. A review article on the benefits of early mobilization following spinal surgery and other medical/surgical procedures. *Surgical Neurology International* 2014; **5**: S66–S73.

4. R. Melzack and P. D. Wall. Pain mechanisms: a new theory. *Science* 1965; 150: 971–979.

5. T. E. Peck and B. Harris. *Pharmacology for Anaesthesia and Intensive Care*, 5th ed. Cambridge: Cambridge University Press, 2021.

6. M. J. Lenart, K. Wong, R. K. Gupta, et al. The impact of peripheral nerve techniques on hospital stay following major orthopedic surgery. *Pain Medicine* 2012; **13**: 828–834.

7. I. Tracey. Persistent post-operative pain: pathogenic mechanisms and preventive strategies. In H. Kehlet (ed.), *Pain 2012 Refresher Courses, 14th World Congress on Pain*. Seattle, WA: IASP Press, 2012, pp. 133–144.

Chapter 35

Recovery of Patients from Anaesthesia and Surgery

Patricia Smedley and Jane Nicholas-Holley

Introduction

The recovery unit, or post-anaesthetic care unit (PACU), is a relatively new concept arising from the high number of preventable deaths due to airway obstruction during the Second World War. Since that time, the need for an area, located near to theatres, where patients can recover safely from the immediate effects of anaesthesia and surgery has been developed to the point where post-anaesthetic care is now recognised as a unique critical care domain requiring a specialist environment and training.

The patient undergoing anaesthesia and surgery experiences profound physiological changes, as normal homeostasis is disrupted. Airway, breathing, and circulation are all affected. The patient may also suffer pain and nausea and vomiting, and experience anxiety. The patient remains within the PACU until they are stable enough to be discharged to the ward or other facility. It is the role of the PACU practitioner to anticipate and manage any complications that may arise during this volatile period. The PACU is a unique location where patients are at high risk from critical incidents. The PACU environment and training are tailored to recognise and enable effective management of emergencies and, if a complication develops beyond the scope of the PACU practitioner, to call for immediate help from the nearby anaesthetic and surgical teams. In the UK, the Royal College of Anaesthetists's guidelines for the provision of anaesthetic services for postoperative care highlight that the management of patients immediately after anaesthesia can potentially be hazardous and that serious complications can occur if adequate standards of care are not provided [1].

Clinical Environment

The PACU is an open plan area, with bays set up to accommodate the flow of patients arriving from theatre at one end and ideally exiting the unit at the other [1]. All bays must be easily observable, well lit to assess patient's skin colour and condition, and well ventilated to remove exhaled anaesthetic agents. The bays should have enough space around them to facilitate swift clinical intervention where complications arise and to comply with infection control policies [1]. There should be an emergency alarm by each bedside to call for help promptly. The PACU should provide a calm and quiet environment, away from the noise of nearby theatres [2]. Curtains or screens ensure that patient dignity and privacy are respected [3].

Patients emerging from anaesthesia can be classified by their care level:

Level 0: A patient whose needs can be met through normal ward care.

Level 1: A patient who is at risk of condition deteriorating, or recently relocated from higher level of care, whose needs can be met on an acute ward.

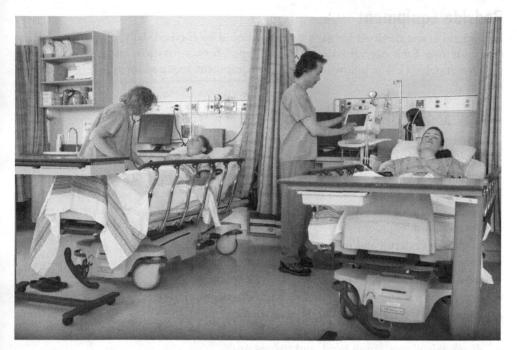

Figure 35.1 Recovery bay: open plan, curtains for privacy, equipment by each bay (image courtesy of Shutterstock)

Level 2: A patient who requires more detailed observation or intervention, including support for a single failing organ system or postoperative care and 'stepping down' from higher levels of care.

Level 3: A patient who requires advanced respiratory support or monitoring and support for two or more organ systems. This includes complex patients requiring support for multi-system failure.

Most patients leaving theatre and arriving in recovery will therefore be initially classified Level 2 and progress to Level 1 or Level 0 before being transferred to ward care. In specialist units such as those undertaking cardiothoracic surgery, Level 3 patients may be cared for in recovery.

As the PACU can provide Level 2 or potentially Level 3 care with suitable clinical support, critically ill patients may on occasion be transferred from the ward or emergency department if an intensive care unit (ICU) bed is unavailable. During the COVID-19 pandemic, some recovery units were called upon to provide full Level 3 care for prolonged periods.

Each bay area should ideally be furnished with several electrical outlets, one medical air outlet, one oxygen outlet, two vacuum outlets, an emergency call bell [1, 2], handwashing facilities. and a dirty utility to dispose linen, clinical waste, and other used items. A central station for computer facilities, telephones to call for outside help in an emergency, and an intercom to communicate directly with theatres are essential. This central area creates a space for staff information exchange, situated in an area where the entire unit can be seen.

Bedside Equipment

Equipment is standardised for each bay and should be checked daily, cleaned, and made ready for use. Each bay area should be equipped for air, oxygen, and suction through pipeline supply [1]. The following minimum equipment required for recovery is outlined below.

Airway and Breathing Equipment

The minimum equipment recommended for airway and breathing is as follows:

- oxygen supply, twin flowmeters, and tubing;
- a wall suction unit with tubing;
- a Yankauer suction tip and a full range of suction catheters;
- for paediatrics, a variety of paediatric equipment for suction, hand ventilation, and oxygen administration;
- Mapleson C circuit and/or bag–mask–valve apparatus;
- anaesthetic face masks with heat and moisture exchange filters;
- fixed- and variable-flow oxygen masks;
- oropharyngeal and nasopharyngeal airways: a selection of sizes;
- gauzes and receivers for laryngeal mask airways;
- syringes to deflate cuffed airway devices;
- disposable gloves, vomit bowl, and tissues; and
- personal protective equipment (where appropriate): goggles, masks, visors, and aprons.

Monitoring Equipment

Each bay will be equipped with a monitor, ECG, pulse oximeter, capnograph [1], non-invasive blood pressure cuffs, and thermometer, to comply with minimal safety requirements laid down by the Association of Anaesthetists [3]. In addition, invasive monitoring equipment for arterial blood pressure and central venous pressure must be available. Facilities for measurement of arterial blood gases should ideally be nearby.

Transfusion Equipment

The following transfusion equipment is recommended:

- syringes and needles;
- intravenous cannulas in a variety of sizes;
- intravenous dressings and adhesive tape;
- intravenous infusion giving sets,
- a wide variety of intravenous fluids, both crystalloid and colloid;
- alcohol wipes;
- tourniquets;
- a sharps disposal bin;
- an intravenous stand;
- infusion pumps; and
- pressure bags.

Drugs

The following drugs should be readily available:

- a selection of analgesics;
- a variety of antiemetic drugs;
- muscle relaxants and reversal agents, sedatives, opioids, and anaesthetic agents.

Miscellaneous

Miscellaneous items include the following:

- a warming cabinet;
- a blood fridge;
- portable suction and oxygen;
- a forced air warming device with blankets;
- an electric fan;
- clean blankets and linen;
- vomit bowls/receivers and tissues;
- gloves and other personal protective equipment;
- various dressings and bandages, etc.;
- a selection of urinary catheters and drainage bags;
- recovery charts; and
- incontinence pads.

Emergency Equipment

The following emergency equipment [3, 4] must be provided:

- an emergency arrest trolley: fully equipped and checked daily;
- reintubation equipment, defibrillator, and emergency drug box;
- a range of airways, supraglottic devices, and endotracheal tubes;
- invasive monitoring equipment and transducers;
- an anaesthetic machine and ventilator;
- a blood warmer;
- a cricothyroid puncture set;
- syringes for arterial blood gas analysis;
- a peripheral nerve stimulator; and
- a chest drain and clamps.

Daily Equipment Checks

All bay equipment, oxygen flowmeters, suction, and monitoring should be tested at the start of the shift. Disposables must be restocked, and a check made that a variety of oro- and nasopharyngeal airways are available. After each patient leaves, the area should be cleaned and decontaminated, and tubing replaced.

Staffing and Skill Mix

Allocation of staff to a changing patient population in the PACU must be flexible. The patient population in the PACU changes constantly, and each patient making a normal recovery undergoes rapid physiological change during this period. The Association of Anaesthetists recommends a minimum of two staff (one a registered practitioner) in the PACU whenever there is a patient who does not fill the criteria for discharge [1, 3].

Stage 1 recovery is where the patient condition may be unstable. Patients arriving in the PACU are cared for on a one-to-one basis until they have met the following criteria [3]. Stage 2 is when the patient is conscious and is:

- maintaining their own airway and breathing spontaneously;
- haemodynamically stable; and
- alert and responds to commands.

At this stage, a one practitioner to two patient ratio is standard. If the patient condition deteriorates, the ratio may change rapidly to two practitioners to one patient until transfer to a high dependency unit (HDU), or the ICU if necessary [5]. At stage 3 patients can be discharged into the care of a competent practitioner who is able to recognise and address any issues or concerns that may arise.

The process of constant assessment, evaluation, and prompt intervention always underpins patient care management in the PACU [6]. In the early stages of recovery, the process repeats rapidly, and observations may be recorded every 10 minutes. As the patient's condition stabilises, observations can be recorded every 15 minutes and, later, 30 minutes. While they remain in the PACU, all patients are under meticulous observation and are kept in the PACU until all discharge criteria have been met. There is no set time period. If complications occur the patient may require discharge to the HDU or ICU [3].

Staffing issues remain a constant problem; many PACUs have a staggered 'relief' system so that support comes in at busy times. Staffing the PACU is dependent on many other variables in the theatre complex, including list allocation [7]. No matter what pressures and constraints are put on the PACU, there should never be a compromise on safe staffing levels.

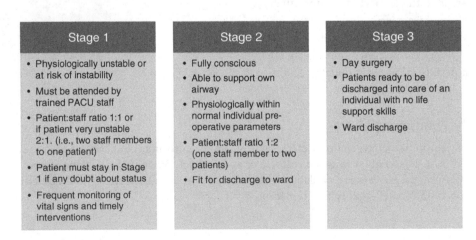

Stage 1	Stage 2	Stage 3
• Physiologically unstable or at risk of instability • Must be attended by trained PACU staff • Patient:staff ratio 1:1 or if patient very unstable 2:1. (i.e., two staff members to one patient) • Patient must stay in Stage 1 if any doubt about status • Frequent monitoring of vital signs and timely interventions	• Fully conscious • Able to support own airway • Physiologically within normal individual pre-operative parameters • Patient:staff ratio 1:2 (one staff member to two patients) • Fit for discharge to ward	• Day surgery • Patients ready to be discharged into care of an individual with no life support skills • Ward discharge

Figure 35.2 Stages of recovery

PACU Staff Training

The qualified PACU practitioner must be either:

- an adult or children's nurse registered with the Nursing and Midwifery Council; or
- an operating department practitioner registered with the Health and Care Professions Council.

PACU practitioners must be trained to local and national standards [1]. Formal training in higher education institutes is offered for post-registration nurses in post-anaesthetic care nursing. Operating department practitioners routinely undertake a 3-year degree in operating department practice, with a significant proportion of the course focused on providing post-anaesthetic care.

Where access to formal training courses in higher education institutes is not always easy, given staff shortages and financial constraints, many PACUs have their own in-house training schemes, which offer orientation programmes and continuing professional development opportunities. In-house training is based on the UK National Competencies for Post Anaesthetic Care [8]. It is important that regular updates and support is given in this acute critical area [3], and the need to review ongoing professional development is now mandatory with the revalidation process for registrants [9].

The practitioner must be trained to understand applied anatomy and physiology of all body systems, together with the principles of airway, respiratory, and circulatory management [1, 3]. Knowledge of fluid management, thermoregulation, pain, and the management of nausea and vomiting are essential. Understanding of the management of emergencies, malignant hyperthermia, laryngospasm, respiratory and cardiac arrest, and suxamethonium apnoea are also needed [10]. The depth and range of knowledge required for working in the PACU is far reaching and encompasses patients of all ages who may have varying degrees of morbidity. Furthermore, there is the need to understand the complications arising from a range of surgical procedures and specialities. PACU practice involves a wide range of clinical skills, which should be highly valued; training in advanced cardiac life support is recommended [3].

Applying theory to practice is part of the ongoing experiential learning in the PACU. Each registered practitioner should be able to take over the patient from the anaesthetist and deal with routine expected problems as they occur. A senior practitioner should be free to supervise all patients, intervene when necessary, and call for anaesthetic help if the patient condition deteriorates. In addition to trained staff, nursing associates, healthcare assistants, and associate practitioners increasingly work in the PACU under supervision of registered staff. Their training is constantly under review and development [11].

Patient Handover

The patient is escorted from theatre to the PACU by the anaesthetist and a member of the theatre team. Oxygen is delivered en route to the PACU and the patient is immediately re-attached to wall oxygen on arrival. Two PACU practitioners receive the patient to ensure a safe handover of care [10]. The handover period represents a complex web of rapid assessment and communication of patient details from the anaesthetist and theatre staff to the PACU practitioner. At the same time, the patient to being attached to monitoring and the first patient assessment made. It is the responsibility of the anaesthetist to ensure that the handover is accomplished safely [1, 3].

Principles of care involve SAFE:

S – supply oxygen;

A – attach monitoring;

F – first assess immediate care needs before

E- effectively communicating; commence verbal handover via SBAR.

SBAR is a tool which ensures a structured verbal handover and can improve communication and patient safety [12]:

Situation:

- the patient's name and age; and
- the operation undergone.

Background:

- any past medical history of note;
- drug allergies;
- the anaesthetic technique (including airway management);
- the analgesia and antiemetics administered;
- the intravenous fluid regime; and
- any surgical or anaesthetic intraoperative event or complication (difficult airway management, blood loss, cardiovascular instability).

Assessment:

- airway: airway status, anticipated airway difficulty;
- breathing: respiratory status, anticipated breathing difficulty; and
- circulation: cardiovascular status, anticipated cardiovascular difficulty.

Recommendations:

- requirement for ongoing monitoring (e.g., central venous pressure, end-tidal carbon dioxide ($ETCO_2$));
- an analgesic plan;
- antiemesis;
- fluid management;
- investigations in the PACU: blood test (full blood count), chest X-ray, blood glucose;
- Additional information: drains, special dressings; and
- postoperative instructions.

The anaesthetist should not leave the patient until satisfied that breathing is spontaneous and that the PACU practitioner is ready to take over care [1, 3].

Planning Patient Care

The PACU practitioner will analyse the patient risk factors from the handover information, the anaesthetic chart, and the patient notes, combined with their initial physical assessment. Understanding the risk factors enables the practitioner to plan interventions to pre-empt risks from becoming complications [13]. For example, the elderly patient having undergone complex prolonged major abdominal surgery may be at risk from hypovolaemia, a delayed return to full consciousness, hypothermia, and so on. If the patient also has a cardiac history, then the risk increases; risk analysis is key to successful outcomes in the PACU.

ABCDE Assessment

The ABCD algorithm underpins patient care management in the PACU [14]. The rationale is simple. The airway (A) must be clear to enable breathing to take place. Breathing (B) ensures that blood is oxygenated for transport to the tissues by the circulation (C). There is no point in focusing first on circulation if the airway or breathing are compromised. D stands for disability and generally describes the patient's neurological status. E is for exposure, which includes thermoregulatory status, wound, dressings and drains. We will consider patient care in this order: ABCDE.

A: Airway

The mix of induction and maintenance drugs given to administer general anaesthesia along with anaesthetic techniques disturbs the normal mechanisms that maintain the open airway. From the onset of unconsciousness, the airway is at risk of obstruction. The pharyngeal muscles holding the tongue in place are weakened and the protective reflexes (swallow, gag, and cough) are lost.

Significant obstruction to free air flow will quickly result in hypoxia and a build-up of carbon dioxide. Total obstruction can result in brain death within around 4 minutes [15].

From the point of induction, the airway must be maintained until the patient is awake and muscle tone returns, together with the protective reflexes. Most often, the anaesthetist will use a supraglottic airway device or endotracheal tube to secure the airway intraoperatively. Ideally, the patient awakens on the table at the end of the procedure and regains airway control. The patient, however, may be brought to the PACU unconscious or semiconscious and thus the airway remains the first priority of care [16].

There are many causes of obstruction immediately following anaesthesia and surgery:

- oral secretions, blood, regurgitation of stomach contents;
- the tongue;
- weakened pharyngeal muscles;
- foreign bodies, such as loose teeth, dentures, throat pack; and
- obstructive sleep apnoea.

Airway Assessment

The Look, Listen, and Feel schema is used to comprehensively assess the patient airway [5] (see also Table 35.1):

- Look: patient colour, saturation of oxygen, misting on mask, respiratory rate and pattern;
- Listen: for sound of breathing; and
- Feel: for breath at nose, and mouth.

In addition to a physical assessment, the experienced practitioner will undertake a calculation of risk factors that may predispose towards obstruction. The unconscious supine patient, with no airway adjunct is a risk. Ear, nose, and throat and dental surgical

Table 35.1 Signs of a clear airway, or partial or total obstruction

Clear airway	Partial obstruction	Total obstruction
Colour pink	Pallor setting in	Pallor to rapid onset cyanosis
Oxygen saturation: 96–100%	Falling saturation/value in low 90s	Saturation falls below 90% or unrecordable
ETCO$_2$ within normal limits	Rising ETCO$_2$	Rising ETCO$_2$
Mask misting	Limited misting	No misting on mask
Feel of air at nose and mouth	Limited feel	No feel of air at nose or mouth
Breathing regular, coordinated	Breathing laboured, irregular, use of accessory muscles	Excessive use of accessory muscles, paradoxical breathing pattern
Breathing quiet, not silent	Noisy breathing, snore, gurgle, crowing noise	Absolute silence – no air passing through vocal cords
Blood pressure and heart rate stable	Tachycardia	Tachycardia, fall in blood pressure Arrhythmias

patients constitute a risk for bleeding or throat packs left in situ, and patients who are obese can obstruct more easily. Immediate pre-emptive intervention will hopefully prevent these risks becoming complications [13].

Intervention and Evaluation

Intervention whether preventative or corrective are considered in three stages [17].

Stage 1 Interventions

Stage 1 interventions are as follows:

- full-flow oxygen;
- use of the oropharyngeal airway to keep tongue away from back of throat;
- use of the chin lift or jaw thrust to lift the tongue away from back of throat (see Figures 35.3 and 35.4);
- suction to clear airway of secretions – a Yankauer suction tip can be used to suction towards the front of the mouth; soft suction catheters are used to penetrate further back into the throat;
- the recovery position to drain secretions; and
- the removal of any foreign body.

A jaw thrust is the most effective way of pulling the mandible forward and releasing the tongue from the back of the oropharynx. The effectiveness of each intervention is evaluated. If there is no improvement, another technique can be tried if a patient's overall status remains stable.

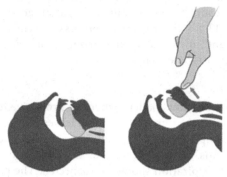

- With one hand on top of head tilt head backwards, while with two fingers of other hand, you lift the chin upwards into the air.

- This manoeuvre should move the tongue forwards to open the airway.

Figure 35.3 Opening up the airway by chin tilt manoeuvre

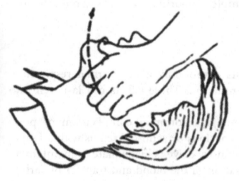

- Grasp the angle of the lower jaw on both sides and lift, moving the jaw forwards.

- If lips are closed, move the lower lip with your thumb to allow air passage.

Figure 35.4 Jaw thrust manoeuvre

Stage 2 Interventions

If the patient deteriorates and obstruction remains a threat, then call for help and deliver oxygen via positive-pressure ventilation using a bag–valve mask or Water's circuit (Mapleson C) while waiting for anaesthetic help. At this stage, the emergency intubation trolley needs to be ready by the bedside, with the appropriate equipment and drugs ready.

Stage 3 Interventions

At this stage it may be necessary to re-intubate the patient, dependent on the anaesthetic assessment. The anaesthetist will need assistance with intubation equipment. Suxamethonium should be drawn up and ready to facilitate intubation. The anaesthetist may need to arrange for the patient to be transferred to the HDU or ICU.

Laryngospasm

This is an airway complication which can lead quickly to serious hypoxia. The vocal cords lie at the narrowest point of the adult airway and allow the passage of air from upper to lower airway. They open and close to produce voice vibrations. They are delicate structures which can go into spasm, where the cords become partially closed. This can be caused by secretions, traumatic intubation or extubation, or surgical manipulation. A tell-tale 'crowing noise' may be heard, unique to the spasm, in association with the other signs of obstruction listed above [18]. See Chapter 33 for the treatment process. Laryngospasm should always be treated as an emergency and, if reintubation is required, it will be the anaesthetist's decision on when to attempt to extubate again.

Aspiration

Aspiration may take place in the semi- or unconscious patient while the protective mechanisms of cough, swallow, and gag are diminished or absent. Vomitus leaves the stomach and travels up the oesophagus and down the unprotected trachea. Acidic vomit reaches the lungs where it can cause dangerous pneumonitis. If there are signs of airway deterioration, or a trickle of aspirate oozes from the mouth, aspiration should be suspected. The patient should be turned on their left side with their head down and suctioned. Careful observation must be maintained for signs of failing respiratory performance. Anaesthetic help should be summoned immediately. A chest X-ray may be indicated [19]. Treatment is dictated by the severity of the symptoms and may range from simple supportive measures to reintubation, bronchoscopy, and ventilation in the ICU.

B: Breathing

Drugs and agents given for general anaesthesia profoundly affect normal respiration, resulting in respiratory depression and hypoventilation. These effects can last well into the recovery stage as seen in Table 35.2 [16].

Also, Table 35.2 shows that hypoventilation is a common complication of post-anaesthetic care, where the patient presents unconscious or semi-conscious with a falling respiratory rate and shallow breathing. The respiratory drive is inadequate to maintain an alveolar ventilation rate that will ensure oxygenation of the blood and transfer of carbon dioxide back into the atmosphere [5]. The airway is at risk of obstruction during this period.

Thoracic or abdominal surgery may cause hypoventilation as breathing can be painful and effort falls.

A full assessment is recommended; it is imperative to look, listen, and feel (see Figure 35.5):

- Respiratory deterioration can happen quickly or in stages.
- Examine the skin for signs of hypoxia from pallor to cyanosis (late stage of hypoxia).
- Falling oxygen saturation to a value in the lower 90s denotes significant hypoxia and hypoventilation along with rising $ETCO_2$.
- Monitor carefully for diminished rate and depth of respiration.
- Diminished misting on mask or feel of exhaled air denotes hypoventilation.
- Pinpoint pupils suggests overuse of opioids.
- These signs usually accompany the unconscious or semi-conscious state where the airway is also at risk [15].

Risk Assessment

A risk assessment enables the practitioner to anticipate problems or identify the root of the problem when it occurs. How long was the procedure? What was total dose of opioids given

Table 35.2 Anaesthetic drug mix and their effect on breathing

Drug group and name	Intraoperative action	Residual effect in the PACU
Induction drugs	Render patient unconscious Airway at risk	Contribute to hypoventilation
Maintenance drugs (triad)		
1. Hypnotic: anaesthetic agents	In combination, hypnotic and narcotics render the patient unconscious and depress the action of respiratory centre, making it less sensitive to carbon dioxide stimulus to breathe	Respiratory rate and depth (i.e., tidal volume) fall, leading to sedation and *hypoventilation*
2. Narcotic: analgesia		If not corrected, it can produce hypoxia and hypercarbia
3. Muscle relaxant	All muscles are paralysed to enable ventilation and tissue handling Breathing must be supported until relaxants are reversed or wear off at the end of procedure	It may leave a residual effect of muscle weakness affecting respiratory muscles and contributing to *hypoventilation*
Sedative	Given to settle the patient intraoperatively	The after effects can last well into the recovery stage and can contribute to sedation and *hypoventilation*

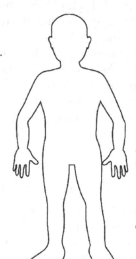

Airway
Noisy breathing indicates obstruction. Silence indicates total obstruction.

Breathing
Severe respiratory distress indicated by
- Shallow or slow breaths or rise in respiratory rate.
- Irregular breathing pattern.
- Use of accessory muscles.
- Unequal chest movement.
- Limited air entry on auscultation.
- Dyspnoea, work of breathing increased.

Sensorium
Agitation, confusion, restlessness are classic signs of cerebral hypoxia. Delayed return to consciousness indicates respiratory depression.

Colour
Pallor – **cyanosis** at lips or conjunctivae are signs of severe **hypoxia**.

Cardiovascular
Raised heart rate indicates compensation.

Figure 35.5 Indicators of impaired respiratory function

and when? Was midazolam used? Was the muscle relaxant reversed? Is the patient elderly, obese, or a smoker? Elderly patients are especially at risk of hypoventilation as their respiratory centre response to carbon dioxide levels is not so brisk [13].

Intervention

Intervention must be directed towards delivering more oxygen to the lungs. Oxygen at full flow is delivered and the airway is managed. The stir-up regime may be trialled by calling the patient and applying gentle massage. If there is no response, and consciousness remains impaired, help must be sought, and the bag–valve mask or Mapleson C circuit used to deliver oxygen via positive pressure [15]. The emergency airway trolley should be assembled including drugs to reverse the effect of opioids.

Specific Antagonists

If naloxone is used to reverse the sedative effect of opioids, the patient may awaken and make an improved respiratory effort, but the analgesic effects will also be reversed, which may cause pain-control difficulties. Furthermore, the opiate effect may outlast the effect of naloxone, leading to a late return of the opiate effect. Flumazenil is a specific antagonist or reversal agent for benzodiazepines, which may improve the conscious level and airway patency, but it should be used with caution as it is not without side effects of its own, ranging from mild (anxiety, tremor, vomiting) to more severe effects such as seizures [16]. The anaesthetist will decide on the treatment, especially whether to use one of these drugs or to provide supportive therapy such as ventilatory support. The effect of antagonists on pain control and patient comfort must be carefully considered.

Residual Paralysis

This is a relatively common complication in patients who have received muscle relaxants that have not been adequately reversed. Typically, the patient displays weak muscle control over limbs and the neck. If asked to grip the hand, the response is weak. Sticking out the tongue and keeping it out is impossible, as is sustained head lift. The respiratory muscles may be weak, and the patient can panic as they feel they cannot breathe properly. Reassuring the patient while eliciting immediate help is vital. The anaesthetist may test neuromuscular blockade with a nerve stimulator, although this can be uncomfortable in the conscious patient. Neostigmine with or without glycopyrrolate may be helpful, or sugammadex may be indicated where rocuronium has been used. In severe cases, sedation and ventilatory support may be required. High-flow oxygen and psychological support are essential [20].

C: Circulation

Anaesthesia and surgery may interfere with homeostasis in the following ways:

- Anaesthetic drugs and agents produce widespread vasodilation and systemic vascular resistance (afterload) falls. If cardiac output is insufficient to compensate, blood pressure will fall. The cardiac output may also be affected by the anaesthetic agents which depress cardiac muscle contractility, resulting in a lowered cardiac output.
- Cardiac arrhythmias can compromise the cardiac output and blood pressure. For example, neostigmine may induce bradycardia (heart rate below 50 beats per minute (bpm)) with a fall in cardiac output and in blood pressure. Conversely, cyclizine may cause a tachycardia (heart rate above 100 bpm).

- Stress caused by anxiety and pain can cause tachycardia. This poses a threat to the cardiac patient as the heart works harder and requires more oxygen, which can challenge the weak heart. Sustained tachycardia also impacts on cardiac output as the period of diastole (during which the ventricles fill) is shortened. Tachycardia can also be caused by volume loss as the heart compensates by beating faster.
- Fluid loss caused by bleeding, or clear fluid loss from open surgery, may cause hypotension. While a haemorrhage will quickly diminish venous return, eventually an interstitial or intracellular fluid deficit will also compromise intravascular blood volume. When venous return (preload) is seriously impaired the stroke volume diminishes, leading to a fall in cardiac output and blood pressure. Hypovolaemia is the most common reason for postoperative hypotension [5].
- In regional anaesthesia, epidural and spinal techniques interfere with the normal state of partial vasoconstriction of blood vessels and cause them to dilate, leading to a fall in afterload and in blood pressure if fluids are insufficient to fill the arteries and veins.
- Myocardial damage due to the intraoperative challenge to a weak heart may be a silent but sinister reason for hypotension. Myocardial contractility diminishes and fails to deliver an adequate stroke volume. Cardiac output and blood pressure falls.

Hypotension is the most common haemodynamic complication in the PACU. It can range from a continuum of mild, residual hypotension caused by the anaesthetic drug mix, to severe hypotension as in shock [5]. Shock is a life-threatening condition of circulatory failure, resulting in inadequate oxygen delivery to meet cellular metabolic needs and oxygen consumption requirements, producing cellular and tissue hypoxia. For more on the cardio-vascular system, see Chapter 8. Table 35.3 demonstrates the impact of continuing haemor-rhagic blood loss on vital signs, urine, and mental status.

What is clear from Table 35.3 is how the heart rate rises steadily with fluid loss to deliver the diminishing stroke volume. Blood pressure remains normal due to increased systemic vascular resistance and tachycardia. However, a point is reached beyond which the blood pressure falls. The respiratory rate increases steadily to hyper-oxygenate the blood in order to compensate for the failing circulation. Urine output falls rapidly to less than 30 mL hourly as the pressure exerted on the renal tubules falls. The patient becomes steadily more anxious and confused as cerebral hypoperfusion occurs. The skin and circulatory changes are not noted in Table 35.3. However, peripheral constriction sets in to preserve fluid for the core primary organs, brain, lungs, and kidneys. Capillary refill time is prolonged and pulses become faint. The skin may adopt a greyish tone, feeling moist, cool, and clammy to the touch [15].

Risk Assessment

As with breathing, understanding the risks ensures that planning includes how to prevent them from becoming complications. Where complications ensue, an awareness of the risk factors helps analyse the contributory factors and effect prompt interventions [13]. Factors to consider include:

- Is there an abnormal baseline BP?
- Is there a cardiac history?
- Was there intraoperative blood or fluid loss and replacement?
- Is pain and stress causing tachyarrhythmias and its treatment?
- Consider the drugs mix – is there a myocardial depressant effect?

Table 35.3 Class of haemorrhagic shock showing changes in vital signs

	Class of haemorrhagic shock			
	I	II	III	IV
Blood (mL)	Up to 750	750–1,500	1,500–2,000	>2,000
Blood loss (% blood volume)	Up to 15	15–30	30–40	>40
Heart rate (per minute)	<100	100–120	120–140	<140
Blood pressure	Normal	Normal	Decreased	Decreased
Respiratory rate (bpm)	14–20	20–30	30–40	>35
Urine output (mL/h)	>30	20–30	5–15	Negligible
Mental status	Slightly anxious	Mildly anxious	Anxious, confused	Confused, lethargic

- Consider the use of regional anaesthesia (e.g., spinal epidural with resultant vasodilation)?
- Is there is widespread peripheral constriction, will there be a fall in pressure when the peripheries open up?
- Is the monitoring sufficient for management? Is there a need for hourly urine measurements, or central and arterial lines?

Treatment depends on the severity of hypotension. Table 35.4 outlines the main treatment lines.

Treatment

Treatment is aimed towards correcting the problem, which should be evident on assessment. High-flow oxygen is given for this condition. Fluid replacement with crystalloids or colloids is indicated in most cases to boost the cardiac output but inotropes may be required. Blood replacement may be required if bleeding is the cause. If the patient is haemorrhaging, then a careful estimate of ongoing fluid loss needs to be kept (monitor drainage: check pads and dressings; measure abdominal girth). Estimate the loss in irrigating fluid for genitourinary surgery, or loss per vagina in gynaecological surgery. Repeat bloods for full blood count and clotting studies. Fresh frozen plasma may be administered [15]. The patient may have to return to theatre. Heart damage may have occurred. A 12-lead ECG and bloods for cardiac enzymes will be taken. The goal must be to relax the work of the heart and allow to heal.

Hypertension

If the blood pressure is 20% above the preoperative normal blood pressure, the patient is considered hypertensive and may require treatment. There are many causes of hypertension

Table 35.4 Causes of hypotension and main lines of treatment

	Residual hypotension	Arrhythmias	Fluid loss	Spinal/epidural	Cardiac insufficiency
Rationale/action	Caused by a mix of drugs on the heart and vessels. Wait and see – the condition may stabilise. Check before sending to ward	Drugs, hypoxia, potassium imbalance. Correct underlying cause	Most common cause of hypotension. Check fluid balance, infuse fluids as per regime. Central venous pressure monitoring may be required	Vasodilation caused by sympathetic nerve interruption. Cardiac depression may result from high block	Myocardial insufficiency from ischaemia – may be irreversible (myocardial infarction). ECG and bloods for enzymes
Oxygen	Yes	Yes			
Fluids	Yes	Yes	Fluid regime may require updating to increase fluid delivery	Fluid regime may require an increase	Fluids with caution
Position	Legs raised to increase venous return (Trendelenburg tilt)	Supine	Legs raised to increase venous return (Trendelenburg tilt)	Apply caution in Trendelenburg tilt as high block may arise and worsen hypotension	Legs raised to increase venous return when required
Drugs	No action may be required. Supportive measures may be necessary	For bradycardia give intravenous glycopyrrolate or atropine	May need vasopressor: metaraminol or phenylephrine	Vasopressor: metaraminol, or phenylephrine. May require anticholinergic (e.g., glycopyrrolate if bradycardic)	Diamorphine, Glyceryl trinitrate, Vasopressors and inotropes may be required
Return to theatre	Not necessary	Not necessary	May be necessary if there is active bleeding	No, but anaesthetic input is required	Transfer to critical care area: ICU, critical care unit, or HDU
Monitor	Ongoing monitoring and assessment →				
Warm	Maintain normothermia →				

including pain, anxiety, shivering, hypoxia, airway obstruction, hypothermia, full bladder, and over transfusion. Treat the pain and allay anxiety, sit the patient up, make them comfortable. If distension of the bladder is causing upset, then catheterise the patient; warm them and if they are overloaded, maintain fluid restriction, and administer diuretics. At all times treat hypoxia. If these interventions do not bring down the blood pressure, then pharmacological intervention may be required.

D: Disability – Neurological Status

Emergence Delirium

Agitation leading to mild aggression is not uncommon in the immediate phase of regaining consciousness from general anaesthesia. Usually this settles within minutes, with careful handling. Delirium may be caused by the residual effect inhalational agents (e.g., sevoflurane and desflurane) or hypoxia, pain, or hypoglycaemia. Young adults can be prone to this, but the elderly are especially at risk. Delirium in children is common and those who were agitated prior to surgery are likely to suffer this postoperatively. Inadequate pain control in children is another contributory factor. Treatment for this condition includes administration of 100% oxygen, which should rectify hypoxia as a contributory or main reason for delirium. Reassurance, reorientation, and ensuring the patient's physical safety are important to calm the patient and prevent injury. The anaesthetist should be notified if these measures fail to improve the situation [15]. Neurological injury should be considered as a possible cause if the patient does not improve.

Delayed Emergence from Anaesthesia

Regaining consciousness after general anaesthesia varies between patients but emergence usually follows an orderly sequence. Look for the return of pupil reaction, return of facial expression, gross movement of limbs. The mixture of opioids, volatiles, and sedatives such as midazolam is the most common cause of delayed emergence. If the cause can be attributed to one of the above, drug therapy may be considered – flumazenil for benzodiazepines or naloxone for opioids. Hypothermia prolongs the unconscious state, increasing the effect of residual volatile agents, and delaying drug metabolism and excretion. Hypercapnia, hypovolaemia, and hypoglycaemia can also cause delayed emergence. These conditions need to be corrected [5].

Neurological damage should be suspected if the unconscious state is accompanied by a new one-sided immobility, rigidity, weakness, drooping on side of face or mouth, or dilated or non-reacting pupil. Imaging such as CT scanning should be considered in delayed emergence, especially in the presence of new neurological signs such as one-sided weakness, seizures, or asymmetrical pupils.

E: Exposure – Thermoregulatory Status, Surgical Dressings, and Drains

Thermoregulatory Disturbance

Exposure is the final stage of the ABCDE assessment and requires a head-to-toe examination of the patient while being mindful of maintaining the patient's dignity throughout. Normothermia is between 36.5 °C and 37.5 °C. Within the perioperative environment body heat can be lost through convection, conduction, radiation, and evaporation mechanisms

[15]. Hypothermia is a core temperature below 36 °C. There are many contributory factors to hypothermia in the operative environment. The patient is starved and placed on a trolley with minimal covering. Heat is normally generated by the metabolism of foods to release energy, and an appropriate ambient temperature reduces the patient's heat loss. The induction of general anaesthesia vasodilates the vessels, enhancing the loss of central core heat to the atmosphere through the above mechanisms. Intraoperatively, the patient is static, with no muscular activity in the form of shivering to generate heat, and is exposed to often low ambient temperatures.

The importance of maintaining normothermia along the perioperative journey has now been well established with recommendations from the National Institute for Health and Care Excellence followed in the UK [21]. Hypothermia can delay recovery by prolonging the action of drugs like propofol and fentanyl, and increasing the concentration of volatiles. It brings discomfort and vasoconstriction leading to poor circulatory flow, delays wound healing, and promotes infection. Shivering increases oxygen consumption, adding to any strain on the cardiovascular system. The use of warming blankets is now an established practice. Ensuring that normothermia is maintained from core to periphery is important. The temperature should be monitored routinely along the patient journey and hypothermia treated at each stage.

Surgical Dressings and Drains

Inspection of the wound site on arrival and at intervals throughout the stay in the PACU is an important part of the assessment. A dry dressing indicates that there is no bleeding from the suture line. Moderate seepage of sero-sanguinous fluid alerts the practitioner to maintain vigilance. It is not necessary to expose the wound site (to possible infection) unless there is fresh blood oozing from the wound. Wound drains should be checked for blood on arrival – and, where possible, the level of drainage marked with the time so that the practitioner can review the speed and volume of drainage. Where excessive, the surgeon should be informed and can decide on further action.

Bladder irrigation following trans-urethral resection of prostate also requires a close examination of blood loss. Pink fluid in the drainage bag is normal, but if the drainage is red, this indicates excessive bleeding from the prostate bed. The surgeon should be called and may advise traction – suspending the irrigation bag to apply traction to the operative site, and blood transfusion may be needed.

Postoperative Pain Control

Pain is activated by tissue damage but is felt only when perceived in the brain. It is therefore a complex subjective experience; it is what the patient says it is [5]. There are many factors that contribute to the individual perception of pain: past experience, age, sex, culture, anxiety, fatigue, and so on. Both pain and anxiety are recognised in the limbic area of the brain and share a close relationship. Uncontrolled anxiety exacerbates pain and makes it more difficult to manage and therefore must be considered in pain control.

Pain assessment is a skill honed with experience. The experienced practitioner will consider many variables: the nature of the surgery, analgesic management intraoperatively, age, sex, signs of stress (raised blood pressure, heart rate, facial expression). However, patient self-report of pain remains the gold standard of assessment. A range of different assessment tools have been developed to elicit patient perception of the intensity of pain [22]. Some examples here:

(1) visual analogue scales;

(2) verbal rating scales;

(3) numerical rating scales; and

(4) verbal descriptor scales.

The aim of pain management is to promote patient comfort during the postoperative phase.

A multimodal analgesic regimen is the norm, with the combined use of opioids, non-steroidal anti-inflammatory drugs (NSAIDs), local anaesthetics, and simple analgesia [22]. This approach avoids heavy doses of opioids in perioperative care and ensures that, using different modes of delivery, the patient is comfortable throughout his perioperative journey.

Multimodal Analgesia

Different delivery methods allow drugs to be taken up at different rates, which means that their effect can be planned to dovetail ensuring continuous pain relief. Local, regional, intravenous, and rectal routes of administration all have their benefits. The use of patient delivery devices such as patient-controlled analgesia (PCA) empowers the patient to manage their pain levels (see Figures 35.6 and 35.7).

Drugs Used in Multimodal Analgesia

Simple Analgesia

Examples of simple analgesics include paracetamol (known as co-codamol when mixed with codeine). Paracetamol given intravenously along with opioids potentiates the effect of the opioids and improves pain control substantially [16].

Non-steroidal Anti-inflammatory Drugs

Examples of NSAIDs include ibuprofen and diclofenac. These drugs act on the local inflammatory response to any painful stimulus. They can be given safely in addition to opioids because they act locally and provide a slow-release background analgesia, which lasts beyond the immediate recovery period. Importantly, they do not cause respiratory depression.

Opioids

Examples of opioids include morphine, fentanyl, and tramadol. They act in the central nervous system to reduce discomfort and can be considered the drugs of choice for severe acute pain in the post-anaesthetic period. Incremental doses are given intraoperatively so that, by the time the patient reaches the PACU, their blood levels are therapeutic. An estimate of the quantity of opioids and time delivering during surgery is important before administrating further doses. Opioids can cause respiratory depression and nausea and vomiting; they must be used with care, and the patient monitored carefully. Tramadol is a relatively new mild opioid with respiratory depressant side effects and it may cause nausea and vomiting.

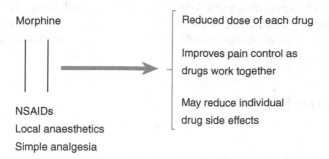

Figure 35.6 Multimodal analgesia rationale

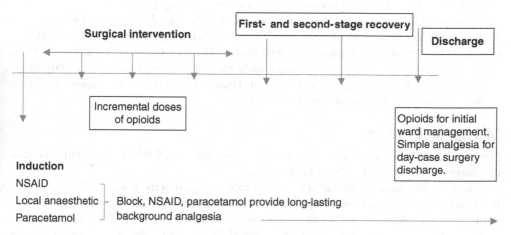

Figure 35.7 Multimodal analgesia in action

Other Strategies

If the above strategies fail to provide adequate analgesia, other drugs such as ketamine may be considered, or regional anaesthesia may be undertaken.

As stated above, pain is associated with anxiety: they exacerbate each other. A calm, reassuring manner is essential to relax the patient and give them confidence that you will relieve them of pain. Warmth, position, and mouth care all play a part in this.

Postoperative Nausea and Vomiting

Postoperative nausea and vomiting (PONV) can be debilitating and prolong recovery. In some cases, the physiological stress of vomiting may cause bleeding at the surgical site. Factors that contribute to postoperative nausea and vomiting include the anaesthetic drugs used, hypotension, hypoxaemia, psychological factors, dehydration, and pain.

Treatment

Pharmacological treatment of PONV may employ more than one antiemetic in targeting the correct receptors. There are many antiemetic drugs available for use including cyclizine, ondansetron, prochlorperazine, metoclopramide, and dexamethasone. The most effective cure for vomiting is to avoid using techniques that cause it. For example, regional anaesthesia or total intravenous anaesthesia could be chosen instead of volatile anaesthesia and emetogenic drugs such as opiates could be reduced or avoided. Always ensure that the patient is well hydrated [5].

Children in the PACU

The care of the children recovering from surgery and anaesthesia is, in principle, the same as for an adult. However, there are important anatomical, physiological, and psychological differences between children and adults. The paediatric range also covers neonates, infants, children, and adolescents all with differing developmental and emotional needs. It is important to understand the normal age-specific parameter ranges. For practitioners not used to caring for children, recovering a child can be challenge [15].

Many units make special provision for the care of children either by having a designated area, with child-friendly décor, or a separate room. Where possible, children should be recovered by a paediatric trained nurse who also is skilled in recovery. This combination, however, is unusual; therefore, units make their own provision to ensure that only those practitioners with experience recover children. Distressed children may respond better to a relative or caregiver being present in the PACU.

Discharge Criteria

National guidelines state that criteria need to be in place in all PACUs to ensure the safe discharge of patients, to wards, or home [1, 3].

The Modified Aldrete Discharge Score is commonly used in the PACU [16] and assesses five discharge factors: activity, respiration, circulation, consciousness, and oxygen saturation (see Table 35.5). Each of the five criteria is awarded a score of 0–2. The total scores can range from 0 to 10 and it is generally accepted that a score above 8 entails that it is appropriate for the patient to be discharged. While discharging a patient is the anaesthetist's responsibility, the use of a recognised discharge criteria allows for delegation of this activity to trained PACU staff. Should the patient not meet discharge criteria, then a medical review is required to determine whether further treatment is required, the patient requires more recovery time in the PACU, or referral to a high dependency setting [3]. The discharge criteria are summarised in Table 35.6.

Handover to Ward

All documentation should be complete and signed:

- anaesthetic record;
- operation record;
- recovery record; and
- prescription chart.

The handover must be thorough using the SBAR approach and including full clinical details, special instructions, ongoing issues, and special instructions. The above documents must accompany the patient (along with their notes) back to the ward.

Table 35.5 Modified Aldrete Discharge Score

Criteria	Interpretation	Score
Activity	Able to move voluntarily or on command:	
	• four extremities	2
	• two extremities	1
	• no extremities	0
Respiration	Able to breathe deeply and cough freely	2
	Dyspnoea, shallow or limited breathing	1
	Apnoeic	0
Circulation	Blood pressure ±20 mm of pre-anaesthesia level	2
	Blood pressure ±20–50 mm of pre-anaesthesia level	1
	Blood pressure ±(>50) mm of pre-anaesthesia level	0
Consciousness	Fully awake	2
	Arousable on calling	1
	Not responding	0
Oxygen saturation	Maintains oxygen saturation >90% on room air	2
	Needs oxygen inhalation to maintain oxygen saturation >90%	1
	Oxygen saturation <90% even with oxygen supplements	0

Maximum score = 10. Low score = 6 or below. High score = 7 to 10.

Table 35.6 Summary of discharge criteria

Criterion	Assessed by
Patient is awake and orientated	Patient knows who they are, where they are and time of day
Maintaining own airway and achieving adequate gas exchange	Pulse oximetry good/appropriate
Cardiovascular status is stable with adequate perfusion to organs	Appropriate heart rate and blood pressure Capillary refill time
Appropriate urine output	Check volume if catheterised
Fluid replacement and loss accurately documented	Ensure fluids are prescribed if necessary
Intravenous cannula secure, patent and free of residual drugs	Ensure intravenous fluids are running well, and the line flushed
Drains patent and wound dressings dry	Visual assessment
Pain well controlled with absence of nausea and vomiting	Scoring system Ensure analgesia and antiemetics are prescribed appropriately
Core temperature should be greater than 36 °C.	Use a temperature monitor such as tympanic or axillary

References

1. Royal College of Anaesthetists. Guidelines for the provision of postoperative care, 2019. Available from: www.rcoa.ac.uk/sites/default/files/documents/2020-02/GPAS-2019-04-POSTOP.pdf.

2. NHS Estates. *Health Building Note 26, Facilities for Surgical Procedures*, Volume 1. London: The Stationery Office, 2004.

3. A. A. Klein, T. Meek, E. Allcock, et al. Recommendations for standards of monitoring during anaesthesia and recovery 2021. *Anaesthesia* 2021; **76**: 1212–1223.

4. Association of Anaesthetists. *Guidelines: Immediate Post-Anaesthesia Recovery* London: Association of Anaesthetists, 2013.

5. J. Yates. Care of the postanaesthetic patient. In K. Woodhead and P. Wicker (eds.), *A Textbook of Perioperative Care*. London: Elsevier, 2005, pp. 181–196.

6. Hatfield, A. *The Complete Recovery Room Book*, 5th ed. Oxford: Oxford University Press, 2014.

7. T. J. Toney-Butler and J. M. Thayer. Nursing process. Available from: www.ncbi.nlm.nih.gov/books/NBK499937/ (accessed February 2021).

8. P. Smedley. Staffing in the PACU: no magic formula. *British Journal of Anaesthetic and Recovery Nursing* 2010; **11**: 3–8.

9. Association of Anaesthetists. *UK National Core Competencies for Post-Anaesthesia Care*. London: Association of Anaesthetists. 2013.

10. Nursing and Midwifery Council. *Revalidation*. London: Nursing and Midwifery Council, 2015.

11. P. Smedley and N. Quine. Postoperative care. In K. Woodhead and L. Fudge (eds.), *Manual of Perioperative Care: an Essential Guide*. Chichester: Wiley-Blackwell, 2012.

12. Nursing and Midwifery Council. What is a nursing associate? Available from: www.nmc.org.uk/about-us/our-role/who-we-regulate/nursing-associates/ (accessed February 2021).

13. NHS England and NHS Improvement. SBAR communication tool: situation, background, assessment, recommendation. Available from: www.england.nhs.uk/wp-content/uploads/2021/03/qsir-sbar-communication-tool.pdf.

14. P. Smedley. Patient risk assessment in the PACU: an essential element in clinical decision making and planning care. *British Journal of Anaesthetic and Recovery Nursing* 2012; **13**: 21–29.

15. A. Waugh and A. Grant. *Ross and Wilson Anatomy and Physiology*, 13th ed. Amsterdam: Elsevier Health Sciences, 2018.

16. J. Odom-Forren. *Drain's Perianesthesia Nursing: A Critical Care Approach*, 7th ed. Amsterdam: Elsevier Health Sciences, 2017.

17. J. Thompson, I. Moppett, and M. Wiles. *Smith and Aitkenhead's Textbook of Anaesthesia*, 7th ed. Amsterdam: Elsevier, 2019.

18. P. Smedley. BARNA learning and teaching resource: airway. Available from: www.barna.co.uk (accessed February 2021).

19. M. Robinson and A. Davidson. Aspiration under anaesthesia: risk assessment and decision-making. *Continuing Education in Anaesthesia Critical Care and Pain* 2014; **14**: 171–175.

20. B. Plaud, B. Debaene, F. Donati, et al. Residual paralysis after emergence from anesthesia. *Anesthesiology* 2010; **112**: 1013–1022.

21. National Institute for Health and Care Excellence. Hypothermia: prevention and management in adults having surgery clinical guideline [CG65]. Available from: www.nice.org.uk/guidance/cg65/chapter/Recommendations.

22. D. B. Gordon. Acute pain assessment tools current opinion. *Anesthesiology* 2015; **28**: 565–569.

The Fundamentals of Emergency Resuscitation

Robert Ayee and Jamie Macpherson

Introduction

Resuscitation is the process whereby attempts are made to control and improve physiological abnormalities to prevent irretrievable organ failure and death. Historically, resuscitation predominantly implied cardiopulmonary resuscitation (CPR) undertaken during cardiorespiratory arrest. Increasingly, the term is also applied to treatments given to stabilise the deteriorating patient and prevent cardiorespiratory arrest.

Since 1983, the Resuscitation Council (UK) has been the authority on setting the standard of care in resuscitation both in and out of hospital. The roles of the Resuscitation Council include the production of evidence-based guidelines, quality standards, and training courses for the resuscitation of adults, children, and neonates.

The 'Sick' Patient

Recognition

Although anyone admitted to hospital could be regarded as 'sick', the word is commonly applied by clinicians as a way of referring to a subset of patients who are identified as at risk of deteriorating if not closely monitored and managed. Although cardiac arrests *can* happen without warning, the majority do not. As many as 80% of in-hospital cardiorespiratory arrests can be predicted by observing the progressive deterioration of the patient over time [1]. It is necessary to reinforce an 'end of the bed' assessment of patients with objective physiological observations, which can be recorded, monitored, and reviewed.

Early Warning Systems

Without systems in place to highlight deterioration, it can be very difficult for busy staff in busy acute hospitals to recognise worsening trends in multiple patients. Early warning systems have been used in hospital settings for over two decades to aid the recognition of high-risk patients. In 2012, the Royal College of Physicians introduced the National Early Warning System (NEWS) to standardise practice; there has since been updated version released in 2017, called NEWS 2 [2].

Cardiorespiratory Arrest

Respiratory Arrest

This is the state where a patient is not breathing (apnoeic) or has severely ineffective respiratory effort. It tends to occur because of problems with either the airway, lungs, or brain. Respiratory arrest causes profound hypoxaemia (low blood oxygen), which starves the cardiac muscle of oxygen and stops the heart beating effectively.

Cardiac Arrest

This is the state where the heart is unable to beat effectively and produce a functional cardiac output. There are many causes of cardiac arrests, which are discussed below. The absence of a cardiac output starves the brain/brainstem of oxygen and, as this controls respiratory function, respiratory arrest will also ensue.

Although described separately, please note that both types of arrest tend to rapidly follow one another. Without effective breathing or circulation, the patient in cardio-respiratory arrest can quickly develop brain injury and irreversible vital organ damage.

Assessment and Resuscitation of the Sick Patient

Objectives of Resuscitation

The objectives of resuscitation are as follows:

- airway patency and protection;
- adequate gas exchange – avoiding hypoxia, hypercapnia, and acidosis;
- haemodynamic stability – maintaining an effective cardiac output, maintaining adequate intravascular volume and control of haemorrhage;
- optimising adequate tissue perfusion;
- preservation of neurological function – avoiding neurological injury, preventing secondary neurological injury (neuroprotection). and the safe control of agitation;
- normalisation of electrolyte/metabolic disturbance; and
- maintenance of normothermia.

ABCDE Approach

When encountering high-pressure situations such as the *sick* or *arrested* patient, it is imperative to work through the clinical problems with a structured approach in mind. The most common approach used in current practice is the ABCDE approach, an acronym standing for: airway, breathing, circulation, disability, and exposure. This approach allows the recognition or exclusion of life-threatening pathology prioritised by how quickly it will lead to death. Airway obstruction will cause a patient to go into cardiac arrest more quickly than hypovolaemia or hypothermia.

Although it is important to follow this sequence, remember that pathology in one domain can impact on the other domains (i.e., depressed conscious level causing airway obstruction). It is also important to be aware that management of pathology in one domain can lead to deterioration in other domains if these are not assessed and optimised. Following the initial assessment, the patient and the effects of any treatment given should be re-assessed regularly.

A: Airway

An untreated airway obstruction can rapidly lead to cardiorespiratory arrest and prompt management is essential.

Objectives

- Establish a patent airway.
- Protect lungs from gastrointestinal contents/blood.

Critical Questions

- Is the airway patent?
- Is the patient at risk of aspirating?

Assessment

- Assess airway sounds:
    - alert and talking – patent airway;
    - noisy airway – partial obstruction:
        - stridor – lower airway,
        - snoring – upper airway;
    - silent airway – complete obstruction.
- Check for foreign objects/material (i.e., vomit/blood).

Management

- Open the airway:
    - airway manoeuvres and/or adjuncts;
    - supraglottic airway device;
    - rapid sequence intubation.
- Remove foreign material:
    - Yankauer suction/Magill's forceps.

B: Breathing

Objectives

- Ensure adequate gas exchange:
    - avoid hypoxia (low oxygen) and hypercapnia (high carbon dioxide).
- Treatment of any immediately life-threatening lung disorders.

Immediately Life-Threatening Pathology

- Respiratory arrest.
- Tension pneumothorax.
- Acute pulmonary oedema.
- Pulmonary embolus.
- Severe bronchospasm.

Critical Questions
- Is there any spontaneous respiratory effort?
- Is effective ventilation taking place?

Assessment
- Oxygen saturation (SpO_2)/end-tidal carbon dioxide ($ETCO_2$) monitoring.
- Respiratory rate and pattern.
- Palpation:
  - tracheal position – midline or displaced;
  - chest deformity.

- Percussion:
  - hyper-resonance/dullness.

- Auscultation
  - air entry/wheeze/crackles.

- Arterial blood gas.
- Chest X-ray.

Management
- Respiratory arrest:
  - support ventilation with self-inflating bag;
  - consider invasive ventilation.

- Any cause of hypoxia – always give high-flow oxygen:
  - non-rebreathing face mask.

- Bronchospasm:
  - nebulised bronchodilators.

- Pneumothorax:
  - chest decompression.

- Oedema:
  - diuretics/ventilation.

C: Circulation

Objectives
- Maintain an effective cardiac output.
- Achieve adequate intravascular volume.
- Treat any immediately life-threatening cardiovascular disorder.

Immediately Life-Threatening Pathology

- Cardiac arrest.
- Major haemorrhage.
- Arrhythmia:
  - tachyarrhythmia;
  - bradyarrhythmia.
- Myocardial infarction.
- Shock:
  - cardiogenic/hypovolaemic/neurogenic/septic/anaphylactic.
- Cardiac tamponade.
- Aorta – dissection/ruptured aneurysm.

Critical Questions

- Is there a carotid or femoral pulse?
- Is the patient haemodynamically stable?
- Is there any evidence of a major haemorrhage?

Assessment

- Heart rate and rhythm:
  - fast/slow;
  - regular/irregular.
- ECG monitoring.
- Blood pressure – consider invasive monitoring.
- Peripheries:
  - warm/cold;
  - capillary refill time.
- Heart sounds.
- Focused echocardiography (if available):
  - left- and right-ventricular function/filling status/tamponade.

Management

- Cardiac arrest:
  - chest compressions plus advanced life support (ALS) algorithm – see below.
- Major haemorrhage:
  - blood products;
  - control of haemorrhage.
- Arrhythmia:
  - drugs – atropine/amiodarone/adenosine;
  - direct current (DC) cardioversion or pacing.

- Hypotension/shock:
  - Intravenous fluid boluses;
  - inotropes/vasopressors.

- Myocardial infarction:
  - angioplasty/percutaneous coronary intervention plus aspirin/morphine.

- Tamponade:
  - may need pericardial drain or surgery.

D: Disability

Neurological dysfunction may result in airway obstruction with or without respiratory arrest.

Objectives

- Preservation of neurological function:
  - preventing secondary neurological injury;
  - safe control of agitation/seizures.

- Treatment of immediately life-threatening neurological disorders.

Immediately Life-Threatening Pathology

- Severe hypoglycaemia.
- Drug overdose.
- Intracranial haemorrhage/stroke.
- Status epilepticus.
- Raised intracranial pressure plus 'coning'.

Note – agitation isn't life threatening, but it can make the patient hard to manage.

Critical Questions

- Is the patient severely hypoglycaemic?
- Is the patient having a seizure?
- Is there an intracranial event happening?

Assessment

- Blood glucose measurement.
- Consciousness level:
  - AVPU (alert, verbal, pain, unresponsive) or Glasgow Coma Scale.

- Neurological examination:
  - pupils:
    - equal/unequal,
    - dilated/pin-point.

- ° muscle tone – decreased/increased;
- ° muscle power – hemiparesis;
- ° reflexes – absent/diminished/brisk.
- CT head.

Management

- Low blood glucose:
  - ° sublingual or intravenous glucose.
- Seizures:
  - ° benzodiazepines → anti-epileptics → general anaesthetic.
- Drug intoxication/overdose:
  - ° reversal agents – e.g., naloxone/flumazenil.
- Raised intracranial pressure:
  - ° mannitol/hypertonic saline (if coning).
- Agitation:
  - ° physical restraint/sedatives/antipsychotics/general anaesthetic.
- Risk of airway aspiration:
  - ° recovery position and consider intubation.

E: Exposure

Are there any clues to explain the patient's condition?

Objectives

- Identification of any other causes for patient's condition.
- Maintenance of normal body temperature.

Life-Threatening Pathology

- Hypothermia.
- Burns/trauma.
- Intra-abdominal emergencies:
  - ° perforated/ruptured organ (i.e., bowel/spleen);
  - ° bowel ischaemia/obstruction.
- Electrolyte or acid-base emergencies:
  - ° hyperkalaemia/hypokalaemia;
  - ° acidosis.
- Pregnancy-related emergencies:
  - ° bleeding – vaginal or abdominal;

   ◦ eclampsia – high blood pressure/seizures.

Critical Questions
- Is the patient severely hypothermic?
- Is there a life-threatening electrolyte abnormality?
- Is there anything else we could be missing?

Assessment
- Skin:
   ◦ colour/rashes/wounds/burns;
   ◦ temperature;
   ◦ needle or 'track' marks.

- Abdomen:
   ◦ guarded/rigid /distended/discoloured;
   ◦ wounds or scars;
   ◦ pregnant?

- Core temperature measurement.

Management
- Temperature management:
   ◦ prevent heat loss – blankets/dry clothing;
   ◦ active rewarming – forced air blankets/invasive warming.

- Correction of electrolyte abnormality:
   ◦ i.e., hyperkalaemia:
      ▪ myocardial stabilisation – intravenous calcium chloride;
      ▪ reduce potassium – nebulisers/intravenous insulin–dextrose.

- Emergency surgery:
   ◦ laparotomy;
   ◦ damage control surgery for trauma/burns;
   ◦ emergency Caesarean section.

- Don't forget analgesia!

Management of Cardiorespiratory Arrest

ALS Algorithm

To help clinicians appropriately manage the patient in cardiac arrest, the Resuscitation Council (UK) designed a standardised protocol for all team members to follow called the ALS algorithm. Using this algorithm results in repeated cycles of CPR separated by rhythm assessments with or without pulse checks. The ALS algorithm is separated into two main loops, *shockable* and *non-shockable*. Defibrillation is delivered after rhythm checks depending on the which 'side of the algorithm' the observed rhythm falls.

The ALS algorithm and guidelines are regularly updated and can be viewed on the Resuscitation Council UK website or in the ALS manual [3]. It can be applied to most cardiac arrest situations, but there may be special circumstances in which additional interventions are required.

Cardiac Arrest Rhythms

Shockable

Ventricular fibrillation (VF):

- Chaotic and dyssynchronised electrical activity of the ventricles leading to lack of coordinated contraction. The myocardium 'shivers' and the cardiac output effectively ceases.

Pulseless ventricular tachycardia (VT):

- Repeated, coordinated electrical activity at an excessively high rate. The ventricle does not have time to fill, and so cardiac output is severely compromised.

Non-shockable

Pulseless electrical activity:

- Any electrical activity (other than VF or VT) in the absence of a pulse. Also known as 'electromechanical dissociation'; electrical activity in the heart may be normal or near normal, but the heart is unable to effectively generate a cardiac output.

Asystole:

- Lack of any meaningful electrical activity in the myocardium. Contraction and cardiac output are absent. All the above rhythms will deteriorate to asystole if left untreated.

Reversible Causes of Cardiac Arrest

These are causes of cardiac arrests that require treatment before the successful return of spontaneous circulation is going to be possible. They can be remembered as the 'four Hs and four Ts':

- **Hypoxia:** low oxygen content in the blood supply to the heart can result in myocardial ischaemia.
- **Hypovolaemia:** low blood volume results in hypotension and reduced cardiac output. This impairs oxygen delivery to the myocardium.
- **Hyperkalaemia:** high potassium destabilises the myocardium, which predisposes to arrhythmias. This 'H' can also refer to hypokalaemia, hypoglycaemia, hypocalcaemia, acidaemia, and other metabolic disorders; these will be identified on point-of-care blood analysis.
- **Hypothermia:** abnormally low core temperature can result in bradycardia and dysfunction of the myocardium.

- Tension pneumothorax: pressurised air in one or both halves of the chest can lead to compression of the great vessels ('mediastinal shift'), blocking blood flow into and out of the heart.
- Tamponade: pressurised blood or fluid in the sac surrounding the heart (pericardium) prevents the heart filling with blood and compromises its blood supply.
- Thrombosis:
  o pulmonary embolus – a large clot in the pulmonary artery can prevent blood flow through to lungs, which impairs oxygenation and reduces cardiac output; and
  o myocardial infarction: a clot in a major coronary artery leads to death of the myocardium, which results in arrhythmias and cardiac dysfunction.
- Toxicity: supra-therapeutic levels of drugs (either prescribed or illicit) can result in a cardiac arrest by several mechanisms:
  o Opiates and sedatives can cause airway obstruction and/or respiratory arrest.
  o Stimulants (e.g., cocaine) can lead to tachyarrhythmias and myocardial ischaemia.
  o Several drugs (including tricyclic antidepressants) increase the QT interval (ventricular depolarisation/repolarisation), resulting in severe cardiac dysrhythmias.
  o Drugs such as beta blockers or calcium channel blockers can affect the heart rate and/or contractility, which can severely reduce cardiac output.

Defibrillation

Defibrillation is the delivery of an electric current through the heart muscle. The aim of defibrillation is to cause synchronous depolarisation of the myocardium that stops erratic electrical activity and allows coordinated electrical activity to resume. Essentially, a defibrillator consists of a capacitor (electrical component that holds charge) shared between two circuits linked together side by side with a switch (see Figure 36.1). The first circuit charges the capacitor, while the second circuit discharges the capacitor through the chest of the patient. An inductor in the second circuit 'slows down' the electrical discharge and makes defibrillation more effective.

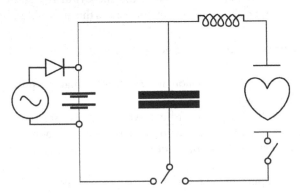
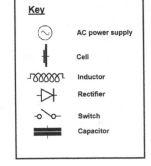

Key	
AC power supply	
Cell	
Inductor	
Rectifier	
Switch	
Capacitor	

Figure 36.1 Defibrillator schematic

Shocks should not be given before CPR is commenced unless it is a witnessed and monitored VF cardiac arrest with defibrillator pads already attached (in which case three back-to-back or 'stacked' shocks are recommended). In all other situations, CPR should be commenced immediately while the defibrillator is being set up. Manual defibrillators allow the selection of increasing doses of energy (starting usually at 150 joules) where successive shocks are required. Shocks should be well planned to minimise interruption to CPR. It is very important to minimise the time where CPR is not being performed; necessary interruptions should be less than 5 seconds.

Pad Position

The shock is delivered via self-adhesive pads (or electrodes) attached to the patient's skin. The position of the pads and the quality of the contact with the skin is critically important in determining the effectiveness of the shock. Usually, the electrodes are applied in the 'antero-lateral' position. One pad is placed below the right clavicle and the other in the mid-axillary line over the V6 position of the 12-lead ECG. These positions are chosen as they can be applied with CPR ongoing and minimise the interruptions to effective CPR.

Safety

It is the responsibility of the person delivering the shock to ensure all staff are clear of the patient; defibrillation of the normal heart can result in a cardiac arrest. Defibrillation can theoretically generate sparks, which can ignite open oxygen sources. However, there have not been any reported instances of oxygen combustion with self-adhesive pads. ALS protocol recommends removing oxygen devices to more than 1 metre away from the patient. Closed circuits such as Mapleson C, self-inflating bags, or circle breathing systems can remain attached. However, if they are removed, then they also need to be removed to more than 1 metre away.

Waveform Capnography

Measurement of the $ETCO_2$ is essential in modern anaesthetic practice. $ETCO_2$ monitoring must always be available and working correctly during the resuscitation attempt.

In the context of CPR, the exact values of the $ETCO_2$ are not as useful as the trend of the waveform (see Figure 36.2), and provides the following information:

- feedback on the patency of the airway and the effectiveness and rate of ventilation;
- a sudden increase in $ETCO_2$, which may indicate return of spontaneous circulation (ROSC);

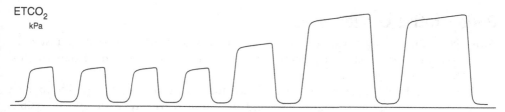

$ETCO_2$
kPa

Figure 36.2 ROSC $ETCO_2$

- a progressively reducing or continuously very low $ETCO_2$, which is related to a poor chance of ROSC.

Outcomes of a Resuscitation Attempt

The term ROSC is used when a discernible cardiac output is established by the patient in the absence of CPR. ROSC is the main initial objective during cardiopulmonary resuscitation. The chances of patients with an initial shockable rhythm surviving to hospital discharge are much greater than those with non-shockable rhythms. Patients presenting in asystole bear the worst chances of ROSC and survival to hospital discharge [4].

If ROSC is not achieved quickly, the likelihood of ROSC and a meaningful outcome for the patient greatly diminishes over time. Therefore, as time passes, regular assessments must be made as to whether continuation of the resuscitation attempt remains appropriate. A decision to stop a resuscitation attempt is highly dependent upon the clinical picture presented to the healthcare team. The duration of 'down-time' pre-hospital, the initial rhythm, the absence of reversible causes, and the patient's pre-arrest co-morbidities and functional status are just some of the factors that should be considered.

It is usually considered appropriate to stop an attempt if there is no untreated reversible cause, and persistent asystole at rhythm check despite ongoing CPR for 20 minutes or more. It is usually considered appropriate to continue when the patient remains in VF or while treating a reversible cause.

Post-Resuscitation Care

ROSC is the only the first part of patient recovery following a cardiac arrest. Additional monitoring and investigations can be undertaken following ROSC to identify any underlying cause and prompt further treatment. Common considerations include the following:

- Antiarrhythmic drugs, inotropes, or vasopressors may be necessary to manage post-cardiac arrest myocardial dysfunction.
- Secondary brain injury can occur after a post-cardiac arrest brain injury. Neuroprotective measures should be undertaken to reduce this injury:
  - ensuring adequate brain blood supply and drainage;
  - sedation and prevention of seizures, which can reduce the brain oxygen requirements; and
  - targeted temperature management in the intensive care unit to prevent pyrexia in the first 72 hours after ROSC.

Perioperative Cardiac Arrest

Although perioperative practitioners will likely come across at least one cardiac arrest in the perioperative environment during their careers, it remains a rare event and accounts for less than 2% of all in-hospital cardiac arrests [5].

The patient should already have standard monitoring attached, resuscitation equipment and drugs are usually quickly available, and the cause is usually acute and reversible. Recognition and initial management of a cardiac arrest is generally much quicker than in a ward or pre-hospital setting.

If the patient is deemed to be at high risk of cardiac arrest, it is common practice for defibrillation electrodes to be applied, to have resuscitation drugs prepared in advance, and to establish more extensive patient monitoring prior to the induction of anaesthesia.

Asystole and the two shockable rhythms (VF/pulseless VT) will be *immediately* apparent from the ECG. Pulseless electrical activity may take slightly longer to recognise in the absence of invasive arterial blood pressure monitoring, but loss of SpO_2 or $ETCO_2$ traces are strong indicators.

Management should follow an ABCDE approach, but with an initial assessment for catastrophic haemorrhage (cABCDE). Unless surgery can treat the underlying cause, the operation should be paused while the arrest is being managed. It is important to consider the risks of cardiac arrest when positioning the patient for surgery. Prone positioning can make CPR ineffective and, if safe to do so, a rapid return to the supine position should be performed.

Non-technical Skills in Resuscitation

Situations with unstable patients that require resuscitation can be complex and stressful, with limited time to assess and treat a patient before their condition becomes unsalvageable. The performance of healthcare professionals is not solely down to their technical skills, but also an array of cognitive and personal ('non-technical') skills.

Situational Awareness

Situational awareness is a complex skill, learned over many years, that allows adaptation to changes in the environment and/or the patient's clinical condition. Situational awareness is comprised of three phases, which constantly feed into each other as the situation changes.

1. Perceiving Information/Changes

Acute care situations are highly dynamic and can change quickly. Healthcare professionals must maintain vigilance and pick up on changes in the environment with all their available senses. For example:

- During a laparoscopy the anaesthetist hears the surgeon requesting the gas to be switched on. Shortly afterwards, the anaesthetist sees the ECG trace slow down.

2. Comprehension and Integration

As information is perceived in the environment, the individual needs to comprehend it in the context of the present situation. Lots of information will be gathered simultaneously and combining information from different sources with prior knowledge is crucial to understand the situation. For example:

- The anaesthetist recognises that there has been a drop in the heart rate and that peritoneal stretch is likely to be occurring, leading to vagal stimulation.

3. Anticipation and Action

By understanding what is happening around them, the healthcare professional can anticipate what may continue to happen if no action is taken or what will happen when various actions are taken. For example:

- The anaesthetist anticipates continued stretch may worsen the bradycardia, which will cause hypotension or even asystole. They locate the atropine and ask the surgeon to reduce the intra-peritoneal pressure

Task Fixation

Task fixation is the state of being entirely focused on an activity at the expense any other focus; it is the antithesis of situational awareness. However, it is not always bad to become task fixated; it may take total focus to perform a high-pressure task well. Situational awareness should be always maintained by the team leader.

Decision Making

Decision making is the skill of identifying all different courses of action available and selecting the most appropriate one for the situation. Good decision making is heavily reliant on good situational awareness. Once options have been identified, the merits and risks of each option must be quickly weighed against each other. The option that has the most appropriate balance of risk and reward should be selected.

Team Working and Leadership

A team is a group of individuals coming together to work towards a common goal. The resuscitation team will be constituted of a multidisciplinary team that has a wide range of different skills and expertise.

For a team to be effective, it requires a team leader who:
- directs and coordinate activities and responsibilities of team members;
- supports all team members, and knows their names and their capabilities;
- is able to take feedback from followers and adapt accordingly;
- maintains good situational awareness;
- is credible and is assertive/authoritative when needed; and
- demonstrates equanimity and helps keep others calm and focused.

Team members need to be:
- effective at exchanging information with the team;
- ready to take on the role allocated by the team leader;
- capable of taking initiative when appropriate and demonstrate active followership; and
- share workload with other team members – such as taking over chest compressions when needed.

Task Management

Task management is the process by which the team leader will coordinate and control the tasks that must be completed. Some tasks happen *sequentially* (i.e., management of an obstructed airway before ventilation), but often tasks can happen *simultaneously* (i.e., vascular access by one team member while another does chest compressions).

Planning, prioritisation, and preparation are essential to the efficient and safe completion of tasks. An example of planning and preparation is identifying what tasks need to happen ahead of a rhythm check. The ABCDE approach is a good example of how to prioritise tasks effectively.

Managing Stress and Fatigue

Recognising signs of stress or fatigue in oneself and other team members is a difficult but important part of working well together as a team. Mild stress is useful in performance as it can increase focus on the task at hand. More intense stress seems to make even well-practiced tasks much more difficult, but this tends to get easier with more experience. Being empathetic and supportive of those that are suffering from the deleterious effects of stress is an important aspect of working together as a team [6].

References

1. Resuscitation Council UK. *Advanced Life Support Instructor Manual*, 8th ed. London: Resuscitation Council UK, 2021.

2. Royal College of Physicians. National Early Warning Score (NEWS) 2. Available from: www.rcplondon.ac.uk/projects/outputs/national-early-warning-score-news-2 (accessed August 2021).

3. Resuscitation Council UK. Adult advanced life support guidelines. Available from: www.resus.org.uk/library/2021-resuscitation-guidelines/adult-advanced-life-support-guidelines.

4. P. A. Meaney, V. M. Nadkarni, K. B. Kern, et al. Rhythms and outcomes of adult in-hospital cardiac arrest. *Critical Care Medicine* 2010; **38**: 101–108.

5. J. P. Nolan, J. Soar, G. B. Smith, et al. Incidence and outcome of in-hospital cardiac arrest in the United Kingdom National Cardiac Arrest Audit. *Resuscitation* 2014; **85**: 987–992.

6. R. Flin, R. Patey, R. Glavin, and N. Maran. Anaesthetists' non-technical skills. *British Journal of Anaesthesia* 2010; **105**: 38–44.

Chapter

37

Human Factors, Ergonomics, and Non-technical Skills

Mark Hellaby

Introduction

Human factors, also known as ergonomics, is an established scientific discipline that has become integral to healthcare in recent years. The catalyst for this in the UK was the Clinical Human Factors group, led by Martin Bromiley. Martin's wife, Elaine, died following errors made during a routine operation when the theatre team failed to respond appropriately to an unanticipated anaesthetic emergency, in part because of a variety of human factors [1]. There is still confusion around the term 'human factors' [2]. This is partly because human factors cannot be explored in isolation but need to be understood in the context of human activity, error, and the culture around error.

Definition of Human Factors

A recognised definition of the term human factors in this context is as follows [3]:

> Enhancing clinical performance through an understanding of the effects of teamwork, tasks, equipment, workspace, culture, and organisation on human behaviour and abilities, and application of that knowledge in clinical settings.

Human Error and Harm

It is recognised that humans will always make errors; indeed, to err is human [4]. Our systems and processes should safeguard against patient harm by anticipating errors. All too often, though, the focus is only on the human error, which reinforces a blame culture by focusing on the individual or team involved. Fortunately, incidents that result in serious patient harm are rare. The different degrees of harm are shown in Figure 37.1.

Much time and effort has been focused on human error and incidents, across a variety of high-risk industries and activities, to understand, categorise, and of course reduce or remove it.

James Reason has led a lot of the work in this field and has demonstrated how we can split the errors that occur in clinical practice into three types: skill-based slips and lapses, rule-based mistakes, and knowledge-based mistakes [5]. Some of these errors are subconscious, due to distraction and other factors, while others involve missing steps though a conscious violation. For example, an active decision not to follow the prescribed rules, process, or known knowledge [6]. Reason also described how errors that come from a strategic level in the organisations – which he referred to as latent errors – can also increase the risk of harm in the clinical area. His work led to his well-recognised Swiss

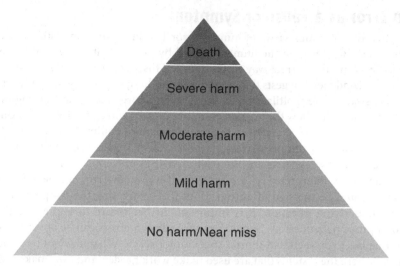

Figure 37.1 Pyramid of harm

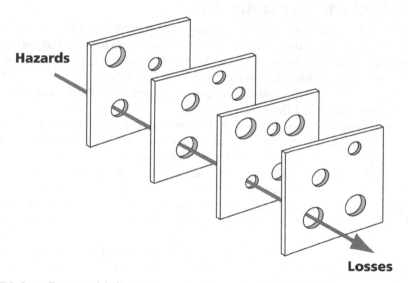

Figure 37.2 Swiss Cheese model of accident causation (licenced under CC BY-SA 3.0)

Cheese model [5], describing barriers to harm resulting from errors as being people but also the systems (see Figure 37.2). Weaknesses in training, tiredness, poor policies, and distraction can all weaken these barriers, which are indicated by the holes in the Swiss cheese slices. Hignett et al. took this work further, following discussions with healthcare staff, and suggested that in the real world we work in these holes and are constantly moving about on the slice and changing size [7]. What is clear, though, from this work is that there are multiple causes of error that form an error chain, some of which may have been around for a long time and started far away from where the incident occurred.

Human Error as a Cause or Symptom

There are two dichotomous views of human error [8]. First, the simplistic view that sees human error as a weakness of the human, caused by poor attention, lack of training, risk taking, and ignoring the correct way to do things. This view sees humans as the risk and variable. The second view suggests that poor design of the systems we work with leads to the errors. These systems are multifaceted and may include organisational training provision, policies, and procedures, how the organisation investigates and learns from previous errors, the layout of the clinical area, and even the procurement of equipment.

This second view sees humans working in a system that is imperfect, with multiple weaknesses, and these weaknesses are often detected, thus preventing harm. As such, human errors can be better interpreted as a symptom of a system error in the same way that hyperthermia could be the sign of an infection. Just as treating the temperature will not address the underlying infection, it is important in healthcare to appreciate the bigger picture to improve patient safety. Sometimes these design errors can be obvious – the drug cupboard that has a top shelf that shorter staff cannot reach. What may not be so obvious is the situation where the systems that are used make work harder, and thus make individuals more likely to fail.

Predictable Variability in Humans

The science of anthropometry looks at the range and limitations of the human body and thus can be used to predict the optimal height of our reach and hence of our shelves. Often, ergonomics is only really considered in healthcare when looking at the position and height of a desk, chair, or computer. There is a presumption that the equipment that practitioners use is well designed, and this fails to recognise the issue of how different equipment is brought together and used differently.

An example of the consequences of not understanding ergonomics has been seen in laparoscopic surgery. There have been concerns over the large numbers of surgeons experiencing pain and injury, linked to the increased use of laparoscopic procedures [9]. While we would expect the design of laparoscopic instruments to avoid injury to the user, one of the identified elements that is often missing is a consideration of how the equipment is arranged in the operating theatre. Often, new equipment is placed around existing equipment, with little consideration given to optimal positioning for staff well-being and safety.

Just as the reach and the range of forces we can exert with different muscles can be measured, so can the function of human cognition and the brain's ability to make decisions, store, and process information. As humans we are all aware of how, in varying situations, we afford attention differently. Those of us who drive cars think about a routine journey, repeating a well-travelled route; but consider how behaviour changes if we observe an incident ahead or the road is icy. Some of us will turn off the radio to limit any distractions so we can fully concentrate on the task in hand. Cognitive psychology offers insight into not only how we store and process information but also how the amount of processing, or cognitive load, affects us in different situations; for instance, when we are stressed or under pressure. Cognitive load describes the mental load that is placed on practitioners by a task or the organisation.

These limitations, just like physical limitations, are quantifiable and should be anticipated by our systems and, importantly, the system designed around these limitations. All these elements require design – not just so we, as humans, can work with the equipment, but so the systems can support us doing our tasks. Human errors are often predictable, and the systems should support them to catch these errors. The systems should aid practitioner's decision making rather than increasing their cognitive load beyond a safe level, which then increases the risk of error. This design expertise goes far beyond understanding the clinical condition; it requires input from a variety of safety scientists, behavioural psychologists, and ergonomists because clinical practitioners can become fixated on the clinical process.

This also explains why human factors cannot be addressed simply by educational processes – we cannot train out the human body's design specification and this should be appreciated and recognised by designing appropriate systems.

Examples of how systems can support staff include automation of medical early warning scores, which are calculated automatically from patient observations and alert staff if the patient deteriorates. Electronic prescribing has the potential to improve patient safety [10] by recognising drug errors and potential adverse drug events.

During the COVID-19 pandemic, many perioperative practitioners supported staff in critical care units. This support included assisting staff from ward areas who were not used to the critical care environment. It is interesting to reflect on this human–equipment interaction. The equipment displays information that the human has to visualise, interpret, and sometimes act on, this is often accompanied by an alarm to draw our attention.

The following is an example of one critical care bed space:

Equipment: ventilator, five syringe drivers, humidifier, bed, mattress, and bear hugger.

Controls: 93 control buttons.

Visual displays: 35 elements on small screens, 22 numerical fields, 21 indicators, 7 waveform fields, 2 digital temperature displays, 2 touch screens.

Alarms: from at least 10 devices with 269 individual alarm messages possible.

There is no inherent communication between the individual pieces of equipment to establish false versus genuine alarms, no standardisation of tones or alarm formats, or even any suggestion to the staff whether one alarm is more important than another alarm or task. Previous studies have suggested over 90% of equipment alarms in critical care units are either false alarms or clinically irrelevant [11].

This is an example where humans' physical and cognitive load is increased by the technology rather than the technology supporting them. This leads to alarm fatigue which can cause staff to fail to respond to alarms [12] as well as causing distraction. Distractions in healthcare, including the perioperative area, are so common [13] that staff can become blind to them. Equipment can cause distractions either through problems finding it or from repeated false alarms and problems with equipment. One observational study suggested that, in the operating theatre, an equipment-based distraction occurred on average every 90 minutes [14]. This is a design issue surrounding how we put the equipment together and manage it; not the individual equipment, but how it is integrated into the system.

Despite several global surgical safety initiatives from the World Health Organization (WHO) and the successes of the Surgical Safety Checklist in reducing patient harm, which have improved communication and culture [15], patient harm rates in operating theatres remain high.

The Working Environment Is Not Simple

There is no quick fix with respect to human factors and anyone who suggests otherwise, understands neither the complexity of the perioperative area nor what human factors are. The perioperative area is an incredibly complicated and diverse socio-technical system, with social, professional, and hierarchical overlapping groups, which connect with other groups in and outside an organisation that uses a variety of software and hardware.

The Complex Clinical Environment

In healthcare, there is often a focus on mandating clinical/emergency processes, and training staff to an observable standard. There is a presumption that if we prescribe and teach a new process to staff, they will perform it correctly. Following harm events, a simple root cause analysis will often be used to identify that a procedure was not adhered to and simplistically arrive at a solution. A human error occurred, and the staff failed to follow policy; they require further education, or a new checklist or a laminated poster to remind them. Let us consider the task of taking a blood sample from a bleeding patient. The task will be described in the organisation along the following lines:

- wash hands;
- obtain equipment and take it to the patient, including a sharps container;
- verbally confirm identity with the patient and check their wristband;
- wash hands and use personal protective equipment;
- draw blood into appropriate blood tube using an aseptic non-touch technique from the median cubital, cephalic, or basilic vein;
- dispose of sharps safely;
- wash hands;
- label the tube at the patient's bedside;
- ensure the form (paper or online) details match;
- complete the request online; and
- send the sample to the laboratory.

In the real world this task is not done in isolation; the performance of the task can be affected positively or negatively by multiple other elements listed in our definition of human factors. For example, think of this potential situation: in a clinical emergency with a high degree of stress, people are making other requests at the same time, the only phone is being used by someone trying to get a critical care bed, the computer in the operating theatre is not working, the drawer where the crossmatch tubes should be is empty, and there are no spares in the theatre storeroom. Consider all those elements which make doing our job harder each day and that we often learn to work around.

One such model that looks at articulating this messy real world is the Systems Engineering Initiative for Patient Safety (SEIPS 2.0) model, which describes the different elements including the tools and technologies that practitioners use (diagnostic and clinical equipment), the organisation (culture, team-working, supervision), internal environment (heating, lighting, noise), external environment (elements from outside, for example, national guidance, packaging of drugs, and design of equipment) as well as the subconscious elements such as social and cognitive ones [16]. Of course, these elements do not work in isolation, or rather should not do. If the system works well, all these different areas should support practitioners to complete the task. In the real world, unfortunately, practitioners often find that the opposite is the case, and the elements are fragmented and not connected, or have a negative impact, making the task more difficult and errors more likely.

Culture

Culture is often a vague concept and distant from people but, in effect, it is often manifested by the values and behaviours of the people [17]. Hence, culture can exist within groups, teams, departments, and the organisation. One of the negative elements around culture that is often discussed is that of a steep hierarchy – where the leader is unquestionable or unapproachable, and this negatively impacts safety. Some key processes that are commonplace in the perioperative area have elements of empowerment. The SBAR communication tool (where the situation, background, assessment, and recommendation is described) uses the recommendation step to authorise more junior staff to make a request to a senior member of staff – supporting communication up hierarchical gradients or across professional or departmental boundaries [18]. The benefit of the WHO Surgical Safety Checklist extends beyond simple compliance with the listed items. Indeed, it has elements embedded in its design to reduce hierarchy and encourage people to speak up. There is discussion around how much of the improvement in patient safety from using the checklist is derived from improving the safety and team culture in the operating theatre [19].

There is international concern that perioperative areas are often a setting where aggression and conflict can occur between professional groups [20]. Additionally, bullying can be common within professional groups and teams [21]. Incivility has a negative effect on performance, both for those it is aimed at and also those who witness it [22], and therefore bullying is a real area of concern.

There is also an embedded culture around error in healthcare where the error is viewed as the fault of the individual or team, with a focus of who did what, rather than why [23]. Interest is building in the work of Erik Hollnagel (and others) into resilient healthcare and Safety II. This work describes Safety I as our typical reactive model of waiting for incidents and focusing on people as the cause of error. Safety II, however, allows us to be proactive and mitigate risk by starting to understand what we normally do to perform the procedure correctly. This involves conversations to identify the elements that make the process harder and recognising the many times humans prevent harm [24]. Safety II sees the human as a resource and positive element of safety. The aim is not to replace our Safety I focus but use Safety II as an alternative lens to help reduce the Safety I events.

Never Events

In England, there is currently a list of 15 events that NHS Improvement defines as 'being serious events that are entirely preventable because guidance or safety recommendations providing strong systematic protective barriers are available at a national level and should have been implemented by all healthcare providers' [25]. Between 1 April 2017 and 31 March 2018 there were 468 events that were provisionally categorised as 'never events' [26]. The three most common never events are wrong site surgery, wrong implant/prosthesis, and retained foreign object post procedure.

What is clear from the data is that not only do these never events continue to happen but, also looking at previous data, there is no significant decrease from year to year. This is despite the widespread use of the WHO Surgical Safety Checklist and the introduction of

National Safety Standards for Invasive Procedures. Does this mean that all the people involved in these never events are poorly trained, reckless, or just careless? Why is it so difficult to reduce the numbers of events despite having clear national processes and guidance? If these events continue to occur, despite all the interventions and national guidance, at some stage we may need to consider that the national guidance is not as robust as first considered, or that the complex causes of these incidents remain misunderstood.

Teams

In acute care, we are used to working in familiar teams, or teams of strangers, which may be rapidly formed for emergencies. These larger teams are then organised into sub-teams: for example, the anaesthetic team, scrub team, post-anaesthesia care unit team, and portering team. Practitioners may know some of the individuals in their direct sub-team but not necessarily all of the others; at times, they may not even be aware of emergencies occurring in another sub-team, even if they are working in the same area. An example of this could be when the anaesthetic team are busy managing laryngospasm in a recently extubated patient in theatre while the surgical team are busy completing paperwork, and unaware of the airway emergency unfolding. Evidence has demonstrated that a lack of familiarity within the surgical team increases morbidity in abdominal surgery [27].

The primary focus of healthcare education has historically been on the clinical (technical) procedures, but equally important is how to turn a team of experts into an expert team [28]. It has been recognised that to support our technical skills we need to learn and develop a variety of non-technical skills. These skills are an important part of human factors – but only a part of it.

Non-technical Skills

Although there is some disagreement and variation in terms – and an overlap from sessions that focus on team and crew resource management – typically, non-technical skills cover elements such as situation awareness, decision making, communication, team working, leadership, managing stress, and coping with fatigue [29]. The lack of awareness and development of team and non-technical skills has been raised numerous times [30]. Compare the training received for a piece of clinical equipment and the need to demonstrate competencies with the ad hoc and sporadic development in non-technical skills, which is often left to a local individual to champion, sometimes using simulation.

Tools have been developed as a metric to help the objective debriefing of specific groups on non-technical skills including anaesthetists [31], surgeons [32], scrub practitioners [33], and anaesthetic practitioners [34]. Healthcare simulation offers a way to build awareness and develop competencies in team working and non-technical skills in the operating theatre [30]. *In situ* simulation in the clinical areas provides an opportunity to work with the real multidisciplinary team and real equipment, and often affords the potential to identify latent (organisational) errors before they are involved in actual patient harm events. Additionally, simulation can be used to test newly built hospitals and departments prior to patients arriving [35].

Of all the elements of non-technical skills, communication is an area that often stands out as a key factor in errors. Reports have highlighted how communication errors are common and avoidable [36]. There are multiple barriers to effective communication in a busy theatre department. These include the ambient noise, multiple specialities with inherent technical language, a steep hierarchy and culture, and a diverse range of ethnic, social, and professional backgrounds. During clinical emergencies, the number of people and ambient noise levels increase, making effective communication even more difficult. The stress of clinical emergencies can result in a variety of physiological responses, including tunnel vision, becoming task focused, and a reduced perception of spoken commands. Conversely, communication itself can increase cognitive load, cause a distraction, and negatively affect patient safety [37]. Learning how to communicate effectively is as important as understanding when to communicate; for example, having an awareness of what the individual you are speaking to is doing and whether that is a critical task.

However, there is more to communication than speaking, which includes empowerment and hierarchy (knowing you are allowed to speak) and developing skills in appropriate assertion. One simple method to improve effectiveness is the routine inclusion of closed-loop communication. This is used to ensure that the thought in one person's head is spoken, heard, and understood by another person.

Sender: 'I need you to ring the blood bank and get this patient [name of patient] urgently crossmatched for two units of packed red cells, and let me know when you have done it.'

Receiver: 'No problem, two units of packed red cells for [name of patient] to be urgently crossmatched – I will come straight back after.'

This may seem like a drawn-out process, but it soon becomes ingrained and less artificial.

Summary

Within the perioperative area, it is crucial to develop effective teams, but there is also a need to recognise the interplay between culture, system design, and technology on individual and team performance and how it affects patient safety. Human factors need to be integrated into healthcare to understand why things go wrong and establish effective system design that helps practitioners do the right thing. The term human error may be one that does more harm to the understanding of human factors; indeed, Sidney Dekker refers to 'human error' as a label and judgement made after the event [8]. Furthermore, the term can support a blame culture within organisations.

References

1. N. White. Understanding the role of non-technical skills in patient safety. *Nursing Standard.* 2018; 26: 43–48.

2. A. Russ, R. Fairbanks, B-T. Karsh, et al. The science of human factors: separating fact from fiction. *BMJ Quality and Safety* 2013; 22: 802–808.

3. K. Catchpole. The Department of Health Human Factors Reference Group interim report, 1 March 2012, National Quality Board. Cited in NHS England, Human factors in healthcare: a concordat from the National Quality Board. Available from: www.england.nhs.uk/wp-content/uploads/2013/11/nqb-hum-fact-concord.pdf.

4. William Richardson. In L. T. Kohn, J. M. Corrigan, and M. S. Donaldson (eds.), *To Err Is Human: Building a Safer Health System.* Washington, DC: National Academy Press, 2000, p. ix.

5. J. Reason. *Organizational Accidents Revisited.* Farnham: Ashgate Publishing, 2016.

6. J. Reason. *The Human Contribution. Unsafe Acts, Accidents and Heroic Recoveries.* Farnham: Ashgate Publishing, 2008.

7. S. Hignett, A. Lang, L. Pickup, et al. More holes than cheese. What prevents the delivery of effective, high quality and safe health care in England? *Ergonomics* 2018; **61**: 5–14.

8. S. Dekker. *The Field Guide to Understanding 'Human Error'*, 3rd ed. Boca Raton, FL: CRC Press, 2017.

9. D. Quinn and J. Moohan. Optimal laparoscopic ergonomics in gynaecology. *The Obstretician and Gynacologist* 2015; **17**: 77–82.

10. Z. Ahmed, S. Garfield, Y. Jani, S. Jheeta, and B. D. Franklin. Impact of electronic prescribing on patient safety in hospitals: implications for the UK. *Clinical Pharmacist* 2016; **8**: 153–160.

11. C. B. Larmee, L. Lesperance, D. Gause, and K. McLeod. Intelligent alarm processing into clinical knowledge. Proceedings of the International Conference of the IEEE Engineering in Medicine and Biology Society, 2006, pp. 6657–6659.

12. J. M. Solet and P. R. Barach. Managing alarm fatigue in cardiac care. *Progress in Pediatric Cardiology* 2012; **33**: 85–90.

13. M, A. Broom, A. L. Capek, P. Carachi, M. A. Akeroyd, and G. Hilditch. Critical phase distractions in anaesthesia and the sterile cockpit concept. *Anaesthesia* 2011; **66**: 175–179.

14. A. Wheelock, A. Suliman, R. Wharton, et al. The impact of operating room distractions on stress, workload and teamwork. *Annals of Surgery* 2015; **261**: 1079–1084.

15. R. Cabral, T. Eggenberger, K. Keller, B. S. Gallison, and D. Newman. Use of a surgical safety checklist to improve team communication. *AORN Journal* 2016; **104**: 206–216.

16. R. J. Holden, P. Carayon, A. P. Gurses, et al. SEIPS 2.0: a human factors framework for studying and improving the work of healthcare professionals and patients. *Ergonomics* 2013; **56**: 1669–1686.

17. T. Singelis and W. Brown. Culture, self, and collectivist communication. Linking culture to individual behavior. *Human Communication Research*. 1995; **21**: 354–389.

18. M. Müller, J. Jürgens, M. Redaëlli, et al. Impact of the communication and patient hand-off tool SBAR on patient safety: a systematic review. *BMJ Open* 2018; **8**: e022202.

19. A. S. Haugen, E. Søfteland, G. E. Eide, et al. Impact of the World health Organization's Surgical Safety Checklist on safety culture in the operating theatre: a controlled intervention study. *British Journal of Anaesthesia* 2013; **110**: 807–815.

20. R. Coe and D. Gould. Disagreement and aggression in the operating theatre. *Journal of Advanced Nursing* 2008; **61**: 609–618.

21. U. A. Halin and D. M. Riding. Systematic review of the prevalence, impact and mitigating strategies for bullying, undermining behaviour and harassment in the surgical workplace. *British Journal of Surgery* 2018; **105**: 1390–1397.

22. C. Porath and C. Pearson. The price of incivility. *Harvard Business Review* 2013; **91**: 114–21.

23. M. F. Peerally, S. Carr, J. Waring, and M. Dixon-Woods. The problem with root cause analysis. *BMJ Quality and Safety* 2016; **26**: 417–422.

24. E. Hollnagel, J. Braithwaite, and R. Waers. *Resilient Healthcare*. Farnham: Ashgate Publishing, 2013.

25. NHS Improvement. Never events policy and framework. Available from: https://improvement.nhs.uk/resources/never-events-policy-and-framework/ (accessed July 2020).

26. Care Quality Commission. Opening the door to change. NHS safety culture and the need for transformation. Available from: www.cqc.org.uk/publications/themed-work/opening-door-change.

27. A. Kurmann, S. Keller, F. Tschan-Semmer, et al. Impact of team familiarity in the operating room on surgical complications. *World Journal of Surgery* 2014; **38**: 3047–3052.

28. E. Salas, J. A. Cannon-Bowers, and J. H. Johnston. How can you turn a team of

experts into an expert team? In
C. E. Zsambok and G. Klein (eds.),
Naturalistic Decision Making. Mahwah, NJ:
Erlbaum, 1997, pp. 359–370.

29. R. Flin, P. O'Connor, and M. Crichton.
Safety at the Sharp End. A Guide to Non-technical Skills. Farnham: Ashgate
Publishing, 2007.

30. S Armenia, L. Thanganathesvaran,
A. D. Caine, et al., The role of high-fidelity
team-based simulation in acute care
settings: a systematic review. *The Surgery
Journal* 2018; **4**: e136–e151.

31. G. Fletcher, R. Flin, P. McGeorge, et al.
Anaesthetists' Non-Technical Skills
(ANTS): evaluation of a behavioral marker
system. *British Journal of Anaesthesia* 2003;
90: 580–588.

32. S. Yule, R. Flin, S. Paterson-Brown, et al.
Development of a rating system for
surgeons' non-technical skills. *Medical
Education* 2006; **40**: 1098–1104.

33. L. Mitchell, R. Flin, S. Yule, et al.
Development of a behavioural
marker system for Scrub Practitioners'

Non-Technical Skills (SPLINTS system).
Journal of Evaluation in Clinical Practice
2013; **19**: 317–323.

34. J. S. Rutherford, R. Flin, A. Irwin, and
A. K. McFadyen. Evaluation of the
prototype Anaesthetic Non-technical Skills
for Anaesthetic Practitioners (ANTS-AP)
system: a behavioural rating system to
assess the non-technical skills used by staff
assisting the anaesthetist. *Anaesthesia* 2015;
70: 907–914.

35. M. Hellaby, S. Wood, and N. Herbert.
Safely moving a hospital. In *The Human
Connection II*. Loughborough: Chartered
Institute of Ergonomists and Human
Factors, 2018, pp. 18–19.

36. A. J. Fowler. A review of recent advances in
perioperative patient safety. *Annals of
Medicine and Surgery* 2013; **2**: 10–14.

37. L. Lingard, S. Espin, S. Whyte, et al.,
Communication failures in the
operating room: an observational
classification of recurrent types and
effects. *Quality and Safety in Health Care*
2004; **13**: 330–334.

Chapter

38

Understanding Intraoperative Death

Daniel Rodger and Heather Hartley

Introduction

It is important to recognise that surgery and general anaesthesia are invasive and inherently risky [1]. An often-unspoken reality of perioperative environments is that, despite best practices, sometimes patients do die during surgery, and many practitioners are left unprepared to handle such an event and its aftermath. Despite the rarity of intraoperative deaths, clinicians' experiences highlight the potential for a long-lasting impact on both individuals and teams [2, 3]. This chapter summarises the incidence of intraoperative death, reviews the potential impact on practitioners, and explores the different approaches to navigate their aftermath.

Incidence of Intraoperative Death

The perioperative environment entails exposure to several potentially catastrophic and traumatic events such as an intraoperative death [4]. An intraoperative death – sometimes referred to as a 'death on the table' – describes the death of a patient in the operating theatre, during anaesthesia or surgery. Most practitioners will experience at least one intraoperative death; those working in regional trauma centres are positioned to encounter a higher incidence of intraoperative deaths during their career compared to those working in ambulatory surgical care [5–7]. A survey of 202 anaesthetists, surgeons, and operating department practitioners working in the UK observed that [8]:

- 82% had experienced an intraoperative death;
- 41% had experienced an intraoperative death in the last 18 months;
- 36% had experienced more than five intraoperative deaths;
- 71% of deaths occurred during an emergency surgery;
- 11% of those who experienced an intraoperative death stated that it had a long-lasting effect on their practice; and
- 55% believed that any additional anaesthetic and surgical work following a death should be cancelled.

In 2009, the World Health Organization launched a strategy to enhance surgical safety, recognising a need to address the global risks and complication rates associated with perioperative care. At the time, they estimated that in industrialised countries the perioperative rate of death for inpatient surgery was between 0.4 to 0.8 percent, and 3–17 percent for major complications; this was expected to be higher in developing countries [9]. Based on the number of surgeries performed in the 56 countries, this would translate to roughly 234 million operations [9] and 900,000 to 1.8 million deaths per year.

Despite this international attention, the exact incidence of intraoperative death remains notoriously difficult to determine due to variable definitions and inaccurate application in the medico-legal literature [10, 11]. This explains the wide variation of anaesthesia-related mortality rates that have been estimated to be between <1 and 6.5 per 100,000 general anaesthetics [12–14]. In paediatrics, the anaesthesia-related mortality rate can be as high as 10 per 100,000 general anaesthetics, and even higher in critically ill children [15]. These rates can differ significantly between countries; it is estimated that the rates of perioperative mortality are two to three times higher in developing countries than in their developed counterparts [16].

A further complicating factor when determining the incidence of intraoperative death is the term 'perioperative mortality', which captures not only deaths in the operating theatre but also deaths that occur within 30 days following a surgical procedure [17]. The National Surgical Qualitative Improvement Program provides risk-adjusted data from over 700 international hospitals, and considers perioperative mortality to be a comprehensive variable, inclusive of the patient's entire hospitalisation [18]. The 30-day mortality is undoubtedly an important quality indicator and, fortunately, only a very small proportion of these cases will have been intraoperative deaths. However, embedding intraoperative deaths into the larger category of perioperative mortality makes it difficult to determine how often patients are dying in the operating theatre.

In one large study of 294,602 admissions for general surgical emergencies at 156 NHS trusts in England between 2005 and 2010, the overall mortality rate was determined to be 4.2% [19]. Nevertheless, it is worth remembering that the death of a healthy patient undergoing an elective surgical procedure requiring general anaesthesia remains extremely rare.

Risk Factors for Intraoperative Death

Anaesthesia and surgery have become increasingly safer and the rates of anaesthesia-related and perioperative mortality in high-income countries has declined for several decades [10, 20]. Despite this, the development of more challenging surgical techniques coupled with continuing to treat older and more medically complex patients means surgery continues to carry a high degree of risk [21, 22]. The possibility of an intraoperative death occurring is dependent on several patient and contextual factors, including: a patient's age, ASA status, and the type and urgency of surgery.

Age

Both infants and elderly patients are at a higher risk of intraoperative mortality. Older patients are more likely to have pre-existing medical conditions or co-existing diseases (e.g., diabetes, hypertension, or ischemic heart disease). In the UK, there is a high-risk patient population who make up 12.5% of surgical admissions but that constitutes over 80% of deaths [23]. This high-risk patient population is commonly older, undergoing major surgery, and has severe co-morbidities. Perioperative mortality rates for neonates and infants under 1 year of age are also much higher compared to older children [24].

ASA Status

While most variables consider intraoperative death retrospectively, there are some strategies used to predict the potential of perioperative mortality for individual patients.

The American Society of Anesthesiologists Physical Status Classification System (ASA) is used by anaesthetists to assess a patient's fitness for anaesthesia. As a rule, the higher a patient's ASA status the greater the risk of mortality, though this is not the purpose of the classification [25]. The relationship between higher ASA status (3 and above) and an increased mortality risk is observed in neonates, children [26], and adults. This means that practitioners working in specialist tertiary centres who perform surgery on more complex patients with a higher ASA status will be more likely to encounter an intraoperative death. More details about the ASA classification are given in Table 38.1.

Table 38.1 ASA status and mortality

ASA classification	Definition	Examples	Perioperative mortality [25]
ASA 1	Normal healthy patient	Healthy, non-smoking, no or minimal alcohol use	0.1%
ASA 2	Patient with mild systemic disease	Mild lung disease, pregnancy, obesity (body mass index < 35), well-controlled diabetes and current smoker	0.2%
ASA 3	Patient with severe systemic disease	Morbid obesity (body mass index ≥ 40), active hepatitis, implanted pacemaker, chronic obstructive pulmonary disease and poorly controlled diabetes	1.8%
ASA 4	Patient with severe systemic disease that is a constant threat to life	Sepsis, life-threatening disease (e.g., unstable angina, poorly controlled chronic obstructive pulmonary disease), recent (<3 months) myocardial infarction or stroke	7.8%
ASA 5	Moribund patient who is not expected to survive 24 hours with or without surgery	Ruptured abdominal/ thoracic aneurysm, massive trauma, intracranial bleed with mass effect and ischaemic bowel	9.8%
ASA 6	Patient who has been declared brain-dead, whose organs are being removed for donor purposes	N/A	N/A

Type of Surgery

Some surgical procedures are associated with increased mortality and morbidity rates. The risk of death in the UK within 30 days of surgery for pericardial procedures and laparotomies was 34.1% and 19% [27], and some of these deaths will have been intraoperative deaths. High-risk surgery includes abdominal aortic aneurysm repair, coronary artery bypass grafting, pancreatectomy, oesophagectomy, major transplant surgery, and craniotomy.

Time of Surgery

There are also contextual risk factors that may contribute to the incidence of an intraoperative death and perioperative mortality more generally. These factors include lower levels of doctor and nurse staffing, fewer operating theatres relative to the number of beds, and a weekend admission [19]. Emergency surgery performed at the weekend has been shown to have 10.5% higher mortality than weekdays and this is likely to be reducible to variances in staffing and sicker patients being admitted at the weekend [28, 29]. This increased risk of mortality at the weekend has become known as the 'weekend effect' and the cause of it remains a topic of debate.

Intraoperative Death as a Traumatic Event

It has been shown that perioperative staff experience physical, emotional, and psychological stress following an intraoperative death [6, 30–32]. These deaths have subsequently been understood as destabilising experiences with the potential to cause a range of symptoms such as insomnia, depression, flashbacks, anxiety, guilt, shame, fear of judgement, loss of empathy, sleep disturbance, and substance abuse [5, 33, 34].

It is not uncommon for clinicians to think about an intraoperative death more than a year later and many express an ongoing preoccupation [32]. Left unacknowledged, symptoms can persist over time, manifesting into difficulty concentrating, a loss of confidence, or emotional instability, effects which can jeopardise a practitioner's professional competence and relationships [5, 6, 33].

Further exploration of these incidences has recognised that clinicians' experiences can be identified on an emotional continuum, ranging from second victimisation to diagnosed post-traumatic stress disorder [35, 36]. Second victimisation is informed by ideas of responsibility: clinicians suffer due to their perception of culpability or fault even when the death was deemed unpreventable [5, 37]. A study examining interdisciplinary perspectives acknowledged that clinicians' experiences of intraoperative death were deeply intertwined with perceptions of responsibility, a perception which shaped future collegial and personal relationships [38].

While intraoperative death is a shared experience, clinicians will have individualised responses and will not inevitably develop the symptoms and conditions outlined above. Historically, patient death was believed to build resilience, but it has been shown that clinicians who have more death experiences are not always protected by the exposure but can experience an accumulation of grief responses [39]. Therefore, following an intraoperative death it can be anticipated that most perioperative clinicians will be affected to some degree – whether it be from that death or compounded by previous death – and will require time to process and emotionally recover [5]. The time to emotionally recover may vary considerably between individuals due to complex interprofessional dynamics and role variability [40]. Because the spectrum of responses can vary significantly between clinicians it is imperative to recognise individual differences and tailor support strategies accordingly.

How symptoms can present or persist after an intraoperative death can also be influenced by contextual factors: the surgical environment, patient features, or type of death. Researchers have identified that effects on clinicians can be exacerbated by the following types of death [8, 34, 41]:

- the death of a child;
- maternal death;
- the death of a previously healthy patient;
- the death of a patient of the same age and sex;
- the death of a patient that is reminiscent of a family member; and
- an unexpected death.

The potential trauma that an intraoperative death can cause is clearly seen in one account from an operating department practitioner [3]:

> Around 10 years ago a young boy (I remember his name to this day) came in for a procedure but went into cardiac arrest. We tried and worked tirelessly to get him back but he died. The whole room was upset and traumatised, and I get emotional about it even now.

In this quote we can see that this experience was more poignant because of the age of the patient and remained vivid even years after.

It also merits recognition that encountering intraoperative death within the context of a pandemic further contributes to the culmination of trauma clinicians experience. In addition to caring for sicker patients and encountering more death, practitioners are at heightened risk of contracting the disease themselves. This is compounded with the difficult reality that clinicians are sometimes faced with caring for and potentially bearing witness to the death of those familiar to them, their colleagues, and community members.

Recognising Intraoperative Death within Surgical Culture

To appreciate the complexity of experiencing intraoperative death, clinicians should be aware of the cultural nuances which shape emotional experiences in the operating theatre. It has been argued that the surgical environment is driven by biomedical ideology, a lens by which clinicians are trained to perceive illness as purely pathological. This discourse prioritises physical illness, justifying invasive and often violent interventions and ascribing physicians with a heightened degree of control [38]. The challenge is that by acknowledging only physical illness, clinicians have difficulty reconciling the emotional and social impacts of a patient death. This ideological conflict is often layered with ideas of fault or perception of professional incompetence. These features contribute to a culture of 'death denial'; this can lead to a reticence among practitioners to discuss an intraoperative death, choosing to avoid it and any associated distress it may have caused [42]. This is further perpetuated by advances in medical technology [43]. Complex surgical techniques and equipment creates an impression that clinicians can 'fight death', raising questions when patients inevitably die. Unfortunately, there remains a hesitancy to discuss or demystify these perceived failures due to fear of professional or legal retribution.

At times it is difficult to ascertain whether the biomedical model informs surgical care or working in a surgical environment necessitates it. Clinicians sometimes psychologically pre-empt potentially traumatising situations in perioperative care using 'functional' or 'mechanistic' dehumanisation [44]. This type of dehumanisation describes how patients are referred to as objects, an example of how 'humanness' in healthcare is commonly denied. This is frequently seen in surgical contexts – practitioners who reference patients by procedure or diagnosis (e.g., the next hip, the 'add-on' laparotomy) rather than by name. In some surgical interventions – for example, the application of sterile draping – while it may be necessary, there is a unilateral focus on illness or injury, and features of 'personhood' are rendered largely invisible [45]. Strategies that unconsciously dehumanise patients put psychological distance between the practitioner and the patient and are perhaps required to protect clinicians from the emotional stress of surgery or intraoperative death [46].

While readers reflect on the support strategies available it is important that they consider these complex, tacit norms which shape how clinicians experience intraoperative death and subsequently how they will access support. There remains a collective unwillingness to raise concerns about the emotional impact of a 'death on the table' [38]. Perhaps this is due to a biomedical mentality – a fear that emotions do not belong in the operating theatre and exhibiting them is a sign of weakness. This, like ideas of dehumanisation, could be a form of emotional insulation; becoming too invested in every patient could lead to empathetic fatigue and burnout.

Intraoperative Death Support

There remains no standardised approach to supporting practitioners following an intraoperative death. This unfortunately often translates to inadequate care for those involved and leaves leaders with limited resources and guidance from which to implement support strategies [47]. An onus lies with organisations, who have a duty of care to their staff and a responsibility to promote clinician well-being. Failure to do so will inevitably diminish their ability to provide safe and effective patient care. Even after the death there may be additional sources of stress, such as a coroner's investigation or inquest. Below we detail some examples of practices that some clinicians have found to be beneficial following an intraoperative death.

Peer Support

Informal peer support remains the primary means of emotional support following a traumatic event such as the death of a patient [35, 41]. It is important to note that peer support is consistently perceived as the most beneficial means of support; peers are perceived to understand and appreciate clinical issues in a way that others may not be able to [5, 33, 46]. Peer support tends to happen organically; clinicians connect with others involved or reach out to a mentor or trusted colleague.

Downtime

This describes time away – perhaps 24 hours or more – from any duties in the operating theatre; the suggestion is that this can provide practitioners with valuable time to process and reflect on the intraoperative death. In response to a survey asking clinicians if procedures should be cancelled after an intraoperative death, 55% agreed it should although this differed between disciplines (anaesthetists, operating department practitioners, and trauma and orthopaedic surgeons felt it should, while other surgeons did not) [8]. Responses to traumatic events and opinions about aftermath care can be informed by the type of surgery and nature of the death [48]. Regardless of whether this is considered a reasonable or required step, it may not always be practicable due to time pressures, staffing issues, and implications of cancelling elective procedures. When human resources are limited – on night shifts or during a pandemic – it is unlikely that additional clinicians will be available to take over responsibilities. However, after an intraoperative death, if practitioners believe their subsequent ability to practice is compromised, every effort should be made to provide them with downtime. Unfortunately, like so many other aspects of addressing intraoperative death, there remains no consensus on whether the anaesthetic and surgical team should continue to work [48, 49]. Any decision to 'down tools' should be individualised and guided by a practitioner's duty of care to their subsequent patients.

Debriefing

Debriefing has been identified as a potentially valuable strategy to address traumatic experiences and mitigate their emotional impact, both inside and outside of the operating theatre. While researchers claim formalised debriefing remains rare in practice, clinicians have stated that they feel the process has merit especially in the immediate post-event period [7]. While many debriefing strategies exist, two approaches have been identified:

- 'Hot' debriefs occur immediately following the event and include the team members involved. The contents of these debriefs vary, but may involve summarising the events that occurred, asking individuals to discuss their actions, and identifying topics for future discussion or education.
- 'Cold' debriefs are scheduled later and are generally associated with patient safety or systems-level improvements. These are often facilitated and generally involve individuals who were not part of the event.

While clinicians and perioperative leadership continue to grapple with how best to navigate debriefing, the literature emphasises three required elements: a consistent process, dedicated resources, and time. One feature on which all stakeholders agree is that debriefing must foster a safe environment, a protected space in which any team member can share freely without fear of retribution [50].

In practice, debriefing occurs on a continuum, ranging from informal discussions focusing on 'what was done right, and what could be done better' to structured formats, inspired by programs designed for first responders and military personnel. One example is the Critical Incident Stress Management (CISM) Intervention, a stepped program focused on addressing mental health challenges after a traumatic event. Embedded within the steps is both a 'defusing phase' and a 'debriefing phase', mirroring the concepts of 'hot' and 'cold' debriefs. The defusing phase occurs immediately after the incident, giving those involved an opportunity to review the case and their initial reactions. The debriefing phase should occur within 72 hours of the event. This phase is facilitated by personnel trained in crisis management and utilises reflection to help identify coping skills and those in need of additional support. The CISM intervention integrates other important support principles, providing participants with pre-crisis education to develop stress-management techniques and post-crisis follow-up, connecting affected members with mental health professionals.

Much is left to be understood about how to appropriately execute a debrief following an intraoperative death in a way that adequately serves the whole multidisciplinary team. Debriefing should be utilised with caution; National Institute for Health and Care Excellence guidance has identified that psychologically focused debriefing is not always beneficial and can be more harmful because it prevents clinicians from accessing helpful resources [51].

Morbidity and Mortality Meetings

Mortality and morbidity (M&M) meetings in the UK commonly occur monthly and are led by a member of the surgical or anaesthetic team [52]. They were first established to review and learn from adverse events, with the purpose of supporting services to attain and maintain a high standard of care. While the original intention was not to provide staff support, reviewing cases that resulted in intraoperative death has been found to be beneficial for those involved [13]. This could be related to the principles used to analyse cases: quality improvement, clinical reasoning, and reflective practice – cornerstones of many existing support strategies. Practitioners involved in traumatic events, including intraoperative deaths, should be encouraged to attend the M&M meeting and to help identify learning opportunities from their experiences. Unfortunately, in many countries outside of the UK, these meetings are mainly reserved for surgeons and anaesthetists, limiting multidisciplinary perspectives, and leaving many members of the multidisciplinary team excluded.

Education

Education can play an important role in developing coping strategies that can help students and practitioners to navigate traumatic events and alleviate the impact of unaddressed stress. This type of education is not only valuable following critical events but can also establish a foundation of resiliency that helps clinicians to endure times of ongoing stress, such as during the COVID-19 pandemic. Higher-education institutions and hospital orientations for new and existing staff – especially those in high-risk environments – should teach the principles of psychological first aid. Such training can provide practitioners with the tools to support others and encourage those that need help to seek it [53].

What to Do When a Patient Dies

When a patient dies in the operating theatre it is essential that the body be treated with dignity and respect. The theatre manager and ward or intensive care staff should be informed immediately and the next of kin should be contacted. Until the need for a post-mortem has been ruled out it is important to leave the tracheal tube, intravenous cannulas, invasive monitoring, drains, and catheters *in situ*. Coroners are independent judicial officers who have the power to request statements, call witnesses, and request post-mortems. Some deaths that occur in a hospital will need to be reported to the coroner and this includes: deaths within 24 hours of admission; a death related to anaesthesia or surgery; and if the death is unexplained [54].

Summary

Intraoperative deaths are fortunately uncommon, but it remains likely that most practitioners will experience at least one during their career. An individual's response will be dependent on an array of patient, clinician, and environment factors – there is no 'normal' response.

Organisational support strategies must be tailored to address individual and team needs. Moreover, each practitioner plays a vital role in contributing to a culture of peer support and recognising the unseen impact and need for appropriate support for those that would benefit from it.

As the anaesthetist George Edwards said in an address to his students in 1938 [55]: ' . . . I hope that what I have said may be useful to you if ever you meet with death on the table, but even more strongly I hope that you never will have that misfortune.'

References

1. A. Pinto, O. Faiz, C. Bicknell, et al. Surgical complications and their implications for surgeons' well-being. *British Journal of Surgery* 2013; **100**: 1748–1755.

2. E. May. Nothing prepared me for my first death in surgery. *The Guardian*, 26 November, 2015. Available from: www .theguardian.com/healthcare-network/ 2015/nov/26/nothing-prepared-me-for-my-first-death-in-surgery.

3. M. Stylianou and S. Johnson. I still remember the boy who died in our theatre. Now I help traumatised NHS. *The Guardian*, 24 October 2019, Available from: www .theguardian.com/society/2019/oct/24/ remember-boy-died-theatre-now-help-traumatised-nhs-staff.

4. D. Rodger and H. Hartley. In the aftermath of a perioperative death: who cares for the clinician? *Evidence-Based Nursing* 2019; **22**: 1–2.

5. F. M. Gazoni, P. E. Amato, Z. M. Malik, et al. The impact of perioperative catastrophes on anesthesiologists: results of a national survey. *Anesthesia and Analgesia* 2012; **114**: 596–603.

6. S. M. White and O. Akerele. Anaesthetists' attitudes to intraoperative death. *European Journal of Anaesthesiology* 2005; **22**: 938–941.

7. R. Soto, J. Kado, B. Kerner, et al. Caring for the care-giver: debriefing following intra-operative death. *The Midwestern Journal of Anesthesia Quality and Safety* 2019; **1**: 1–4.

8. J. Haslam. Death on the table. *UK Casebook* 2005; **13**: 7–10.

9. A. B. Haynes, T. G. Weiser, W. R. Berry, et al. A surgical safety checklist to reduce morbidity and mortality in a global population. *The New England Journal of Medicine* 2009; **360**: 491–499.

10. J. H. Schiff, A. Welker, B. Fohr, et al. Major incidents and complications in otherwise healthy patients undergoing elective procedures: results based on 1.37 million anaesthetic procedures. *British Journal of Anaesthesia* 2014; **113**: 109–121.

11. A. Argo, S. Zerbo, A. Lanzarone, et al. Perioperative and anesthetic deaths: toxicological and medico legal aspects. *Egyptian Journal of Forensic Sciences* 2019; **9**: 20.

12. A. Lienhart, Y. Auroy, F. Pequignot, et al. Survey of anesthesia-related mortality in France. *Anesthesiology* 2006; **105**: 1087–1097.

13. F. M. Gazoni, M. E Durieux, and L. Wells. Life after death: the aftermath of perioperative catastrophes. *Anesthesia and Analgesia* 2008; **107**: 591–600

14. A. Gottschalk, H. Van Aken, M. Zenz, et al. Is anesthesia dangerous? *Deutsches Ärzteblatt International* 2011; **108**: 469–474.

15. L. Cronjé. A review of paediatric anaesthetic-related mortality, serious adverse events and critical incidents. *Southern African Journal of Anaesthesia and Analgesia* 2015; **21**: 147–153.

16. M. S. Avidan and S. Kheterpal. Perioperative mortality in developed and developing countries. *Lancet* 2012; **380**: 1038–1039.

17. J. S. Ng-Kamstra, S. Arya, S. L. M. Greenberg, et al. Perioperative mortality rates in low-income and middle-income countries: a systematic review and meta-analysis. *BMJ Global Health* 2018; **3**: e000810.

18. American College of Surgeons. ACS National Surgical Quality Improvement Program. Available from: www.facs.org/quality-programs/acs-nsqip.

19. B. A. Ozdemir, S. Sinha, A. Karthikesalingam, et al. Mortality of emergency general surgical patients and associations with hospital structures and processes. *British Journal of Anaesthesia* 2016; **116**: 54–62.

20. D. Bainbridge, J Martin, M Arango, et al. Perioperative and anaesthetic-related mortality in developed and developing countries: a systematic review and meta-analysis. *Lancet* 2012; **380**: 1075–1081.

21. D. M. Gaba. Anaesthesiology as a model for patient safety in health care. *British Medical Journal* 2000; **320**: 785–788.

22. R. S. Lagasse. Anesthesia safety: model or myth? A review of the published literature and analysis of current original data. *Anesthesiology* 2002; **97**: 1609–1617.

23. R. M. Pearse, D. A. Harrison, P. James, et al. Identification and characterisation of the high-risk surgical population in the United Kingdom. *Critical Care* 2006; **10**: R81.

24. L. P. Gonzalez, W. Pignaton, P. S. Kusano, et al. Anesthesia-related mortality in pediatric patients: a systematic review. *Clinics (Sao Paulo)* 2012; **67**: 381–387.

25. G. Cavill and K. Kerr. Preoperative management. In T. Smith, C. Pinnock, and T. Lin (eds.), *Fundamentals of Anaesthesia*, 3rd ed. Cambridge: Cambridge University Press, 2009, pp. 1–24.

26. L. de Bruin, W. Pasma, D. B. M. van der Werff, et al. Perioperative hospital mortality at a tertiary paediatric institution. *British Journal of Anaesthesia* 2015; **115**: 608–615.

27. T. E. F. Abbott, A. J. Fowler, T. D. Dobbs, et al. Frequency of surgical treatment and related hospital procedures in the UK: a national ecological study using hospital episode statistics. *British Journal of Anaesthesia* 2017; **119**: 249–257.

28. R. Ricciardi, P. L. Roberts, T. E. Read, et al. Mortality rate after nonelective hospital admission. *Archives of Surgery* 2011; **146**: 545–551.

29. J. Sun, A. J. Girling, C. Aldridge, et al. Sicker patients account for the weekend mortality effect among adult emergency admissions to a large hospital trust. *BMJ Quality and Safety* 2019; **28**: 223–230.

30. B. M. Gillespie and S. Kermode. How do perioperative nurses cope with stress? *Contemporary Nurse* 2004; **16**: 20–29.

31. R. Michael and H. J. Jenkins. Work-related trauma: the experiences of perioperative nurses. *Collegian* 2001; **8**: 19–25.

32. J. Todesco, N. F. Rasic, and J. Capstick. The effect of unanticipated perioperative death on anesthesiologists. *Canadian Journal of Anesthesia* 2010; **57**: 361–367.

33. T. W. Martin and R. C. Roy. Cause for pause after a perioperative catastrophe: one, two, or three victims? *Anesthesia and Analgesia* 2012; **114** (3): 485–487.

34. S. D. Pratt and B. R. Jachna. Care of the clinician after an adverse event. *International Journal of Obstetric Anesthesia* 2015; **24**:54–63.

35. M. A. M. Baas, K. W. F. Scheepstra, C. A. I. Stramrood, et al. Work-related adverse events leaving their mark: a cross-sectional study among Dutch gynecologists. *BMC Psychiatry* 2018; **18**: 73.

36. Å. Wahlberg, M. Andreen Sachs, K. Johannesson, et al. Post-traumatic stress symptoms in Swedish obstetricians and midwives after severe obstetric events: a cross-sectional retrospective survey. *BJOG* 2017; **124**: 1264–1271.

37. A. W. Wu. Medical error: the second victim. The doctor who makes the mistake needs help too. *British Medical Journal* 2000; **320**: 726–727.

38. H. Hartley, D. K. Wright, B. Vanderspank-Wright, et al. Dead on the table: a theoretical expansion of the vicarious trauma that operating room clinicians experience when their patients die. *Death Studies* 2019; **43**: 301–310.

39. E. M. Rickerson, C. Somers, C. M. Allen, et al. How well are we caring for caregivers? Prevalence of grief-related symptoms and need for bereavement support among long-term care staff. *Journal of Pain and Symptom Management* 2005; **30**: 227–233.

40. H. Hartley. Intraoperative death: the untold stories of perioperative teams. Master's Thesis, University of Ottawa, 2018. Available from: http://dx.doi.org/10.20381/ruor-21489.

41. J. Wilson and M. Kirshbaum. Effects of patient death on nursing staff: a literature review. *British Journal of Nursing* 2011; **20**: 559–563.

42. C. Zimmermann. Denial of impending death: a discourse analysis of the palliative care literature. *Social Science and Medicine* 2004; **59**: 1769–1780.

43. T. Tucker. Culture of death denial: relevant or rhetoric in medical education? *Journal of Palliative Medicine* 2009; **12**: 1105–1108.

44. N. Haslam. Dehumanization: an integrative review. *Personality and Social Psychology Review* 2006; **10**: 252–264.

45. A. Barnard and M. Sandelowski. Technology and humane nursing care: (ir) reconcilable or invented difference? *Journal of Advanced Nursing* 2001; **34**: 367–375.

46. E. J. O. Kompanje, M. M. van Mol, and M. D. Nijkamp. 'I just have admitted an interesting sepsis'. Do we dehumanize our patients?. *Intensive Care Medicine* 2015; **41**: 2193–2194.

47. H. Edrees, C. Connors, L. Paine, et al. Implementing the RISE second victim support programme at the Johns Hopkins Hospital: a case study. *British Medical Journal Open* 2016; **6**: e011708.

48. A. R. Goldstone, C. J. Callaghan, J. Mackay, et al. Should surgeons take a break after an intraoperative death? Attitude survey and outcome evaluation. *British Medical Journal* 2004; **328**: 379

49. S. Jithoo and T. E. Sommerville. Death on the table: anaesthetic registrars' experiences of perioperative death. *Southern African Journal of Anaesthesia and Analgesia* 2017; **23**: 1–5.

50. I. Clegg and R. MacKinnon. Strategies for handling the aftermath of intraoperative death. *Continuing Education in Anaesthesia, Critical Care and Pain* 2014; **14**: 159–162.

51. National Institute for Health and Care Excellence. Post-traumatic stress disorder. Available from: www.nice.org.uk/guidance/ng116/resources/posttraumatic-stress-disorder-pdf-66141601777861.

52. Royal College of Surgeons. Morbidity and mortality meetings: a guide to good practice. Available from: https://www.rcseng.ac.uk/standards-and-research/standards-and-guidance/good-practice-guides/morbidity-and-mortality-meetings/ (accessed 29 May 2020).

53. F. Gispen and A. W. Wu. Psychological first aid: CPR for mental health crises in healthcare. *Journal of Patient Safety and Risk Management* 2018; **23**: 51–53.

54. S. Bass and S. Cowman. Anaesthetist's guide to the coroner's court in England and Wales. *BJA Education* 2016; **16**: 130–133.

55. G. Edwards. Death on the table. *British Journal of Anaesthesia* 1938; **15**: 87–103.

Chapter 39

Extended and Advanced Roles in Perioperative Practice

Sally Stuart

Introduction

The roles of the surgical first assistant (SFA), surgical care practitioner (SCP), and anaesthetic associate (AA) have been introduced into perioperative care over the last few decades. This chapter highlights the history, educational pathways, role boundaries, and the professional and legal implications of each. It clarifies the nature of each extended or advanced surgical care team role, and the scope and limitations of their practice.

Surgical First Assistant

History

The SFA, previously known as 'first assistant' [1] and 'advanced scrub practitioner' [2], was first formally introduced to meet the rapidly changing needs of perioperative healthcare delivery due to the reduction of junior doctors' working hours [3, 4].

The current definition is [5]:

> The SFA is the role undertaken by the registered practitioner who provides continuous, competent and dedicated surgical assistance to the operating surgeon throughout the surgery; surgical first assistants practice as part of the surgical team, under the direct supervision of the operating surgeon.

In the early days of the role, there were concerns that the traditional role of the scrub practitioner would be diluted and in the absence of a national framework, with defined parameters for the role, lacked standardisation. Perioperative practitioners were concerned regarding the legal and professional implications of acting in a dual role [6].

In 2003, the newly formed Perioperative Care Collaborative (PCC), reviewed and redefined the role to advanced scrub practitioner; this change both acknowledged the expert nature of the role and highlighted the role as open to both registered nurses and operating department practitioners. The aim of the position statement was to clarify expectations and implications of the role, especially the legal and ethical implications of undertaking a dual role. The title changed to SFA in 2012 [7], following a decision from the Royal College of Surgeons [8] for greater clarity of perioperative titles, and roles and responsibilities, in an ever-changing healthcare system. For the first time, the PCC introduced nationally recognised competencies which were to be achieved through a programme of study, and employing organisations would be responsible for the training and scheduling of SFAs in practice. Further recommendations from the PCC supported the SFA role as an addition to the surgical team, and that it should not be carried out in conjunction with the scrub role unless for minor cases, and policy and risk assessment supported this in practice.

The latest recommendations from the PCC updated the definition recognising the SFA as part of the surgical team [5]. The nationally recognised competencies and underpinning knowledge and skills were to be achieved through the successful completion of a validated university programme of study for SFAs to meet nationally recognised standards (see Box 39.1). In relation to dual roles, risk assessments and policy are the responsibility of the employing organisation to decide the appropriateness of the dual role. For the first time the PCC introduced the SFA extended scope of practice (see Box 39.2).

Education

There are various university short courses available throughout the UK. On successful completion of the course, the trainee SFA is expected to demonstrate the underpinning knowledge and skills to competently assist for surgical procedures specifically listed by the PCC [5].

Entry requirements include:

- registered healthcare professionals with post registration experience in perioperative care;
- support from a manager, mentor, or consultant surgeon; and
- a risk assessment of the role.

Role Boundaries

Pre- and Postoperative Phases

The SFA role primarily involves intraoperative tasks; however, as a member of the surgical team, the SFA may visit the patient pre- and postoperatively. This can improve the communication between the patient, the ward, and the operating theatre. Furthermore, due to previous experience of the perioperative setting, the SFA may liaise with the scrub team to communicate any specialist equipment requirements prior to surgery.

Intraoperative Phase

Box 39.1 lists the intraoperative skills which may be performed by the SFA. The skills are not exhaustive, and any additional skills must be risk assessed and must not involve any surgical intervention [5].

Box 39.1 Roles and responsibilities of the SFA

Assisting with patient positioning, including tissue viability assessment
Skin preparation and draping prior to surgery
Superficial skin and tissue retraction with cutting of superficial sutures
Handling tissue and manipulation of organs for exposure or access
Nerve and deep tissue retraction (the SFA can only move or place retractors under the direct supervision of the operating surgeon)
Cutting deep sutures and ligatures under direct supervision of the operating surgeon
Assisting with haemostasis in order to secure and maintain a clear operating field including indirect application of surgical diathermy by the surgeon
Use of suction as guided by the operating surgeon
Camera manipulation for minimal invasive access surgery
Application of dressings as required

Box 39.2 SFA extended skills

Administration of prescribed local anaesthetic in superficial layers
Suturing skin layers
Suturing and securing drains
Superficial haemostasis including surgical diathermy

The SFA may extend their scope of practice through the addition of knowledge and skills through a university-accredited course. In addition, completion of an intercollegiate basic surgical skills course is mandatory and will provide the necessary nationally recognised training and assessment [8]. It is a legal requirement that any additions to the SFA's scope of practice must be risk assessed to protect the patients, the practitioner and the organisation [9]. Box 39.2 demonstrates skills which may be completed under the direct supervision of the surgeon. It is the SFA's responsibility to ensure all skills are included in a logbook and monitored through annual appraisal.

Professional and Legal Implications

As a registered practitioner, the SFA has a professional obligation to maintain accountability for their own acts or omissions. Any breach of professional standards could, first and foremost, harm the patient and could result in misconduct proceedings, potentially resulting in dismissal [10, 11]. The SFA must never work outside of the parameters of the role which has been risk assessed by their employer and defined in the job description. Therefore, as long as the SFA works to departmental policies, the employing organisation will provide vicarious liability on behalf of the SFA. The SFA should ensure appropriate enhanced indemnity insurance to satisfy the requirements of their professional body; this is particularly pertinent when working in the private sector.

Fundamentally, the SFA should always work to the limits of their competence and should ask for assistance if any task is beyond the limits of their competence [10, 11].

Surgical Care Practitioner

History

The SCP, formerly known as the surgical assistant [12], has a more advanced role than the surgical first assistant, which extends beyond the perioperative environment. An SCP is defined as [13]:

> a registered non-medical practitioner who has completed a Royal College of Surgeons accredited programme (or other previously recognised course), working in clinical practice as a member of the extended surgical team, who performs surgical intervention, preoperative care and postoperative care under the direction and supervision of a consultant surgeon.

A landmark publication, *The Role of the Nurse as Surgeon's Assistant in the Operating Department*, first formalised the expanded role over 25 years ago [12]. This document raised issues of accountability and how competence should be achieved and maintained. The SCP role initially emerged locally and in an often informal and unplanned way [14].

The UK's Department of Health, through the National Practitioner Programme which led the drive to expand and modernise the workforce needs of institutions, introduced the first SCP curriculum framework [15]. A working party with representatives from the Royal College of Surgeons of England and patient representative groups developed national standards of practice to reduce variable standards and confusion.

The second edition of the curriculum re-affiliated the Royal College of Surgeons, patient representative groups, and other organisations' commitment to the education and training of SCPs [13]. The curriculum embraced the changes in the role of the SCP in the wider surgical setting due to the diminished surgical workforce.

The following specialities are currently available within the SCP curriculum programme:

- urology surgery;
- trauma and orthopaedic surgery;
- cardiothoracic surgery;
- plastic and reconstructive surgery;
- paediatric surgery;
- general surgery;
- vascular surgery;
- maxillofacial surgery;
- otorhinolaryngology; and
- gynaecology.

Education

The entry requirements for SCP training are determined by each individual higher-education institution. However, the Royal College of Surgeons stipulates that any applicant must be able to demonstrate the academic ability and clinical aptitude for the rigors of the course and the role [13]. The course can currently be completed either part or full time at level 7 via one of two pathways – the postgraduate diploma or master's degree in surgical care practice in the chosen speciality.

The course will comprise of core and speciality modules which encompass the underpinning theory and practice of the following:

- the principles and practice of assisting;
- legal and professional issues in advanced practice;
- clinical history taking and assessment;
- anatomy and physiology relating to surgery;
- research studies; and
- an advanced project (if following the master's degree pathway).

Milestones must be completed at specific points throughout the programme, these are achieved through formative assessments completed by the trainee SCP's clinical supervisor. There is currently no exit examination required by the Royal College of Surgeons.

Entry requirements include:

- having evidence of a minimum of 18 months' post-registration experience, although some SCP programmes may ask for more;
- being currently registered with either the Nursing and Midwifery Council (NMC) or Health and Care Professions Council (HCPC);

- satisfactory Disclosure and Barring Service security check;
- showing evidence of the ability to undertake level 7 study; and
- being appointed as a trainee SCP with an employer.

Role Boundaries

The scope of practice for the qualified SCP is supported directly by the specific education and training presented in the curriculum framework and is based on the principles of the good medical practice guidelines [17]. These principles are based on knowledge, skills, responsibility, and accountability rather than just performing specific tasks.

The SCP role encompasses the following aspects of surgical care:

Preoperative Phase

The SCP will assess new patients and perform diagnostic investigations and surveillance within the clinic setting. They will carry out a preoperative assessment of risk, including investigation and interpretation. The SCP may also be responsible for consenting and surgical site marking patients for specific surgical procedures.

Intraoperative Phase

They will provide skilled assistance and perform surgical intervention; for example, wound opening, wound closure, tissue dissection, and the insertion of drains.

Postoperative Phase

They will assess patients and manage the surgical patient postoperatively.

Additional Roles/Advanced Roles

In some surgical specialities, the SCP may perform specific surgical procedures under the direction and proximal supervision of the responsible consultant surgeon. SCPs performing such roles must adhere to clinical governance processes to ensure patient safety and should work within the limits of their competence.

Opposition to the Role

Over the years there has been opposition to the role from some members of the medical community, who believe that such roles may hinder the training of surgical trainees and consider it unethical for anyone other than a doctor to carry out surgical intervention [17–19]. However, the experienced SCP can enhance the experience of the transition to proximally supervised operating for the surgical trainee [20]. The SCP uses a blend of experience and personal qualities, in addition to knowledge and skills, to gain the necessary trust of their clinical supervisor to provide training of medical students and junior surgical trainees [21].

Professional and Legal Implications

The SCP role goes beyond the scope of their current regulatory bodies, with many practitioners independently performing surgical procedures and running outpatient clinics under the direction and proximal supervision of their clinical supervisors. Within these settings, the SCP undertakes skills which were previously carried out by medically trained professionals; unless the boundaries are clearly set, this could expose the SCP to a multitude of professional and legal liabilities [22]. As with the SFA role, the SCP must act within the boundaries of their scope of practice, and always consider their duty of care to their patients and themselves [23].

Anaesthesia Associate

History

The AA, formerly known as physician's assistant (anaesthesia), role was first introduced in 2004. This was in direct response to the predicted workforce shortage following the reduction in junior doctors' hours and to support the National Health Service plan [3, 4]. The Royal College of Anaesthetists and the Department of Health worked together to formulate a new model of care, which would develop a non-medical practitioner to provide advanced anaesthetic care [24]. They perform highly specialist skills for anaesthetists in a variety of situations and perioperative settings, in the absence of a medically qualified anaesthetist.

The AA is a member of the anaesthetic team and, working to the medical model, provides skilled anaesthetic care under the medical direction and supervision of a consultant anaesthetist [25]. This may involve one consultant anaesthetist supervising two AAs or one AA and one anaesthetic trainee. It has been suggested that the role could improve theatre efficiency and throughput of patients without compromising patient safety [26].

Education

The postgraduate education programme of study is 27 months in duration and most of the programme involves clinical practice. On completion of the programme, the successful AA will be awarded the Anaesthesia Associate Postgraduate Diploma [27].

The course comprises 12 modules, which encompass the underpinning theory and practice of the following:

- clinical practice of anaesthesia;
- physics in anaesthesia;
- the anaesthetic machine and monitoring;
- anatomy and physiology relating to anaesthesia and surgery;
- clinical history and examination;
- management of life-threatening emergencies; and
- advanced practice.

Assessments are through nationally recognised examinations developed by the Royal College of Anaesthetists, at 8 and 24 months. The final exit examination takes place at the Royal College of Anaesthetists in London.

There are two entry routes to the programme of study:

- a registered practitioner: for example, a nurse or allied health professional with 3 years post-registration experience within perioperative care and recent successful academic study; or
- direct entry through a biomedical science background with the achievement of at least a second-class honours degree and demonstrating a clear commitment to a career in healthcare.

Role Boundaries

The role encompasses all aspects of anaesthetic care.

Preoperative Phase

The AA will assess patients preoperatively to check their health status and discuss the planned pre-, intra-, and postoperative care. To optimise the patient for surgery, the AA may organise additional investigations. In agreement with their consultant anaesthetist, who will be responsible for patient care, the AA may be responsible for planning aspects of anaesthetic care.

Intraoperative Phase

The AA may deliver the anaesthetic or sedation under the direction of the anaesthetist.

Postoperative Phase

The AA may assess the patient postoperatively in the post-anaesthetic care unit.

Additional Roles/Advanced Roles

The AA may participate in the resuscitation of patients during an emergency.

Post qualification, and with further education, skills training and assessment, the AA may undertake additional treatments, including regional anaesthesia, cardiopulmonary exercise testing, research, and teaching. Any activity which is beyond the basic scope of practice of the AA should be appropriately managed through clinical governance, appraisal, and audit.

Opposition to the Role

As for the SCP role, there has been some opposition to the development and implementation of the role. Initially, there were concerns from anaesthetists surrounding reduced training opportunities and career prospects [28]. However, in the United States there is evidence that non-medical anaesthetists are not only cost-effective but produce the same safety and quality care as their medical colleagues [29]. With this in mind, the Royal College of Anaesthetists are envisaging that modern anaesthesia will involve greater collaboration with AAs to improve patient outcomes [28].

Professional and Legal Implications

AAs who are already registered practitioners such as operating department practitioners and nurses have statutory regulation through either the HCPC or NMC. Although this provides some level of assurance, the current structure does not reflect the advanced role undertaken and there are concerns that the regulatory body would find it difficult to fully support the AA [30]. Moreover, direct-entry AAs do not have this assurance.

Medical Associate Professionals

The AA and the SCP roles falls within the Medical Associates Professions group, a move made by Health Education England in 2014 to place some professions under a single umbrella, with the intention to work towards a common education and training programme and to support the move towards statutory regulation [31].

Currently, the General Medical Council in the UK is working towards becoming the regulators for AAs. It is expected that legislative processes will be completed in the summer of 2023 [32]. This union will provide universal standards for continuing professional development, appraisal, and assessment of competency and capability for all registered AAs. This will maintain and improve the quality of care given to patients and the standards within teams. It will track areas of new knowledge, skills, and behaviours and address areas requiring improvement. In line with all practicing professionals, AAs will be required to provide confirmation of their qualifications and that there are no outstanding concerns about their fitness to practice [33].

References

1. National Association of Theatre Nurses. *The Role of the Nurse as First Assistant in the Operating Department.* Harrogate: National Association of Theatre Nurses, 1993.

2. Perioperative Care Collaborative. The provision of the non-medical perioperative practitioner working as first assistant to the surgeon. Available from: www.aodp.org/Files/PCCFirstAssistant_submenu_200.pdf.

3. Department of Health. *The NHS Plan: A Plan for Investment, a Plan for Reform.* London: Her Majesty's Stationery Office, 2000.

4. National Health Service Employers. *Working Time Directive: Frequently Asked Questions for Trust Implementation Teams.* London: NHS Employers, 2009.

5. Perioperative Care Collaborative. *Surgical First Assistant: Position Statement.* London: Perioperative Care Collaborative, 2018.

6. M. G. Fisher. Considerations of the dual role. *Journal of Perioperative Practice* 2015; **25**: 153–154.

7. Perioperative Care Collaborative. *Surgical First Assistant: Position Statement.* London, Perioperative Care Collaborative, 2012.

8. Royal College of Surgeons. *Position Statement: Surgical Assistants.* London: Royal College of Surgeons, 2011.

9. Health and Safety Executive. The health and safety toolbox: how to control risks at work. Available from: www.hse.gov.uk/pubns/priced/hsg268.pdf.

10. Health and Care Professions Council. *Standards of Conduct, Performance and Ethics.* London: Health and Care Professions Council, 2016.

11. Nursing and Midwifery Council. *The Code.* London: Nursing and Midwifery Council, 2015.

12. National Association of Theatre Nurses. *The Role of the Nurse as Surgeon's Assistant in the Operating Department.* Harrogate: National Association of Theatre Nurses, 1994.

13. Royal College of Surgeons of England. *The Curriculum Framework for the Surgical Care Practitioner.* London: Royal College of Surgeons, 2014.

14. J. Thatcher. Assistants in surgical practice: what's in a name? *British Journal of Perioperative Nursing* 2003; **5**: 210–213.

15. Department of Health. *The Curriculum Framework for the Surgical Care Practitioner.* London: Her Majesty's Stationery Office, 2006.

16. General Medical Council. *Good Medical Practice.* London: General Medical Council, 2013.

17. R. Moorthy, J. Grainger, A. Scott, et al. Surgical care practitioner: a confusing and misleading title. *Annals of the Royal College of Surgeons of England* 2006; **88**: 98–100.

18. R. Ballweg, E. Sullivan, D. Brown, and D. Vetrosky. *Physician Assistant: A Guide to Clinical Practice.* Philadelphia, PA: Elsevier, 2013.

19. D. Scholfield. How will the introduction of surgical care practitioners affect future surgical training and practice? *Surgery* 2016; **34**: 484–486.

20. A. Jones, H. Arshad, and J. Nolan. Surgical care practitioner practice: one team's journey explored. *Journal of Perioperative Practice* 2012; **22**: 19–23.

21. S. Hall, J. Quick, and A. W. Hall. The perfect surgical assistant: calm, confident, competent and courageous. *Journal of Perioperative Practice* 2016; **26**: 201–204.

22. M. Nicholas. The surgical care practitioner: a critical analysis. *Journal of Perioperative Practice* 2010; **20**: 94–99.

23. G. R. M. Campaner. The presence of a surgical care practitioner in the perioperative team is of benefit to the patient and the consultant-led extended team. *Journal of Perioperative Practice* 2019; **29**: 81–86.

24. Royal College of Anaesthetists. *The Role of Non-Medical Staff in the Delivery of Anaesthesia Services*. London: Royal College of Anaesthetists, 2002.

25. Royal College of Anaesthetists. Anaesthetic Associates (AAs) information for patients. Available from: www.anaesthesiaassociates.org/wp-content/uploads/2019/12/AnaesAssociate-patientinfo2019web.pdf.

26. M. Gwinnutt and C. L. Gwinnutt. *Clinical Anaesthesia*, 5th ed. Chichester: Wiley Blackwell, 2017.

27. University of Birmingham. Anaesthesia Associate Post Graduate Diploma. Course details. Available from: www.birmingham.ac.uk/postgraduate/courses/taught/med/physicians-assistant-anaesthesia.aspx (accessed 3 May 2020).

28. S. Bampoe. Physicians' assistants in anaesthesia: colleagues or competitors? *British Journal of Hospital Medicine* 2015; **76**: 610.

29. B. Dulisse and J. Cromwell. No harm found when nurse anesthetists work without supervision by physicians. *Health Affairs (Millwood)* 2010; **29**: 1469–1475

30. Department of Health and Social Care. *The Regulation of Medical Associate Professionals in the UK: Consultation Response*. London: Her Majesty's Stationery Office, 2019.

31. Health Education England. *Working Towards a Common Education and Training Programme to Support a Route to Statutory Regulation for Physicians' Assistants (Anaesthesia), Physician Associates, and Surgical Care Practitioners in England*. London: Health Education England, 2014.

32. General Medical Council. Dates are changing but our commitment to PAs and AAs remains. Available from: www.gmc-uk.org/news/news-archive/dates-are-changing-but-our-commitment-to-pas-and-aas-remains.

33. General Medical Council. Bringing physician associates and anaesthesia associates into regulation. Available from: www.gmc-uk.org/pa-and-aa-regulation-hub/map-regulation (accessed 16 December 2020).

Index